THE HURRIED WOMAN

THE HURRIED WOMAN

Conquer Fatigue, Achieve Successful
Lifelong Weight Management, and
Rekindle the Fire in Your Relationships

Brent W. Bost, M.D., F.A.C.O.G.

VANTAGE PRESS
New York

FIRST EDITION

Copyright © 2001 by Brent W. Bost, M.D., F.A.C.O.G.

Published by Vantage Press, Inc.
516 West 34th Street, New York, New York 10001

Manufactured in the United States of America
ISBN: 0-533-13619-9

Library of Congress Catalog Card No.: 00-91580

0

To my wife and best friend, LaNell,
who has stood by me in
good times, bad times, and worse times . . .

My four children, Amanda, Neal, Stephen, and Thomas
who had to give up more of their time with
Dad than they should have . . .

My patients, whose suffering inspired this book . . .

And to God, who loves me in spite of who I am (and am not)
and, fortunately, also has a sense of humor

Contents

Acknowledgments

There are several people who helped in the preparation of *The Hurried Woman* and deserve a special "thank you":

Gigi Fontenot and Dana Knippa, RN, who put up with a lot of the difficult early work in developing the ideas and ultimate organization of this book.

Susan Becker, RD, LD, and Amy Dean, RD, LD, CNSD, who provided much of the research and technical assistance in developing and validating the weight maintenance strategy proposed here.

Dr. Raymond McHenry and Lyn Brown, MA, for their spiritual guidance, as well as practical advice, in getting the book published. Lyn also did a great job in proofreading the first manuscript.

A very special thanks to my brother, David, for his constant encouragement, bordering on nagging (and sometimes, harassment!) to finish what I had started.

Finally, to all of my family, friends and patients who told me their woes, listened to my endless babbling, responded to my countless questions, and offered words of encouragement, let me say "thank you"—you deserve it!

Introduction

Are you a Hurried Woman? (You probably aren't if you have time to stop and read this! But you obviously thought you *might* be; that's why you're here. Perhaps the title sounded like something "familiar" in your subconscious mind.) Well, you're here now; read on and see if you are or you aren't one.

As I am an obstetrician/gynecologist, my day is filled with Hurried Women. But they usually don't complain about being "hurried"; in fact, the office visit usually starts out something like this:

"Hello, Mrs. Culpepper [the names have been changed to protect the innocent]. How are you doing?"

"Oh, I'm fine, Dr. Bost." (She sounds sincere, but her speech trails off a bit at the end—a hint that there's more than meets the ear here.)

"Now, Connie, don't say it unless you mean it. You know you can tell me the 'real untold story.' "

"OK, doctor. I just haven't been feeling myself lately. I'm tired all the time, I can't seem to get this weight off, and . . . well . . . I . . . "

"You have no sex drive?"

"Right! [She sounds relieved to finally have it out in the open.] Zip! Nada! None! I just don't *feel* like having sex most of the time. Once we get started it's OK, but I'm not the one who initiates things anymore. What do you think is wrong?"

"There are tests we need to run to rule out other medical explanations for your symptoms, but I suspect from what you're telling me that you are suffering from the Hurried Woman Syndrome."

"Hurried Woman Syndrome! What's that?" (Some doubt has begun to creep into her voice.)

"Let me explain it to you first, and then I think you'll begin to understand. . . . "

The Hurried Woman usually has complaints in one or more of three major areas:

1. **Fatigue or "down" mood**—"I'm tired all the time and I don't know why."
   "I feel 'down' a lot of times even when things are going OK."
   "I just can't seem to get a good night's sleep."
2. **Weight gain**—"I eat like I used to, but I keep gaining weight."
   "I exercise a lot, but I can't get this weight off."
   "I'm too tired to exercise." (Triggered by #1.)
3. **Low sex drive**—"It's not that I don't love my husband, *but . . .* "
   "I'm too tired to have sex most nights." (Number 1 strikes again!)
   "I don't *feel* sexy anymore." (The old "2–3 combo.")

Do any of those sound familiar? You may have said or thought about one or a combination of them more than once lately. If these complaints are becoming *your* complaints, and particularly if they are starting to drain the fun out of life, then you probably are a Hurried Woman.

I chose the title *The Hurried Woman* because it describes the major underlying cause of the problem. Besides, I thought it was a catchy phrase and it's a lot easier to say than "The Fatigued, Overweight, Undersexed Woman," which wouldn't have fit on the cover anyway. (I also thought about calling it *Weary Women*, but can you imagine an interview with Barbara Walters?) However, the relationship among these three areas—fatigue, weight gain, and loss of interest in sex—may not be clear to you at first. In fact, it took me a long time to discover the link among them, and I have been a practicing obstetrician/gynecologist for over fifteen years! Once I figured it out, though, I was amazed at the number of patients who suffer with this condition. In fact, it's estimated that over 60 million American women suffer from these symptoms. Believe me, you're not alone!

Over the last five or six years, I began to notice that the three most common troubles my patients complained about were not pregnancy, bleeding, and pain, as my formal medical training had led me to believe.

No, the three most common complaints were fatigue (sometimes described as feeling "down" or "blah"), weight gain, and low sex drive—often in a combination of two or all three (what I call "the works"). As I talked with these women about their symptoms and circumstances, I began to see a common thread that linked these problems together for the vast majority of patients—stress.

There are many causes of stress, and they often vary from patient to patient. Sometimes the stress can't be avoided, such as that of a sick child or a high-powered career. However, for the majority of women I treat, much of the stress is avoidable or at least could be managed better. The avoidable stresses are those that come from a busy, hectic schedule and lifestyle choices that many of us have embraced as completely "routine." Yet the effects of this kind of stress, what I call "hurry," can have very significant long-term and wide-reaching consequences for the woman who labors under it and those around her who suffer along with her.

The woman who is burdened by the Hurried Woman Syndrome is just that—she's hurried (or "harried" as the English might say) by the many struggles that complicate her life. She's usually fairly young, between twenty-five and fifty-five, and has two or more children. Most often, at least one of her kids is between the ages of four and sixteen. Her spouse (or perhaps lack of one), her children, and her work all tend to pull her in different directions, causing a lot of internal stress. This constant conflict of needs, both hers and theirs, can wear down even the strongest women and ultimately lead to physical as well as emotional problems, even depression.

The effects of these life stresses are primarily manifested in three areas: fatigue or perhaps a "down" mood, weight control, and sex drive (or libido for you Freudian types). The symptoms of hurry often begin in one area (particularly fatigue and/or depressed mood) and then spill over into the other two. Sometimes these stresses are virtually impossible to avoid, but oftentimes the pressure comes in areas that appear to be low-stress at first but then build steadily until they overflow and become a problem. Like a cup under a dripping faucet, at first each drop seems to have little or no effect on the amount of water in the cup, but eventually the cup fills up and then spills water over the edges.

Many of the activities that bring stress or hurry into your life are "good" things in themselves: family events, entertainment, children's activities, volunteer work, and church activities. But when they overwhelm you, they can be dangerous to your health and to your relationships. Water is an essential element for life, but too much water is called *drowning*! Moderation is important.

Well, you've probably decided by now that there may be something here for you—some help, finally! You may not be complaining about trouble in all three symptom areas, but you know that something's wrong and you want to feel better. But, you may ask, why read *The Hurried Woman* when there are so many other self-help books available? Two reasons: First, and most important, *The Hurried Woman* has the right strategy for each of the three problem areas—fatigue, weight control, and improving your marriage both physically and emotionally. Second, *The Hurried Woman* is the only integrated approach to overcoming these common, but very important, problems. You could go out and buy a diet book, a book on fatigue, a self-help marriage guide, and a book on getting the stress out of you life—four books—and probably get a handle on some of your problems. However, *The Hurried Woman* addresses the *underlying cause* of these symptoms and offers a unified approach to conquering fatigue, putting in place lifelong weight management, and rekindling the fire in your relationships. No other single book can help you do all of these things as effectively.

The Hurried Woman is laid out in four parts. The first part will discuss the effects of ''hurry'' or stress on the modern woman and how it attacks her physically, leading to fatigue, mood problems, and even depression. In the second part, heavy emphasis (no pun intended!) will be placed on weight gain and how it can be caused by and contribute to problems in the other two areas. I will also line-out a very sensible approach to losing weight that works—*for the long run.*

Sex will be the topic of the third part. Don't skip over the first two parts and read it first—that would be cheating. Plus, you really need to read the first part to fully understand the third, so be patient. I also encourage you to have your husband read this part. Even though he may suffer from osteocephaly (from *osteo* [bone] and *cephalos* [head], i.e., boneheadedness!), it will help him to better understand your needs and I hope, make your love life as a couple more satisfying. Actually, I encourage husbands to read the whole book, but good luck with that one! Most men can't stay awake through the Sunday comics, much less a book on women's problems.

The fourth and final part will attempt to "tie it all together" and make sense out of the first three parts. In addition, the last part will offer suggestions to take the hurry out of your life and allow the joy back in. I encourage you to spent some quality time looking at the last part.

Each of the first three parts ends with answers to frequently asked questions (FAQS) related to topics in that section. I recommend that you study these questions and the responses given, as they may make more sense to you than the textbook approach the chapters take. You may even find that someone else has already asked your question. This should make it easier to come away with something that's helpful to you.

After reading the titles of each part, you may not feel that all four of them apply to you. However, I think you'll find useful information in each one. You may be shocked to find that you actually *do* have symptoms in each of the three symptom areas and, I hope, also be able to see that these problems are really interelated. Besides, knowing all about the Hurried Woman Syndrome may enable you to help a friend or family member who comes complaining to you about struggling with symptoms of the syndrome.

Well, since you're in a hurry to get started—a bad habit I hope to help you recognize and correct soon—turn to chapter 1 and let's begin.

THE HURRIED WOMAN

Part I
Fatigue

"Life Must Go On—But I Can't Remember Why"

1

Fatigue and the Hurried Woman

Fatigue is the most common complaint of the Hurried Woman, and it's usually the first sign of the Hurried Woman Syndrome. Most women realize that they should be tired after a long day at work or with the kids and expect that they will feel better after they rest. This type of fatigue is predictable and temporary for most of us. However, the fatigue that the Hurried Woman feels is pervasive, hard to shake: it doesn't ease up much even after a good night's rest. (Do you even remember getting "a good night's rest" lately?) Things that used to be easy to do are a lot harder now, they wear you out more quickly; your batteries take longer to recharge for some reason. Eventually, this chronic tiredness begins to blunt your mood. It can make you crabby or disagreeable. Perhaps you just don't feel as "perky" as you did before. (My wife hates the word, *perky*—sounds like something only Barbie could be!) Maybe you don't look forward to things that previously brought you pleasure, like shopping. (No, I'm sorry. That's a bad example. My wife would get off an autopsy table to go shopping!) But overall, life just doesn't seem as pleasing as it once was, and your energy levels are just "not right somehow." This feeling of "not rightness" is one of the earliest symptoms of the Hurried Woman Syndrome.

"In the Beginning . . . "

The fatigue starts subtly at first. Most women describe it as a nagging lack of energy. Sometimes it's a feeling of uneasiness, that something's wrong . . . but what?

"I don't know why I was so tired last night. It was just a routine day."
"I just don't feel 'myself' lately."

3

Then the tiredness builds into an obvious lack of energy but, more important, a lack of desire to participate. Things that were previously interesting or even fun to do are no longer interesting or fun. In fact, these activities often come to be dreaded.

"I don't want to do that *today* (or maybe *ever again*, for that matter!)."

The eagerness to engage life that she relied upon as a source of strength in the past has now left her, leaving a vacuum—the life has been literally sucked out of living for the Hurried Woman. Those events in her life that she previously embraced eagerly and the problems that she used to attack with full force are becoming harder to handle. They seem to sap the energy right out of her—much more so than in the past. Yes, she still plods along, feeling too guilty to quit now—she's "committed," you know! (or soon will be committed; to the "funny farm," that is!)—but she is beginning to realize that it hurts a lot worse now than it used to and it's getting harder and harder to keep going day in and day out.

Continual fatigue leads to other problems, such as being in a "down" mood because you can't get things done or maybe anxiety about what you've got to do but don't have the energy to do. It may keep you from exercising regularly, which, as we will see later, is critical for good health, both emotional and physical. Because men and women often are very different in how they approach life and particularly their sex life, chronic tiredness also leads to low sexual performance in women more so than men.

Most important, the long-term effect of unchecked fatigue is guilt. Guilt about not wanting to participate anymore or pulling back from activities and the friends involved with those activities. Guilt about snapping at your family because you're on edge and tired all the time. Guilt about not being the wife and mother you were before all this tiredness began to overwhelm you. Guilt leads to more guilt, sometimes anger, and finally depression if not stopped.

If your fatigue levels seem exaggerated out of proportion to the work you do, then you should go see your primary care doctor (internist, family practitioner, or ob/gyn) and get it checked out. Don't just keep suffering in silence hoping it will go away by itself. You and those who love you are suffering with you, believe me. Go see your doctor. This is important.

2

Medical Causes of Fatigue

Many medical conditions cause fatigue or present with fatigue as an early symptom. But before I go any further, let me say something extremely important to your understanding of fatigue and the Hurried Woman:

Don't forget that raising a family is work—*hard work!*

Motherhood

There is a sign in my office that says: MOTHERHOOD AIN'T FOR SISSIES, and believe me, it *ain't* neither! Raising a family is hard work particularly if it's your *second* job. Let's say on an average day you crank out eight or nine short, fun-filled hours at "the plant," then come home to prop your feet up and read the newspaper. Right? *Wrong!* Instead, you now begin your second shift, *at home*—cooking, cleaning house, washing clothes, doing homework, paying bills, shuttling kids from baseball, to gymnastics, to band rehearsal, to soccer, to a friend's house, to the movies, and to who-knows-where-else they want to go! Oh, yeah—and you also need to be a sex machine for "Big Dog" a few nights each week. Are you tired yet? Even moms who stay at home get tired, too.

Being an ob/gyn doctor is not particularly hard physical work—of course, snatching a baby from the "jaws of death" can be a harrowing experience, but fortunately that doesn't happen every day! The majority of my workday is spent talking with patients about their problems and helping them arrive at solutions they can live with. It does require a lot of mental energy, but let's face it; the job doesn't really burn up a lot of calories with *physical* effort. However, after about twelve or fourteen hours at the office and hospital each day, I get tired and really need a break from work for a while. (Twenty years or so would be nice.) Mom, however, if she stays at home starts her day out early, and it just keeps

5

"rolling along" like a weenie down a steep hill. Yes, she gets sixteen or more hours a day of uninterrupted joy at her chosen profession—motherhood (or child ranching, as we call it here in the countryside). What a deal, huh? No wonder she's tired at the end of the day . . . week . . . decade . . . well, whenever her work finally ends.

I love my four children dearly, but if I had stayed at home with them every day, sixteen hours a day, seven days a week, for about 358 days a year (as my wife has), they would be stuffed and mounted on the wall of my living room or buried in a shallow grave in the backyard by now. I don't have the mental and emotional stamina to do my wife's job, and believe it or not, my kids are really good children. (Don't tell them I said that or they'll want more allowance.) My wife, LaNell, has a gift (or maybe, she's a little crazy) that allows her to do her job well, and with style, I might add. Either way, gifted or crazy, she has a tough job to do sixteen-plus hours every day, seven days a week. And don't forget, she's on-call every night, too—for fever, nightmares, upset stomachs, snakes in the house, etc. (We live in the country and I'm away from home on-call some nights.) Frankly, being on-call wears me out at times. In fact, there are some call nights when I don't get a single phone call after I get to bed, but I still wake up tired the next day. I guess the knowledge that I have to be available "at a moment's notice" to jump in the car and run to the hospital keeps me from resting soundly. Well, moms have the same problem and it's harder for them because they are on-call *every night*. It has got to wear a woman down after a while.

I have one last thought on this subject before we move on: "Mother" is a lifetime job. You can never retire from motherhood. The title is yours, forever—*FOREVER!* Indeed, once you are crowned as "Mother" you may never abdicate the throne. I have a great deal of respect for mothers. It's a *neverending job*. Well, really, it's not just a job—it's an adventure!

Going to the Doctor

The following discussion cannot replace a conference with your doctor, but I include it here to help you organize your thoughts *before* you see him/her. You can't expect to become a doctor by reading one or two self-help books and visiting the health food store. If it were that easy, why did I waste fourteen years after high school to become a board-certified ob/gyn specialist? You've got to trust your doctor to help you sort this stuff out. However, you can help your doctor get to the bottom of this problem quickly by having your thoughts organized and writing your symptoms down *before* you go in for a visit.

Anemia—a very common cause of fatigue in women, particularly because of menstruation. If your periods are particularly long or heavy or if your fatigue seems much worse during and immediately after your menstrual cycle or if you've been anemic in the past, be sure to relate these facts to your doctor. A complete blood count (CBC) is a simple and inexpensive test to screen for anemia. Besides checking your iron status, it may also give a hint to nutritional problems like deficiencies of folic acid (folate) or vitamin B_{12} (cyanocobalamin) or underlying problems with blood cell formation that can also cause anemia.

It is important to check for other sources of blood loss if you have iron-deficiency anemia. Most physicians will use a urinalysis to check for blood cells in the urine and a guaiac test for blood hiding in the stool. If you've had frequent kidney infections, kidney stones, rectal bleeding, or dark stools that are almost black, like tar, you need to tell your doctor, since these may signal abnormal blood loss from other places. People with a history of stomach ulcers also tend to be anemic.

Thyroid disease—many women with either overactive (hyper) or underactive thyroid (hypothyroidism) will complain of fatigue. Other symptoms associated with hypothyroidism (low thyroid) are weight gain, cold intolerance, constipation, and menstrual irregularities. Hyperthyroidism (too much thyroid hormone) causes agitation, racing pulse, heat intolerance, and weight loss. However, if hyperthyroidism is untreated for an extended period of time, the patient will "burn out" from the excessive thyroid levels and begin to tire out and complain of fatigue and sometimes weight gain. The *only* valid test for thyroid disease in women, particularly women on estrogen (birth control or estrogen replacement pills in menopause) is a TSH, or thyroid-stimulating hormone. Estrogen increases the levels of the protein in the blood, called thyroid-binding globulin, or TBG, that binds up thyroid hormone in the bloodstream. The simple test for thyroid hormone (T4) measures **all** thyroid hormone in the blood, both bound and unbound. However, *only the unbound* hormone is available for use by the body. Patients on estrogen have more TBG and therefore more bound-up thyroid hormone than patients who don't take estrogen. Because of this confusing set of facts,

7

patients on estrogen may have a normal thyroid hormone test (T4), but much of that hormone is bound up by TBG and is **not** available to regulate metabolism. So a T4 test can be misleading in a woman on estrogen.

TSH, however, measures how much thyroid the brain is receiving (unbound) and is a more reliable test of true thyroid functioning in women. Simply put, a woman *must* have a TSH level to know whether her thyroid hormones are in balance, *period!* End of discussion! I will go so far as to say to get another doctor if yours doesn't know this fact, because if (s)he doesn't know this little "pearl of wisdom," what else about how women are "fearfully and wonderfully made" does he/she not understand?

Menopause—most women have heard a lot of information about menopause in the past few years and are much more aware of it now than they were a few years back. Symptoms include irregular to absent periods, hot flushes (often called flashes), night sweats, insomnia or rest-lessness, emotional lability (the technical term for moodiness), and de-creased ability to concentrate, as well as fatigue. FSH, or follicle-stimulating hormone, is the test used to detect menopause. Unfortunately, FSH can only detect whether a woman is in menopause or not and cannot predict when in the future it will occur. Many women experience the same symptoms as menopause but with worse emotional changes and fatigue in the few months to even years prior to menopause. This condi-tion is called peri-menopause and can often be treated with low-dose birth control pills. Peri-menopause will be discussed later in this chapter and in the part of this book on sex drive. (Don't jump ahead to part 3 yet; be patient!)

Auto-immune diseases and arthritis—lupus, rheumatoid arthritis, ankylosing spondylitis, polymyalgia rheumatica, and polyarteritis nodosa are all unusual diseases that tend to cause arthritis, muscle aches, skin rashes, fatigue, and many other symptoms too involved to discuss in great detail here. Most doctors will screen based on your symptoms with perhaps an anti-nuclear antibody (**ANA**) screen and sedimentation rate (sed rate) as a bare minimum. These screening tests often lead to more sophisticated testing if they turn up positive or you have other symptoms peculiar to one of these ailments.

Infections—most infections cause fatigue as a symptom. Acute in-fections, both viral and bacterial, are typically recognized by the patient because the associated symptoms of the infection are readily apparent. Most patients get tipped off that something's wrong when they have fever, chills, nausea, vomiting, etc. However, some more chronic viral infections, low-grade upper respiratory or urinary tract infections, and allergies can drag you down over time. Also, many viral infections can be followed by an extended "post-viral syndrome," which may persist for several weeks to months after the acute infection is gone. Sometimes the time elapsed is so great that the patient doesn't see the connection anymore. Broad-based screening tests are often used to pick up the telltale signs of low-grade or persistent infections.

In addition to a CBC, TSH, FSH, ANA, sed rate (and perhaps, serums B_{12} and folate level), several commonly used screening tests are listed here with the conditions they seek to diagnose:

Test	Condition
Mono spot test	Mononucleosis
Epstein-Barr viral titers	
Liver function tests	Hepatitis from any source—viral,
(SMA 12 or 20, or comprehensive	post-viral, chemical or drug
metabolic profile)	toxicity, cancer
Hepatitis profile	Specific tests for Hepatitis A,B,
	and C
CMV titer	Cytomegalovirus infection
HIV	AIDS and "pre-AIDS"
RPR	Syphilis—on the rise of the United
	States
TB skin test	Tuberculosis—on the rise in the
	United States

Other illnesses—many other conditions can cause fatigue as a symptom, including heart disease, lung disease, kidney failure, diabetes, high blood pressure, Addison's disease (adrenal gland insufficiency), multiple sclerosis, cancer, and Parkinson's disease, to name a few. Since fatigue is such a pervasive symptom for a wide variety of ailments, you need a doctor to help you sort all of this stuff out!

Be Prepared

The main benefit of this discussion will be to help you organize your thoughts and create a time line of your symptoms and any over-the-counter medicines or home remedies you may have tried. Gather up a little family history about cancer, neurologic diseases such as Parkinson's and multiple sclerosis, and depression. Think about your menstrual history, weight gain or loss over the last year, change in appetite or diet, etc., and *write it down* in note form so you can take it with you for your appointment. Most doctors are not intimidated by this, and it makes the visit go smoother. However, you can get carried away with this, such as listing every bowel movement you've had since 1978 (I've had 3,822; how about you?) or dating your symptoms from events rather than dates. A statement like "I've gained thirty pounds since my sister's wedding" will have to be followed by a question from your doctor, who hasn't the foggiest notion of when your blessed sister tied the knot; "Well . . . how long ago was that?" Don't waste time for both of you by speaking in eccentric terms. Instead, tell the doctor "I've gained thirty pounds *over the last eight months.*" Organizing your thoughts into a list of symptoms and a time line saves time for more important discussion and helps your doctor focus on you and your health, not trying to unravel your confusing history.

Now, after spending all this time going through the medical causes of fatigue, I wonder if you can guess which one is the most common cause. I'm sure that you'll be disappointed to learn that only about 10 percent of patients who go through this medical work-up find anything wrong. The majority of patients have normal lab work. Don't be disillusioned; I'll give you the answer to this mystery later.

The most common abnormal lab finding is anemia, followed by thyroid disease and auto-immune diseases like lupus and polymyalgia rheumatica. But the complaint of fatigue is the most common complaint (other than pregnancy) that I see every day in medical practice. To give you an idea of how common this complaint is among women, let me give you some statistics from my practice. I see about thirty to thirty-eight patients each day in my office, and on any given day I will see about five to six women complaining about fatigue or fatigue and the other problems associated with Hurried Woman Syndrome. If you do the math, you'll figure out that almost twenty-five or thirty women come to me each week complaining about fatigue. Another way of looking at this is that almost 20 percent of the patients in my practice are complaining about fatigue at any given time! I find that phenomenal. In fact, that's the main reason I began researching this problem and, fortunately, found the link between fatigue and the Hurried Woman Syndrome—so many of my patients were suffering from it with no organized medical approach

10

to the problem(s) available. I also got tired (no irony intended!) of not being able to spend the twenty to thirty extra minutes necessary to explain to each of these women why they feel so bad, how the fatigue relates to the other problems they are experiencing, and how to fix it. That's why I felt compelled to write this book.

Well, if the medical causes of fatigue (or at least those that you currently think of as "medical") are usually not found to be the problem, what is the reason for the overwhelming tiredness? And why do so many women suffer from it? Before I give you the final answer to these questions, we need to talk about depression.

3

Depression and the Hurried Woman

Depression is quite common in women. In fact, almost 30 percent of all women will suffer from some form of depression or anxiety disorder during their lifetimes. Although I'm not a psychiatrist, I have to help patients decide whether they are clinically depressed or just responding normally to a stressful life. Now, I'm not saying that you are depressed; in fact, you probably are not depressed. But if you are, you need more help than this book can provide. That's why it's important to know whether you are or are not depressed before we go much further.

Major Depression

The symptoms of major depression are:

Group 1
Sad or irritable mood (dysphoria)
Loss of interest/capacity for pleasure (anhedonia)

Group 2
Sleep problems (too much or too little)
Appetite/weight (increase or decrease)
Impaired concentration/decision making
Suicidal thoughts (particularly planning it)
Feelings of guilt, self-blame, worthlessness
High fatigue levels
Psychomotor agitation/retardation (fidgeting or slouchiness)

A diagnosis of major depression requires at least one symptom from Group 1 and four or more symptoms from Group 2. I know what you're thinking: *Looking at this list, I'm depressed and so are all my friends! Everyone* has these symptoms at some time or other. But before you become depressed about being depressed, let me explain that the difference between not being depressed and being depressed is the duration of these symptoms and how severely these complaints keep you from functioning normally.

Depressed or Not Depressed? That is the Question!

The symptoms of depression are often experienced by normal people. These symptoms usually spring up when we are under pressure. We can usually recognize the cause of the stress, fix it (or at least live through it), and then get back to normal. This is not depression. The duration of symptoms and the degree to which they mess up our functioning are not long enough or bad enough to qualify as depression.

Sure, you're more tired than you used to be (of course, you are also *older* than you used to be), you've gained a few pounds over the last year or so (I've eaten a few bowls of Blue Bell ice cream this last year, too—Homemade Vanilla is still my favorite, but my wife likes Pralines and Cream, oh yeah!), and you have noticed that you have more restless nights or an unexpected nap occasionally while watching the news, but you are not depressed—at least not yet, anyway. Why? Because you can still go to work every day, take care of your family, and muster up the energy to get up early and go shopping with the girls *when you want to.* Although you do have some of the symptoms of depression, they are not severe enough to stop you from doing what you need to do and much of what you want to do. This is why you are not depressed. But it may be getting more difficult to keep going.

I have a test I want you to take to see if you are depressed. You'll find it in Appendix A in the back of the book. Stop for a moment and take it to see where you are on the depression scale. If you find that you are depressed or have thought about a plan to kill yourself, you *must* consult your doctor immediately. That's right; set the book down and call your doctor *now!* I should interject here that most normal people have *thought* about being dead or even killing themselves as a possible solution to a tough situation. A fleeting thought of running your car off the road or taking a handful of pills is not a suicide threat, but *dwelling* on the thought or *making plans* to "off" yourself is not healthy. If that's where you are, GO GET HELP *NOW!* Otherwise, you're OK for the moment. Now, go take the test and I'll wait here for you.

After the Test

Since you are still reading the book, you must not have been depressed enough to stop and go see your doctor (a score of 65 or greater), but if you are a Hurried Woman you probably scored higher than you expected (between 20 and 65). Well, if you're not depressed, but you're not happy with how you feel, what are you? You are experiencing what I call pre-depression. A psychiatrist would probably call it minor depression or dysthymia, but I am not willing to debate the point. Practically speaking, you are somewhere between depressed and normal—whatever that is! Let's see how it works.

Brain Chemistry and the Rebalancer System

Depression is caused by a chemical imbalance in the brain and has nothing to do with being a "wimp" or a "weenie" or "not trying hard enough to get happy," although many of us heard these stories about depression when we were younger and can't seem to let go of them. Serotonin and dopamine are the two major "mood chemicals" that can get out of balance in the brain and cause depression. The brain has its own rebalancing system that keeps the levels of serotonin and dopamine from getting too far out of kilter.

There are three basic types of rebalancer problems. (Have you noticed how most things come in threes? Weird, huh!) First, some people have a genetically defective rebalancer and are plagued by depression most of their lives—essentially, a long-term rebalancer problem. Second, many women experience a short-term rebalancer problem—premenstrual syndrome (PMS), which will be discussed briefly at the end of the chapter. However, the Hurried Woman is affected by the third type of chemical rebalancer problem—chronic stress or "hurry." You could have PMS in addition to the Hurried Woman Syndrome, which will make both of them worse when you are in the premenstrual time, but I would like to focus now on the Hurried Woman Syndrome alone. Research clearly shows that stress, particularly the chronic stress experienced by the Hurried Woman, can cause physical illness—ulcers, high blood pressure, heart disease, even cancer—and, yes, depression.

Depression versus Pre-depression

You don't go to bed one night with your chemicals 100 percent balanced and "feelin' great," then wake up the next morning with your chemicals way out-of-balance (say, 65 percent balanced) and depressed. There is a level between being depressed and being normal—I call the space between the two pre-depression. Look at the following diagram:

Brain Chemistry

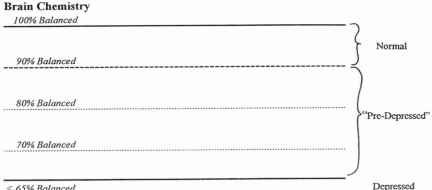

The chemicals in our brain obey the law of entropy—that all things in the universe tend toward disorder. This is one of the many natural laws of physics (or maybe thermodynamics?). Anyway, it's one of those "laws" that annoyed the heck out of me back in college that really do apply to us. Because of entropy, the brain must constantly rebalance the serotonin/dopamine levels in its different compartments for us to remain feeling normal (well, as normal as we can be). Stress causes our rebalancer to function at less than 100 percent efficiency, and more stress causes even less efficiency. When the inefficiency gets bad enough, the chemical balance becomes severe enough for us to begin to see symptoms.

For example, let's say your chemicals are at least 90 percent balanced (or only 10 percent out-of-balance) and you are functioning well on a daily basis but feel more fatigued than usual if you dip below the 90 percent level. After a vacation or a few days away from work, the kids, your in-laws—whatever it is that adds stress to our life—you feel better. Most experts would call this normal. The following diagram shows someone in this situation:

Brain Chemistry

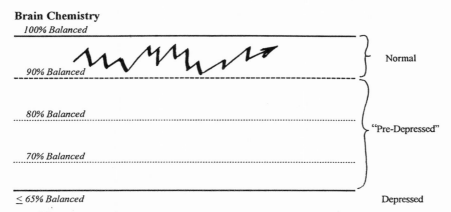

If stress continues to worsen and your chemical balance drops down to the 80 percent level, then you are more fatigued, but your overall mood also changes to being more irritable (can we say crabby?), and perhaps you stop exercising because you're "just too tired." Maybe you do like a lot of us and begin to "comfort" yourself with food. The combination of decreased activity and increasing food intake causes—duh!—weight gain. The following diagram demonstrates what this situation might look like graphically:

Brain Chemistry

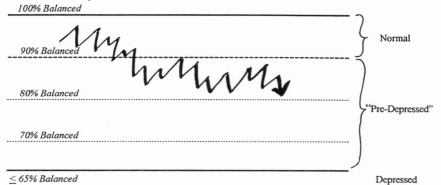

Let's say that the stresses in your life continue to push your brain's chemical balance further down to the 70 percent level (30 percent out-of-balance). At this point, you begin to see sleep disturbance, particularly

16

what the pros call terminal insomnia—no, that doesn't mean you're going to die from it! Terminal insomnia means you wake up before the alarm goes off and can't go back to sleep again. Everyone does this once in a while when they have a big day ahead of them or are worried about some upcoming event. However, if this type of insomnia is a frequent happening, it can be a sign of depression or perhaps pre-depression. Trouble falling asleep (sleep initiation) is more the sign of anxiety and a busy life. When you go to bed you get still and no one is bothering you (except you!) and you begin to sort through the events of the day and plan for tomorrow. This is a normal reaction. But, back to our example, the chemical balance would now look like this.

Brain Chemistry

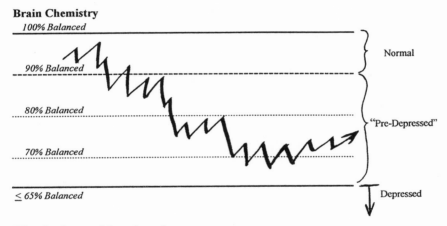

What's the problem here?

You've got too much on your mind.

Why?

Because you are trying to do too many things! Simple, right? (Your grandmother could have told you the answer to that one! But since she doesn't charge for her advice, you don't tend to believe her.)

But . . . what's the solution?

Read on!

The Effects of Stress and Hurry on Brain Chemistry

You can see from the previous section that as your chemicals become more and more unbalanced, the symptoms of pre-depression get worse and worse. Proof that stress, particularly chronic stress, can lead to depression comes from studying death and the grieving process.

If your spouse dies (stop cheering; this is serious!), you should feel down and have low energy levels for some period of time (no, not "just until after the funeral," behave!). However, if you couldn't get over the grief after six months, you would be diagnosed with depression and placed on antidepressants . . . *and they would work!* You would get well, usually very quickly. This is strong proof for stress being a cause of depression, and hurry is a form of stress. Chronic stress in your life can cause the chemicals in your brain to become unbalanced, causing first, pre-depression (part of the Hurried Woman Syndrome) and, eventually, depression, if left untreated.

So, if stress can cause depression and depression can and should be treated with antidepressants, doesn't it also make sense that pre-depression can be treated successfully with medication? I think it can, and many of my patients would agree with me, as do most experts in the field.

It is completely logical to assume that the main difference between depression and pre-depression is the degree to which the chemicals are out-of-balance—you're OK if your balance is greater than 90 percent, but if the balance is less than 65 percent you're depressed and treatment will rebalance you up to 90 percent, where you will feel normal again. That's easy to see. But if your balance is between 65 and 90 percent, then you are pre-depressed and the same treatment will probably rebalance you up to 90 percent, where you will feel normal again. Doesn't that make sense? You don't have to suffer at 70 percent efficiency if you don't want to—there are medicines to help you feel normal again. The following diagram describes the woman who is pre-depressed with the Hurried Woman Syndrome:

Brain Chemistry

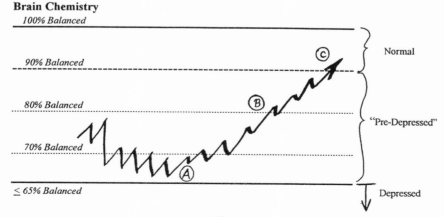

18

Her serotonin/dopamine levels fluctuate between 65 and 90 percent balanced. If she begins treatment at point A, she will see noticeable improvement by point B and feel essentially normal again at point C. Rebalancing her brain chemistry will improve and eventually reverse her symptoms of pre-depression.

What's amazing is the fact that these new anti-depressants don't sedate you and are not addictive. Our mothers took Valium for stress back when we were kids (and dinosaurs roamed the Earth) and it caused them to be "chemically absent" from a lot of their (and our) lives. Even though you feel rotten being a Hurried Woman, you don't want to be non-functional (the technical term is *gorked*) from medication or get hooked on something. These concerns are unwarranted with the newer anti-depressants, which are well-suited for the treatment of pre-depression. Obviously, you will need to discuss this with your doctor to get a prescription. And remember, your doctor will also need to screen you for the other medical conditions discussed earlier in the chapter that cause fatigue—such as anemia, vitamin deficiencies, electrolyte (salt) imbalances, abnormal thyroid functions, chronic infections, and auto-immune diseases. After further investigation, your doctor may want to test for other conditions as well.

Warning: the surgeon general has determined that Brent Bost is not your doctor and does not want to become your doctor for this problem! At least not through your reading a book anyway. There is no substitute for the eyeball-to-eyeball, stethoscope-to-chest personal interaction between patient and physician. You must discuss *your* symptoms and circumstances with *your* doctor and together agree on a treatment plan that's right for you. (Of course, if I *am* your doctor, we will do that, too.)

4

Treatment of Fatigue and
the Hurried Woman Syndrome

If your medical work-up for fatigue shows no other causes and your score on the depression scale shows that you are not depressed (and your doctor agrees that you are not depressed), then I propose that you are suffering from the Hurried Woman Syndrome (or pre-depression) and that your fatigue is treatable in several ways. Certainly you may prove to not need all of the treatments outlined here. Start with the simple things and work up as needed. Hopefully, after you consult with your doctor, he or she will be able to offer some additional guidance, particularly if medications are needed.

1. Vitamins

Most everyone can benefit from a good multi-vitamin. Multi-vitamins fill in the gaps of our often hurried and sometimes missed meals. I recommend Theragran-M, Centrum, and One-a-Day Plus Iron, although I am sure there are many other good vitamins out there. I also recommend a little extra vitamin C (500 milligrams per day), particularly for allergy and cold sufferers.

In addition, vitamin B_6 (pyridoxine) has been shown to help PMS sufferers with mood symptoms in double-blinded placebo studies. The current recommendation is 50 to 200 milligrams per day. Excessive doses of Vitamin B_6 can cause your hands and feet to go numb, so don't take too much of a good thing.

Women over thirty also need calcium to help prevent osteoporosis later in life. The current recommendation is 1,500 to 2,000 milligrams per day. I won't debate whether or not you need a supplement with vitamin D, but there is no compelling medical evidence that it makes any difference, except in cave dwellers and people who don't drink milk or get any sun exposure.

I would also recommend iron, which is available over-the-counter in low dose, to any woman who has heavy menstrual cycles or feels faint or dizzy or short of breath or has chest pain around her cycle. It would be wise to get your doctor to check you out to be sure you don't have anything worse than a mild anemia should you experience any of these symptoms.

2. Exercise

Aerobic exercise is very helpful in correcting mild fatigue and critical to the successful treatment of the Hurried Woman Syndrome. Exercise releases chemicals in the brain, called endorphins, that make us feel better. These chemicals give us a sense of well-being. Exercise also improves our physical stamina, allowing us to run faster and jump higher. (Wait a minute; that was Keds tennis shoes!) Just as in the saying "you have to spend money to make money," you have to spend energy to get energy. Exercise gives us more energy. I sometimes have trouble convincing myself to go walk on the treadmill when I get home after a particularly tiring day at work. But I have proven to myself over and over again that if I can make myself do it, I feel better the next day.

"I'm too tired to exercise," starts a vicious cycle and probably is the most common excuse people give for not following through on an exercise program. If you don't exercise today, you will be more tired tomorrow, which will further discourage you from exercising and make you even more tired the next day. This continues until you give up on exercise altogether. You must say to yourself, "I'm too tired to *not* exercise. If I don't do it tonight, tomorrow will be a worse day than today was." It's a bit of a psychological challenge to convince yourself of this fact at times, but if you can do it you will be rewarded in the end.

Exercise is also critical for successful weight loss, particularly for people over thirty. This is especially true for women. The minimum amount of exercise to maintain body weight is three, thirty-minute sessions of exercise each week. This is a "maintenance dose" of exercise. To lose weight many women must exercise more; some authors feel that most women need up to three hours of exercise per week to effectively take weight off and keep it off. Every women has to find her own level, which makes it tough to "prescribe" exercise. I will discuss this in more detail in the next chapter on weight loss.

3. <u>Un-hurry Your Life</u>

You've got to get the pressure off the brain's chemical rebalancer system if you want to feel better. Exercise encourages other chemical systems to help lift energy levels, but you must seek to take some of the unnecessary stress out of your life if you really want to get back to feeling normal.

You need to simplify your life. Get rid of the "clutter." Analyze your schedule and the activities you participate in and allow your kids to participate in. Set priorities that reflect the *long-term goals* you have for you and your family. Organize those activities into a reasonable schedule that you can live with while reserving some time each day for you. You are important enough to deserve time to yourself. Time alone, or at least time to do the things you want to do, helps make you feel rewarded for working hard and gives you time to stand back and reflect on your goals and priorities. It gives you the perspective you need to see what's important in your life and the lives of those you love and order things appropriately. Sometimes the time that you spend exercising is perfect for accomplishing this goal as well. This is the main topic of the fourth chapter and probably the most important one for you to grasp in your efforts to become an Un-Hurried Woman.

4. <u>Counseling and Supportive Therapy</u>

Many patients respond to counseling. A psychiatrist, psychologist, or counselor may be able to help your identify the things that cause stress in your life and help you find a better way to cope with them. Even if you can't eliminate the cause of the stress, learning how to take charge of it and control its effects on you will be helpful. Other supportive therapies can provide additional relief from symptoms. These programs go by such interesting names as resilience training, cognitive behavioral therapy, and stress management. Massage therapy may also be helpful.

22

Your counselor or doctor can direct you to one of these programs if he or she feels you might benefit from one or more of them.

5. Limit Caffeine and Sugar

Several studies have identified excess caffeine and processed sugar as culprits in worsening PMS symptoms. As in most things, moderation is the best approach. Limit your caffeine intake to three or four eight-ounce servings of caffeine-containing drinks each day. Also, remember that chocolate has caffeine in it. Stay away from candy bars, frosted doughnuts and other pastries that are loaded with sugar.

There have been recent concerns raised about Aspartame (Nutrasweet), the artificial sweetener found in many diet drinks and used as a sugar substitute. The manufacturer assures the public that unless incredibly huge amounts are taken (like ten two-liter bottles of diet drinks each day), there should be nothing to worry about. I'm not sure the final word is in yet on Aspartame. It seems that when I drink a lot of diet drinks I get bloated and actually seem to gain weight—or maybe have more trouble losing it. Whatever the final conclusion, I think using Aspartame in moderation makes sense. Perhaps limiting yourself to three or four, eight-ounce servings of diet drinks a day makes sense for now. (Consider two packets of the Aspartame sugar substitute equal to one serving.)

5. Hormones

Certainly if you are in menopause you should consider estrogen replacement therapy to prevent osteoporosis and lower heart disease risks. Besides that, you will likely feel better without all the hot flushes and night sweats, experience a better attitude toward sex, have better energy levels, and think more clearly. All of these benefits have been scientifically validated in well-designed studies.

Patients in peri-menopause may well benefit from birth control pills to control irregular menstrual cycling and prevent the wide hormone swings that worsen the emotional symptoms associated with PMS and menopause.

6. Medications

From the previous discussion you can see that I am not an advocate of Valium and other anti-anxiety drugs for treatment of PMS. Nor do I feel that stimulants like Metabolife or its cousins (largely caffeine and ephedrine) are the right answer, either. Some patients do benefit from these treatments, but these patients are in the minority.

Recall that the moderate to severe fatigue of pre-depression is caused by a chemical imbalance of the serotonin/dopamine system in the brain. Therefore, the most appropriate treatment for patients with this degree of imbalance will be to help the rebalancing system function more effectively. That is precisely what the new line of antidepressants do.

These medications are divided into two categories. The first group are what I call the new antidepressants (creative, eh?) to distinguish them from the "old antidepressants." This former group rebalances the serotonin/dopamine chemical system in the brain, but the exact mechanism by which they do it is not clearly understood. The older antidepressants have some effect on the serotonin/dopamine system, but they do it through an indirect mechanism that produces unwanted side effects, particularly sedation. Some patients still need the older type of antidepressant, particularly in treating insomnia, but I don't routinely use them in treating Hurried Woman Syndrome because the new medications work so much better. Medications in this first group include:

Medication (Generic)	Manufacturer
Welbutrin *(bupropion)*	Glaxo-Wellcome
Effexor (*venlafaxine*)	Wyeth-Ayerst
Desyrel *(trazodone)*	Apothecon
Serzone *(nefazodone)*	Bristol-Meyers Squibb
Remeron *(mirtazapine)*	Organon

Welburtrin *(bupropion)* is also marketed under the name Zyban, which is used to help people stop smoking. It helps cut cravings and what I call hand-to-mouth reflex, which can be either cigarettes or food. Because of this potential extra benefit, I prefer to start patients who are also trying to lose weight (or stop smoking for that matter) on Welbutrin. Plus, this medication has very few side effects and can be used virtually forever, if needed.

The second group of antidepressants, which are well suited for the Hurried Woman, are called selective serotonin reuptake inhibitors, or SSRIs for short. The SSRIs work specifically on the serotonin/dopamine system and are chemically similar to one another, so that their action and side-effect profiles are very similar. These medicines include:

Medication (Generic)	Manufacturer
Zoloft *(sertraline)*	Pfizer
Paxil *(paroxetine)*	Smith-Klein Beacham
Prozac *(fluoxetine)*	Dista
Celexa *(citalopram)*	Parke-Davis

This second group of medications works very much like the first group but also has, in my opinion, more mood-elevating capacity. In addition they have been shown in clinical studies to be very effective in treating the mood symptoms of PMS.

Prozac, the first medication produced in this category, got some bad press when it first became available. One early study said that Prozac might increase the rate of suicide when used in depressed patients. But remember, depressed people *do* commit suicide more frequently than other people, and the worse the depression is, the higher the risk of suicide. Whenever a brand-new, "better than all the rest" medicine comes to market, the first patients to get it are the ones who haven't done very well on the medicines available up to that point. In other words, the patients with the toughest cases of depression got Prozac because it was new. More recent studies show Prozac to be good medicine for depression, as well as PMS, with no increased risk of suicide. I have had good experience with it in treating Hurried Woman Syndrome, too. Prozac also causes weight loss in 20 percent of patients who take it, so I will often try it first in situations where weight gain is also a problem.

The patient response to these new medications has been, to put it in a word, phenomenal. Almost 80 to 90 percent of patients in my practice have gotten better with treatment. Some have more remarkable results than others, but on the whole, the response has been phenomenal. The best thing about these new medications is that they simply do what they are supposed to do—rebalance chemicals in the brain—and little else. That's why there are so few side effects compared to the older treatments, like Valium and the old-style antidepressants. The new medicines have a "pure" action in the body and are therefore better tolerated.

These medications are not addictive and they are rarely sedating, so patients can take them and work, sign contracts, drive a car, take care of children, etc., without fear of being "out of it." Plus, these drugs can be taken indefinitely because of their low toxicity and rare side effects. In contrast to Valium, these medications are not "feel-good pills." You don't take them on a bad day and skip them on a good day. You must take them every day in a steady dosing pattern to get the maximal effect and avoid side effect. These medications work with your body's natural rebalancer system to stay in balance, rather than artificially taking over the system or putting extra chemicals into the system to try to balance it artificially. This is the main reason that you can't take the medicines just when you feel like it. If you take them off-and-on-again you are "bumping" the rebalancer system rather than helping it work more smoothly and are likely to have side effects like agitation and sleeplessness.

I ask my patients to take these medications for at least two to three months to see what kind of response they get. Remember, these medicines work slowly and smoothly to rebalance your chemicals, so it takes a while to see how well they will work for you. Because of their similar actions, the side-effect profiles of these medications are very similar. The most common complaints are: GI upset (nausea, diarrhea), insomnia, and dry mouth.

Fortunately, most of these complaints are gone within a week or two of starting the medication and occur in only about 5 to 10 percent of patients. Occasionally some patients will complain about decreased sex drive or perhaps some difficulties in achieving a climax on the medication. Obviously, this is *not* a welcome side effect, and it occurs in about 10 to 15 percent of women. This side effect will often go away after a few weeks. However, if it persists for very long, most patients will choose to get off the medicine, which is understandable. A good rule to follow when taking any medical treatment is: If the treatment is worse than the problem, don't take the treatment.

Don't be discouraged if the first one of these medicines you try doesn't seem to work or if you experience side effects, because you may find that another one works great. These medications are a lot like sport shoes: all sport shoes cover your feet and can be used in several activities, but one brand may fit you better than another one and some styles are better suited for one use than another. Whenever we ask a patient to try one of these medicines, the first one we pick will usually work in nine out of ten cases, but if the first one doesn't work right, I will generally recommend trying another one. Most patients can find one that helps them feel better.

One final word about the medical treatment for Hurried Woman Syndrome. Although these medications are helpful in restoring a more normal balance to the complex chemical systems in the brain, they don't fix the underlying cause of the chemical imbalance—hurry. You will probably feel better and can cope better with treatment, but you are still suffering from the stresses that brought you to the doctor in the first place. In other words, the new antidepressants help make the symptoms better, but the "disease" is not really being cured. When someone gets pneumonia, he or she get a cough, fever, and chills and complains about being short of breath. If the person takes something for the fever and some cough medicine and breathes with an oxygen mask he or she will feel better. This is called supportive therapy—it makes the patient more comfortable. But until he or she gets on an antibiotic and kills the bacteria that is making him or her sick, he or she will not get well—cured. I would propose that the patient with Hurried Woman Syndrome is in a similar predicament. Until she decreases the stress and hurry in her life, she will never really get well. Oh, certainly she'll feel better on "supportive treatment"—antidepressants, vitamins, hormones, exercise, etc.—but until the stress is relieved (or at least lessened to some extent), she will never be cured. As I said earlier, some stresses in this life are truly unavoidable—these we must learn to deal with. However, much of the hurry in our lives is self-inflicted. We sign up for it ourselves or allow those around us to draw us into it. Many of these situations are not bad things in themselves, but the sheer burden of meeting the obligations day-in-and day-out for weeks, months, or years on end eventually takes its toll and causes the symptoms of the Hurried Woman Syndrome—fatigue, weight problems, and waning sexual energy.

Getting at the root cause of the syndrome—hurry—will be the main thrust of the last part of this book. I hope you will read it with an open mind and see the potential remedy offered there. Although I sincerely advocate the supportive treatment previously outlined for the Hurried Woman to help her cope with her disease, I more strongly advocate going for a "cure" rather than just a "patch."

Pre-Menstrual Syndrome

Another condition in which the serotonin/dopamine rebalancing system is important in pre-menstrual syndrome (or PMS, if you've been locked in a time capsule!). PMS is quite common. About 40 percent of adult women complain of having PMS at some point in their lives. Historically, PMS has been around for a long time, having been described in the Bible—remember ''Mary rode Joseph's ass all the way to Jerusalem.'' (I know, osteocephaly strikes again! Even doctors get it.) Patients in peri-menopause often describe intense worsening of their PMS symptoms, probably due to the wide hormone swings that occur with ovaries that are beginning to ''sputter.''

PMS causes a sudden short-circuit in the brain's rebalancing system, which produces the crabbiness and/or crying spells patients often complain about. By definition, these symptoms can occur only after ovulation (mid-cycle) and improve quickly within twenty-four to forty-eight hours of starting menstruation. If the symptoms occur at other times in the cycle, then there must be something acting along with the PMS or the problem is not simply PMS. Fortunately, most people who suffer with PMS describe their symptoms as mild and those with more severe symptoms can be treated effectively with a combination of dietary restrictions (limiting caffeine and processed sugar), vitamin B_6 (400 to 600 milligrams per day), regular aerobic exercise, and medications including birth control pills, which smooth out the hormone fluctuations, and the new antidepressants (like Zoloft, Paxil, Prozac, and Welbutrin). These medications are 80 to 90 percent effective in controlling the mood symptoms of PMS.

Another little-known fact about PMS is that men can get it, too. In fact, I suffer from it. I get moody and irritable and have frequent crying spells at the end of the month when my house note is due—it's called *Pre-Mortgage Syndrome.*

5

FAQS and Statements

"Alright, I made my appointment with the doctor. What can I do now before I go?"

I advocate doing just what your grandma would have told you to do if you'd asked her this question: get some rest, take a good multi-vitamin with iron, exercise regularly, change your underwear, and eat sensibly, cutting back on sugar and caffeine. Simple, right? Most likely, you already have tried some of these things and just haven't seen results yet—or at least, not the results you expected to see.

At this point, you owe it to yourself to get the medical work-up for fatigue. Remember to organize your thoughts about when your symptoms began, what makes them better and worse. Is there a pattern to your symptoms or are they "willy-nilly"? Write down a time line of symptoms and severity. Some people even find that keeping a symptom diary is helpful. Be certain to mark your periods on your diary also.

"Stress can't be causing me to be this tired. I'm not under any stress."

Yeah, right! And the pope is not a Catholic, either. When women throw this defense up I often ask them to describe their typical day or maybe a week. They will usually proceed to tell me about getting everybody ready for school, making breakfast and lunches, getting homework into backpacks, cleaning up the endless piles of stuff lying around the house, and then shuttling the kids to school, pre-school, day care, etc.

Then if they stay at home, the laundry begins and cleaning up the house—because every mom knows that you can't really clean the house right if the dirty little people who live there are at home at the time. Or if Mom goes to work, she gets to do these other duties when she returns home from her first job—only to start the second one, at home. Then her afternoon and evening are usually spent restfully shuttling kids between activities, such as baseball, soccer, basketball, gymnastics, etc., and then doing (hush!) homework with the kids and, oh yeah, supper, often on-the-run. Then baths and bedtime rituals, catching up with the latest news from friends and family via the phone message center (a tool of the Devil!), soon follow.

What did we do before telephone answering machines? Live a little slower—and a little longer—I suspect. I've grown to hate the blasted thing at times. Before I had an answering machine I used to worry about missing my calls; now I worry about getting messages! I think that missing a few calls here and there was actually better somehow. More about this later. Usually by the time we finish reviewing a typical day, most women begin to understand that they are a lot busier and rushed than they realized.

"Why am I getting so tired now? I've been doing this for years."

I think that Hurried Women are often deluded by the notion that just because they were able to juggle all this mess a year or two ago, they should be able to continue juggling it flawlessly and (since they are so well trained) perhaps they can add a little more on the side without noticing any loss of performance. Obviously, we all have limits, and most of us come up to our limits slowly. Sometimes we are able to expand those limits, but eventually even a marathon runner has got to take a break. No one can keep going and going and going (except the Energizer Bunny, of course!).

Motherhood is a lot like running a marathon. Runners who train for a marathon don't ever run the whole twenty-six miles until the day of the race. They train by running twelve to sixteen miles one day a week and by running four to eight miles two other days each week. They never actually run the seventeenth to the twenty-sixth mile until they have to, because no amount of training can make the last ten miles of the marathon any easier to endure. It is beyond the athlete's ability to train for this last leg of the race. Indeed, most marathon runners admit that the last ten miles of the race are painfully cruel. A lot of women live their lives like a marathon. They train up to run the first sixteen miles and are success-fully able to keep up the pace for a long time. But, after several years of struggling, they find themselves in mile twenty or twenty-two, where the pain is getting too great to ignore, wondering why they are having trouble. Even the best-trained athlete gets tired and needs rest after a long race.

Why do moms think they are any different? Even the best mom needs a break now and then. It makes sense.

"What about Chronic Fatigue Syndrome?"

A great deal of interest has been given to this "disease" in the last few years. It causes an almost intractable fatigue, with some sufferers complaining that they can't even get out of bed without fear of collapsing. In its most extreme stages, work is out of the question and even everyday activities become impossible for some patients. The cause of chronic fatigue syndrome is unknown. Chronic viral infections (like mononucleosis), some type of auto-immune process (like lupus), and possibly "unknown chemical disturbances" in the body have all been proposed as causes, but nothing definitive has yet been proven.

Interestingly enough, the disease is almost exclusively described in women and the only therapy that helps is—surprise—exercise and antidepressants. My unscientific opinion (even a scientist can have an unscientific opinion now and then!) is that Chronic Fatigue Syndrome is probably a form of chronic depression and that's why antidepressants work and why no other tenable explanation for the condition has been found yet. In fact, chronic fatigue in women is nothing new; it's just been described in different ways in the past. We had hypoglycemia (which affected mostly women) in the 1980s, Chronic Fatigue Syndrome in the '90s, and I think that Hurried Woman Syndrome will carry us into the next decade. The difference now is at least we are beginning to understand (and I hope, treat) the underlying cause and not just the symptoms.

I'm not saying that hypoglycemia and Chronic Fatigue Syndrome are not real diseases—they are. But I suspect that they have been and are continuing to be overdiagnosed. "Pure" cases of Chronic Fatigue Syndrome are probably more rare than rocking horse manure! In my opinion, the real cause of the fatigue that many of these patients complain of is a stress-induced depression or a milder "pre-depression," which can be treated by exercise, diet, antidepressants, and most important, de-stressing one's life *if you catch it early enough.* However, once the fatigue has "set in deep" for several months or even years, simple treatments don't work anymore.

"Are there other medical conditions associated with the Hurried Woman Syndrome?"

Interestingly enough, there are several very important illnesses in which stress seems to play a pivotal role. Recent studies indicate that almost 50 percent of migraine sufferers, 70 percent of patients with fibromyalgia, and about half of the patients who have Irritable Bowel Syndrome also suffer from some degree of depression—often the pre-depression that haunts the Hurried Woman.

In fact, studies have shown that many patients who present to their primary care doctor with symptoms like vague abdominal or chest pain, fatigue, dizziness, nausea, headaches, back pain, insomnia, shortness of breath, and numbness have no detectable organic cause, even after years of thorough investigation. Most experts now believe that these patients are probably suffering stress-related symptoms from either depression or pre-depression. Therefore, many women who suffer from the Hurried Woman Syndrome may also have additional complaints other than the fatigue, weight gain, and low sex drive that are common to the syndrome.

"What about over-the-counter treatments and 'natural' remedies like St. John's wort?"

There are several effective over-the-counter treatments for PMS symptoms. Most women have heard about and even used these products before. I think over-the-counter medications should generally be tried first before going to the doctor. If Midol or ibuprofen controls your menstrual cramps and pre-menstrual bloating, then you can and should use it. Always follow instructions and stay within the label's dosing guidelines and warnings. And don't hesitate to call your doctor for approval, particularly if you take other medications.

All drugs, whether over-the-counter or prescription, are regulated by the Food and Drug Administration (FDA) for both effectiveness and safety. This also includes quality controls on the product itself. In other words, each regular-strength acetaminophen (Tylenol) tablet has exactly 325 milligrams of pure medication—no more and no less, with nothing added. Manufacturers of regulated medications, whether prescription or over-the-counter, must satisfy the FDA that their products work, are safe, and are exactly the same from pill to pill. This is an expensive and time-consuming process, but since the thalidomide tragedy of the 1960s Washington and U.S. consumer groups have, for the most part, been happy to keep things the way they are.

However, there is no such regulation of the nutritional supplement and herbals market. No one is watching to see if the product does what it says it does, is safe for you to use, or is made with enough quality control to be the same from bottle to bottle. Makers of herbal products can make any claim they want about their product without any scientific research to back it up because they are not policed by the FDA. Of course many of them do try to substantiate their claims as part of their marketing effort, usually by giving a few patient testimonials ("I used Blue Ear Cream and it worked for me. Just look how blue my ears are, Connie!") or quasi–research statements like "three out of four doctors recommend Dung Fu Root Powder to their patients with underarm dingle-dangle." What you don't hear is that they only asked a total of *four doctors,* all of whom are on the company's payroll and who are actually not even M.D.s but rather are DSHTTRDWWAHAs (Doctors of Strange Herbal Treatments That Really Don't Work Worth A Hoot Anyway). So, how much faith should you place in this kind of "proof"?

Even more fortunate for consumers, there are misled, sometimes stupid, and even (gasp!) corrupt M.D.s who tout products in which they are financially involved and that are no more effective than snake oil. In my opinion, these doctors should be forced to give up their licenses to practice medicine (or at least be publicly flogged), because not only have they violated the public trust by lying to patients, but they are often lying to themselves—the worst lie of all.

In addition to trying to fool the public with weak proof of their product's effectiveness, many herbalists are now packaging them like real medications. Many have gone so far as to produce a label that looks very much like the FDA label of active ingredients and nutritional values. The big difference is that the nutrition product manufacturers will list their ingredients in terms that only a witch would appreciate: "Rose hips, *Angelica archangelica,* black cohosh, squirrel scrotums, and eye of newt." What is the active ingredient (chemical substance) in "black cohosh" that we're giving to *humans?* Might I have offered you "dirt from the southwest corner of my backyard" and been just as precise and perhaps as therapeutic, too? ("I don't know what's in that dirt that makes it so good, Jimmy Don. But it shore does work good! At least, gooder than that dirt from over by the outhouse, where the grass is always so green.") Since I have been trained as a scientist, this stuff drives me crazy!

I think it's no coincidence that many makers of herbals and nutritional products want to keep the ingredients in their products "secret." That way, no one will study them scientifically and prove them to be ineffective. Once that happens, they're out of business and must move on to another snake to extract the oil from. Now, before you think I am totally against searching for "natural" remedies, don't forget that over one-third of the prescription medications in use today are from plants and other natural sources. In fact, the best therapies available today encourage the body's natural mechanisms either to perform better (like the new antidepressants) or replace something the body needs but can no longer make for itself (such as human insulin, thyroid hormone, and estrogen). Medicine and pharmaceutical manufacturers are constantly searching out new and better treatments for patients. Let's face it. They can make a lot of money if they find one that works. But (and this is a big "but") scientifically proven effectiveness, patient safety, and uniform product quality are extremely important when trying to decide between a new treatment and an old one that has been effective in the past but could be improved upon.

Finally, a word about the concept of "natural." Many people in our culture have an almost knee-jerk reaction that "natural is better," particularly when it comes to medical treatments. But before we go much further, let me remind you that death is absolutely natural (and it's inevitable, too). Even though death is the natural alternative to illness, most of my patients aren't signing up for it! Another myth about "natural is better" is that if the medicine comes from a plant it must be better. Nothing could be further from the truth.

On the one hand, the estrogen replacement hormone, estradiol, is the exact same estrogen women make prior to their menopause—exactly the same. On the other hand, the soy protein, phytoestrogen, may have some estrogenic action in women but is certainly not normally found in humans and may not even be effective at preventing osteoporosis and heart disease risk. Now, which of these two treatments seems more "natural"? I think it's pretty obvious which one is more natural to the human condition, yet many patients run away from proven estrogen treatments toward plant products that they erroneously perceive as "better" somehow. Don't forget that hemlock comes from plants and that's the stuff that "socked it to Socrates."

Back to the original question: is St. John's wort effective? The answer is unclear at present. This herbal is being tested against antidepressants and placebo in blinded trials. My suspicion is that it may do better than the placebo for a short while, but in the long run I doubt it will prove to be as effective as the new antidepressants. In addition, St. John's wort can cause an increased bleeding tendency and should be stopped two weeks before any type of surgery and should not be used with an antidepressant or some types of blood pressure medicine.

Part II
Weight Control

"God Must Love Calories—That's Why
He Made So Many of Them"

6

Weight Control 101—The Basics

Statistics

Weight gain is a huge problem (no pun intended—really!) for my patients and for a growing number of people in this country. It can be one of the cardinal symptoms of the Hurried Woman Syndrome, or it can simply be an isolated problem. Either way, being overweight can have serious health consequences, both physically and emotionally. According to recently published statistics from the National Health and Nutrition Examination Survey II, about 25 percent of American woman are classified as "overweight," with a Body Mass Index, or BMI, between 25 and 30, and another 25 percent are "obese"—their BMI is greater than 30. You can look up your BMI using your height and weight in Appendix B at the back of the book. This table will also provide a range of "ideal" weight for your height. I assume Moses got these numbers from the burning bush on Mount Sinai along with the Ten Commandments; that's why we've adopted them as "ideal." Obviously, the ranges are pretty wide, so you'll have to decide if you're "small-framed" and pick a number in the lower portion or if you're "large-framed" and pick a number at the high end of the range to suit you. Yes, and if you're Baby Bear, you can pick the one in the middle that's "just right."

Find your height on the left-hand side of the table, then move to the right in the row with your height until you find your weight or the number that is closest to it. Then look at the top of that column to find your BMI. If you BMI is between 19 and 24, you are within the normal weight range for your height. If your BMI is between 25 and 30, the government considers you "overweight," but you can still pay taxes. If your BMI is greater than 30, you are considered "obese" and may soon have to pay more taxes! Actually, women who are obese by these standards run some really significantly increased health risks. Some weight-related diseases that have been identified and widely publicized are:

Heart disease: If your BMI is 29, you are twice as likely to die of a heart attack than if your BMI is less than 22. That risk of death *doubles again* if your BMI is 32 and goes up steadily as your BMI rises further.

Diabetes: Women with a BMI of 24 (still considered normal) are 350 percent more likely to develop diabetes than women with a BMI of 22! Even more incredible, women with a BMI of 31 are 3,000 percent (or 30 times) more likely to develop diabetes than that thin little twit with a BMI of 22!

Infertility: Women who are classified as obese (BMI greater than 30, or more than 20 percent above their ideal body weight) are two to three times (200 to 300 percent) more likely to have cycle irregularity and infertility than women who are mildly overweight or in the normal range.

Cancer: Many experts believe that cancers of the breast, gallbladder, cervix, uterus, and ovaries are linked to obesity, as women who are obese suffer higher death rates from these tumors. I'm not certain whether obesity actually causes the cancers or perhaps makes them harder to detect early, which leads to higher death rates because the treatments are usually less effective in more advanced cases. (For example, women with very large breasts are more likely to die from their breast cancer than women with smaller breasts, but this is probably because the woman with smaller breasts can usually find her lump earlier and therefore get treated earlier than the woman with large breasts who has more trouble with self-examination.) Whatever the real reason behind these statistics, it is clear that obesity is truly a disease and needs to be addressed medically just like chest pains, diabetes, or a screwdriver stuck in your forehead!

You may not have a weight problem and I hope you never have one. However, I would still encourage you to take the time to read through this information. You most likely have a family member or a friend who is continually struggling to lose weight and desperately needs some guidance on how to best go about this difficult process. As you can see from the preceding discussion, it's important! With all of the conflicting and competing information and misinformation bombarding the public, you might be able to help a friend, parent, or child finally succeed at one of the most difficult and yet important tasks facing almost half of American women.

Dr. Barry Sears in his book *The Zone: A Dietary Road Map to Lose Weight Permanently; Reset Your Genetic Code; Prevent Disease; Achieve Maximum Physical Performance* (Regan Books, 1995) presents some interesting insights into what he calls "the fattening of America." I will share some of his ideas with you here and augment them with other opinions, some widely accepted and others not. Of course, it doesn't matter whether the information is widely accepted or not as long as it's helpful to you, because the one certain thing about our scientific understanding of human nutrition is that we really don't understand a whole lot about it yet.

Since we "didn't build the machine and don't have an owner's manual" for humans it's little wonder that medicine is still somewhat in the dark about exactly how "fearfully and wonderfully" humans are made.

Nutrition—a Science?

The major problem with studying individual nutrients in isolation is that they never really exist in true isolation in a *living* animal. In other words, a scientific experiment cannot control and keep all of the other nutrients, bodily functions, and chemical reactions in a living animal constant while manipulating only the nutrient under study—at least, not for very long. Living animals, and particularly humans, constantly find themselves in a changing set of circumstances. That's why there are many "facts" about nutrition that seem to be in conflict at any one time and why very well respected nutritionists are constantly in disagreement about the best way to diet, optimally maintain the body's many intricate functions, and promote general good health. The conflicts over dietary fiber, cholesterol, and what constitutes "the perfect diet" are all good recent examples of the problems with getting a firm handle on weight loss.

Another major problem with past scientific research in the field of nutrition has been the reliance on a faulty assumption—that all humans are created nutritionally equal, endowed by their creator with certain inalienable properties including life, liberty, and the uniform pursuit (and handling) of happiness (calories!). Nothing could be further from the truth. Our genes control to a great extent what our individual daily calorie needs are, what we do with excess protein, carbohydrates, and fats if we get too many of one or more of these (and we usually do!), and what our biochemical reaction will be to imbalances of these main nutrients. There is no one uniform human response to a high-cholesterol diet or to a high-protein, low-carbohydrate diet or a high-carbohydrate, low-fat diet, although scientists have conducted much of their past nutritional research with this thought in mind. Little wonder so many similar experiments have come out with conflicting results and caused an almost constant debate among nutritionists about the proper diet for humans and the best diet technique to use for the most efficient weight loss. Dr. Sears points out in *The Zone* "that in the world of nutrition nobody's really wrong. They just aren't quite correct" (p. 72). And I suspect that this will remain the case for many more years. If only God had sent the Ten Nutritional Commandments along with the other admittedly more important ten, we wouldn't be in such a daze about diet and weight control.

One truth that comes out clearly from studying the available research, and the bookstore shelves for that matter, is that there are about as many diets recommended by nutrition experts as there are nutrition experts! And most of them actually work to accomplish weight loss—in the short run. But I would propose to you that short-term success in a weight loss program is *not* the important part. Short-term weight loss is a physiologic certainty of starvation and is generally pretty easy to accomplish, no matter what diet you start. Most women can lose a few pounds of water weight whenever they begin a diet program. And although this initial success is well received and encouraging to the new dieter, it is often quickly followed by a "plateau" (or stable weight) that is really hard to get below. No, the real test of a successful diet effort is *long-term*—**keeping the weight off** is the big challenge. Most fad diets simply cannot do this for you, for a variety of reasons we will discuss later. For now, let's discuss the genetic truths about nutrition and weight control and how they impact your efforts to diet, then talk about a diet plan that will work for you—*in the long run.*

Medical Causes of Weight Gain

If you've only got ten pounds to lose, you probably could lose it any number of ways, including the method I offer you here. If you've got more than that hanging over you (or off of you, as the case may be), I think you should consult your doctor. If you've gained more than ten pounds in the last year, you need to be certain there is no underlying medical condition that needs treatment, including depression. Thyroid disease is also quite common in young women, as many develop thyroid problems in their childbearing years. As discussed in chapter 2 on fatigue, you must at least have a TSH (thyroid-stimulating hormone) to check your thyroid function. I additionally like to check a fasting blood sugar and hemoglobin A-1-C or glycosylated hemoglobin, to screen for diabetes, and a cortisol level to look for Cushing's Syndrome (an adrenal gland problem). Your doctor may wish to test for less common problems or do further screening than this, but this is what I do at a minimum for women who complain of significant weight gain.

Polycystic Ovary Syndrome

This special condition, estimated to be present in about 5 to 10 percent of young women (in other words, it's pretty common!), is associated with obesity in well over half of the women who have it. If you read older information on Polycystic Ovary Syndrome (PCOS), originally referred to as Stein-Leventhal Syndrome when it was first described in 1935, you will get a rather confusing picture of the condition. I will give you the most current information available at the time of this writing, but some new and exciting research will be coming out soon that will, we hope, help this select group of women, particularly when it comes to weight control.

PCOS is "officially" diagnosed when a woman of childbearing age presents with: (1) irregular menstrual cycles called oligo-ovulation (her cycles are typically seven or more weeks apart or she has fewer than eight cycles a year, which may sound good at first, but believe me, it's more trouble than triumph): (2) signs of "male-type" hair grown on chin or beard area, breasts, and the line between the pubic hair and bellybutton (called hirsutism) *and/or* significant acne *and/or* abnormal blood levels of male hormone, specifically testosterone; and (3) the exclusion of other medical problems that can look like PCOS. These unusual conditions include tumors that secrete prolactin, thyroid disease, tumors that produce male hormones, and adrenal gland malfunction. You probably recognize this list of diseases from the medical work-ups of fatigue and obesity that were discussed earlier, but if you think you may have PCOS you need to discuss it with your gynecologist or endocrinologist (an internal medicine specialist who specifically treats hormone and metabolism problems, most often diabetes and thyroid disease). Unfortunately, most general practice doctors just don't have a lot of experience with this condition.

The symptoms of PCOS and the percentage of patients with each are as follows:

Irregular periods (oligo-ovulation)	≥90 %
Hirsutism (not just a few "wild hairs")	75%
Polycystic ovaries (on an ultrasound)	70%
Obesity	60%
Male-type balding (receding hairline)	20%
Acne (the real "deep" pimples)	15%

The fat distribution in women with PCOS is more like that of men—the majority of the weight is focused at the waist and above (like a man with a pot belly and broad shoulders, sometimes referred to as "apple-shaped"), rather than in the hips and thighs or "saddle bag" area (or "pear-shaped") where most women complain of weight gain. Like a lot of conditions described earlier, if you have some of the symptoms, but they're mild, you're probably normal. But if you've got a lot of the symptoms and some of them are pretty noticeable, then you may have something that needs fixing. When in doubt, go see your doctor—that's why he or she went to school all of those years (a minimum of fourteen years to be a board-certified obstetrician/gynecologist, to be precise!), so he or she can help you sort this kind of stuff out.

Although most women with PCOS first present their problems to the doctor in the childbearing years, many of these women were actually considered skinny or too thin as teenagers. The weight problems seemed "to grow on them" over time (no pun intended—really!), many times after their first or second child was born. The weight gain associated with PCOS comes at a different time for each woman.

These young women with PCOS also get older each year just like everybody else, which means that about 5 to 10 percent of *all* women from age twenty to eighty have this condition; they just don't necessarily fit into the new definition of PCOS that has been adopted only recently. In other words, a lot of women who are obese today have PCOS, even women who are in their forties, fifties, sixties, and older. We just "missed" the diagnosis when they were younger because the nature and definition of PCOS have only been recognized recently.

The actual cause of the weight gain associated with PCOS is unknown, but the best theory at present is that the fat cells somehow become insulin-resistant in PCOS and therefore don't respond appropriately to exercise and diet changes. In other words, women with PCOS are diet-resistant. This is one of those good news/bad news deals. The good news is: I can now explain why many women who diet faithfully and exercise hard can't lose weight—they probably have PCOS. The bad news is: the only way they're going to lose weight is to eat even less and exercise harder than the average woman—which, of course, your grandma could have told you. Before you get too discouraged, though, there is some additional "good news": there is a lot of ongoing research to try to solve this mystery, and I predict that within five years we'll have some better tools to help you control your weight. But for now, diet and exercise are the keys to successful weight management and a healthier future.

Weight Gain and the Hurried Woman Syndrome

When it comes to weight gain and the Hurried Woman Syndrome, it is often difficult to tell which is the cart and which is the horse. Did the weight gain come from stress and the loss of physical activity associated with fatigue or did the patient gain weight, then get frustrated and "down" about being overweight, which caused her to lose her self-esteem and begin to withdraw from her normal activities, including her sex life?

When a woman gains weight, it often changes the way she perceives her body—she may not feel "sexy" and may not want to participate in sex as much as she did in the past. She may also perceive, rightly or wrongly, that her husband is not as interested in her when she's feeling fat. Whether she is or isn't fat is irrelevant to how she feels about her weight and how she looks—if she *thinks* she is fat, then *she is fat* and no amount of convincing from her husband (who she knows will lie to have sex!) will change her opinion on the subject.

Whatever the order of events, if you have problems with fatigue and/or low sex drive in addition to your concerns about weight, you may be suffering from the Hurried Woman Syndrome and should read the other chapters in the book to see what you can do to get better. Women with these three problems often benefit from a complete medical work-up and possibly hormones or other medications along with the diet and exercise program outlined here.

7

Your Survival Genes Are Killing You

Genetics and Weight Regulation

For the most part, we all tend to become like our parents, both in our attitudes and in our physical attributes. You might be much more like one parent than the other, but the trend to be like our ancestors is one we've all noticed. (It's also funny how our parents tend to become like *each other* through the years, but I think that's more of a learned behavior rather than genetic—in fact, a lot of people even start to look like their pets, but that can't be genetic—can it? Let's get back to the subject at hand.)

Most people who struggle with weight will have at least one parent with a weight problem. This certainly points to a genetic basis for weight regulation. Although it is clear that our attitudes about food, our preferences for different styles of foods and spices, and the way we eat our meals are all influenced by the way we were brought up, I think it's important to remember that, for me anyway, many of these things have changed dramatically since I left home twenty-plus years ago and have even changed remarkably in the last five years. In other words, my eating style and food selections have been constantly changing through the years since I left my mother's direct culinary influences, yet the trend to be like her physically has not. The way your body handles food and your overall ''style'' are determined by your genes. Let's face it, statements like ''I have my mother's thighs'' are all too familiar to most women. Obviously, a lot of women would agree that they tend to put weight on like their mothers did.

Your genetic code determines how you handle the calories you put into your body as well as the efficiency with which exercise burns those calories. This is how your genes set your weight balance. It is important to understand that not everyone responds to food and exercise the same way. After all, each human is genetically different, yet there are obvious similarities, too. According to Dr. Sears, about twenty-five percent of Americans won't gain weight on a high-carbohydrate diet, whereas about 25 percent will gain a lot more weight than expected and about 50 percent will gain weight as expected, based on their insulin response to carbohydrates. This explains why a one-size-fits-all approach to dieting doesn't work. It's impossible to prescribe the exact calorie "dose" for optimum weight management that always works for everyone, because not everyone handles the calories they eat in the same way. Each patient has to find the right balance of calories and exercise by trial and error to a certain extent. It might be interesting to know which group of "carbohydrate responders" you fall into, but practically speaking, it doesn't matter. You cannot change the way your body responds; you have to learn to cope with it.

If you can lose weight when you diet but just find it difficult to stay on a plan, you are probably in the normal-response group—that's about half of all people. If you really can't seem to lose weight in spite of really cutting down on calories, even below the levels of most diets, then you may be in the "over-responder group," which is where one-in-four Americans find themselves. Unfortunately, you're going to have to do a lot more cutting back on calories and increasing exercise than most people to get control of your weight. If, however, you are one of those lucky people (about 25 percent of the population) who just can't seem to *gain* weight, you are probably in the "under-responder" group, are lucky beyond belief, and are also probably not reading this chapter anyway! Since that's true, let me take this opportunity to say that one-in-three American women *hate your (little) guts!*

Survival Genes

Actually, people who have trouble losing weight are genetically superior to those who can't seem to gain weight and even those with what would be called a normal carbohydrate response. Why? Remember that the primary drive for any animal species is survival—to stay alive as an individual, as well as propagate the species through reproduction. Thousands of years ago, our ancestors lived on a pretty harsh diet compared to today—estimated by experts at less than 1,000 calories per day. During a bad winter or times of drought (and if all of the convenience stores were closed, of course), the calories available for consumption dropped off to starvation levels very quickly. In such harsh times, those people who can "eat anything" and never gain weight would be *dead!* You, however, would be dancing on their narrow little graves, running off with their grieving menfolk, and looking like a centerfold for *Cave Queen* magazine. In other words, the same genes that confound you now by causing you to struggle with weight gain would protect you from starvation in harsh nutritional circumstances—you have superior survival genes! The only problem is: you don't need them now and you can't shut them off when you want. They are constantly there, protecting you from the ill effects of starvation. And remember that most diets, particularly fad diets, are simply that—starvation—for one class of nutrients or another to force your weight down. When you get on a diet, your survival genes see your decreasing nutritional input as impending starvation—a bad winter—and begin to turn on metabolic safety mechanisms in your body to prevent you from losing weight! Ouch! Unfortunately, the genetic news gets worse.

In the early stages of starvation (or any diet), the body causes shifts in its metabolic pathways too keep glucose levels stable. These mechanisms are rapidly deployed and involve mostly water shifts between "compartments" inside the body. Indeed, most of the early weight loss in any diet, particularly the high-protein, low-carbohydrate ketosis diets, is from waterloss. For most dieters, this is the first five to ten pounds, which usually come off in the first two weeks of any diet. This lost water is also the first weight to come back when the fad diet fails, so it's really false encouragement. Of course, some encouragement beats no encouragement at all, but it's important to realize that this water weight is not the real weight you are wanting to get rid of, but it's a start.

As the diet continues, your survival genes start to realize that this may not be just a bad winter but a bad year (or two) and crank up some very powerful long-term changes in metabolism that will protect you from dying under these new harsh circumstances. Theories abound as to what these exact changes are in response to starvation. Some people believe that the intestinal tract improves its absorption of nutrients under diet conditions, while some experts believe that the body's storage capacity increases with dieting and that fat cells become stingy—Dr. Sears reports that high-protein ketosis diets make fat cells ten times more efficient at holding onto fat than they were before starting the diet. This effect probably doesn't last a lifetime, but I suspect it does last a long time. Gee, that's great news, isn't it? Not only do you already have genetically the most efficient fat cells on the planet; they're also trainable. That's right, ladies! Not only does your adipose tissue have an *attitude;* it also has a *memory!* (Sound like your mother-in-law?) This ability of fat cells to adapt to change probably accounts for the yo-yo effect that plagues women who attempt to diet frequently. And although I don't have a lot of scientific proof, I think pregnancy is a metabolic reprogramming event for a lot of women also. The effects may not be too noticeable after the first baby, but many women don't begin to have weight trouble until their second or third pregnancy. Of course, it's impossible to factor age out of the equation, because everyone is older after their last pregnancy than after their first one! But it is clear that gestational diabetes tends to worsen in each successive pregnancy, and more so in pregnancies that are less than a year apart.

I have also noticed that when women who have previously lost a lot of weight (more than thirty pounds) do get pregnant, those who lost the weight recently tend to gain it all back within the first two or three months of pregnancy, whereas those who lost the weight more than a year earlier seem to be able to keep it off more easily. I know that there can be a lot of alternative explanations for this observation, but I still believe that it will ultimately be proven that pregnancy, through some physiologic mechanism, sets up a lot of women for weight troubles in the future. It certainly makes sense when looking at the survival gene model that God would have given pregnant women an added measure of protection against starvation. Regardless, it is absolutely clear to me that pregnancy creates *children*, and having them around sets up a whole set of social and environmental circumstances that lead to weight gain for a lot of women!

In summary, your genes determine for the most part what you look like as well as the way your body handles the "calories in minus calories used up equals your weight" equation. You cannot change your genetic makeup but must learn how to deal with it effectively to get your weight where you want it *and keep it there.* Understanding how your body's system of weight regulation works can help you avoid common mistakes as well as learn how to successfully manipulate a diet and exercise plan to fit your physiology as well as personality and schedule. However, it is extremely important for you to realize now and admit that you must become committed to a program of weight management *for the rest of your life.* Weight gain is a "forever" problem for you. If you refuse to see it that way, it will continually defeat you. Sure, you may be one of those women who pick up a diet for two or three months, lose the weight, and then be content to go back to "business as usual" afterwards. But the weight will always come back when you stop the diet, unless you change your "business as usual" to include effective weight management. And each successive diet attempt will become more and more difficult until it doesn't work anymore and you're stuck with a much more difficult problem to fix. Trust me on this one: I've seen many women succeed and hundreds more fail multiple times on this one point. *Make a life-long commitment to mange your weight now* and be successful—forever. Dodge the commitment now and you will ultimately fail. The choice is yours.

8

Exercise and Weight Loss—The Real Untold Story

The Calorie Equation

In its simplest form, the balance of calories going into and out of our bodies determines any weight gain or weight loss we experience.

Calories in − calories expended = weight gain (or loss)

When the calories in are more than the calories expended, we gain weight. If we expend more calories than we take in, *over time* we will lose weight. Remember, it does take time for these changes to take place, but for now, I want to stress *the balance* between calories and your weight.

Simply put, your weight is determined by the balance of calories that go into your body versus the calories you burn up in physical activity. If you put more calories in than you burn up, you gain weight. If you cut back on the calories going in or increase the calories you get rid of through exercise, you will lose weight. Simple, huh? Actually, it *is* quite simple. I think that's what makes it so difficult to accept for many people. They are looking for some "magic trick" or "secret twist" to the equation that will make it easier to manipulate their weight, but the basic facts are immutable: you are what you eat (minus what you can work off through exercise). Most women who want to lose weight will focus a great deal of attention to the "calories in" part of the weight equation, and this is critical to successful weight management, yet it's only half of the story. For a lot of my patients, the "calories expended" portion is relatively neglected, but I assure you it is equally important to successfully controlling your weight, particularly for women over thirty.

Unless you've been preoccupied the past few years perfecting "auto-proctoscopy" (the art of looking up your own rear end), you've no doubt heard that exercise is good for you. It promotes less heart and lung disease, lowers blood pressure and cholesterol, helps counter diabetes, improves energy levels, and helps fight depression, osteoporosis, and obesity. It even helps with low sex drive, the topic of the next part of the book. Not only is exercise good for you, it is also the primary regulator of your metabolism—how your body handles the "calories in" part of the calorie-balancing equation—and, ultimately, your weight.

Virtually every body function, including reading this book, expends calories. Obviously, the more physically taxing the activity, the more calories will be expended. Some common activities and the amount of calories expended per hour are listed in Appendix B. When you analyze the activities and the amount of calories expended, a few facts leap out at you:

1. The more vigorous the activity, the more calories expended—duh! Walking up stairs for an hour (1,100 calories) burns almost three times as many calories as walking briskly for four miles (400 calories). Running for an hour or about eight miles (800 calories) burns about twice as many calories as an hour of walking (400 calories).
2. Exercise that forces you to carry your weight, rather than floating in water or sitting on a bike, expends energy at a much faster rate. An hour of swimming burns about 500 calories per miles, whereas an hour of running (about eight miles) burns about 800 calories.

However, there are several very important points about exercise that you won't get from the table in Appendix C. The most important ones are as follows:

1. There is a minimum amount of exercise that every woman needs to maintain her body weight

Once that level is reached, additional exercise will improve her ability to lose weight, but only to a point. This maximum exercise benefit tops out for most women at around six hours of aerobic activity per week. Marathon runners, high-endurance swimmers, and other "extreme athletes" train to the level of *anaerobic* conditioning, which burns off a lot more calories and changes metabolism in such a way as to allow for more weight loss, but this level of training, in my opinion, is not really healthy for most women, particularly those who are interested in childbearing. This type of training often pushes body fat levels too low and disturbs menstrual functioning and bone metabolism, among other things.

You may have also realized that the flip side of the exercise "pearl" is that if you don't at least exercise at the required minimum level, you will *gain weight* unless you diet much more intensely. I think a lot of "diet failures" are actually "exercise failures." Most women and even some diet experts don't understand the critical importance of exercise in a long-term weight management program.

2. There is no one "prescription" for exercise that will work for everybody.

The kicker about this minimum level of aerobic exercise is that every woman must find her own unique level. A one-size-fits-all approach to exercise leads to failure for a large number of women. I will give you a few guidelines to help you get started, but most women must go through some trial and error to find the level of activity that's right for them. Most experts recommend starting out at three half-hour sessions per week and adding a session after two to three weeks if results are less than satisfactory. An alternative to adding a session each week would be to push up the time in each session by ten minutes each week until you see improvement. A one-hour session would be the maximum I would recommend. Besides, going longer than an hour may be impractical and increase your "hurry" if you've got kids to shuffle around or any real schedule constraints—the heart of the Hurried Woman Syndrome. Also, if you are starting from "couch potato" levels of activity, you must build up slowly and progressively so you won't injure yourself and give up on exercise. Exercise is an essential element of long-term weight management. You've got to have it to be successful, so be patient and build up to your level of exercise carefully. Besides, this is a lifetime commitment to exercise, so if it takes a few more weeks to get your exercise level up where it needs to be, big deal! You've got the rest of your life to work on it. Be patient! Injuries are one of the major reasons committed women give up on exercise programs and then ultimately fail at weight control. Be careful and do it right the first time.

3. Exercise reprograms your metabolism to discourage fat storage and help improve energy levels.

Whenever we take in extra calories (those we don't need for immediate use) the body must make a choice where to store them. Obviously, we all wish the body would let us flush them down the toilet, but it doesn't work that way. Once the calories are in the body, they've got to go somewhere. If you are a couch potato, the body doesn't see any immediate need for these calories to supply energy and puts them into long-term storage or fat. If, however, you routinely exercise for three or four half-hour sessions each week, the body will see the probable need for these calories to provide energy in the near future and place them into short-term storage, or muscle and liver glycogen. The short-term storage area does link some water to the calories in it, but nowhere near the levels of water that are associated with fat storage. Fat tissue is 97 percent water, and that's where the weight of fat comes from: its water content. So, encouraging any extra calories in to go into short-term storage through regular aerobic exercise rather than fat storage produces less weight gain in the long run. Exercise makes fat cells less resistant to giving up their stored energy, too. This allows you to burn fat more easily when you do exercise. The short-term storage area can also quickly convert these "extra" calories into energy. Converting fat back into energy takes time—ask anyone on a diet how slow this can be, right?! Therefore, exercise helps improve energy levels while also discouraging fat storage.

4. Exercise burns calories. Adding exercise to a diet plan allows you to eat more (or diet less) and still maintain your caloric balance (weight).

This fact is what makes exercise so appealing to me. I absolutely hate to diet. Even worse, I love Blue Bell Homemade Vanilla Ice Cream. I mean I *love it!* In fact, it's almost better than sex—almost. I eat a bowlful of that delicious, mouth-pleasing pure white, creamy, dreamy dessert almost every night. I have discovered that if I run three miles, three days a week, I can eat my Blue Bell and not gain any weight. I have also found that if I eat Blue Bell every other night, I only have to run two days a week to keep the weight down. (But this would cost me about 180 bowls of Blue Bell each year!) Knowing these facts about my exercise response and my diet allows me to choose between diet and exercise to keep my weight stable. If I want to diet less, I must exercise more. If I don't want to exercise or perhaps if I miss running for a week because of the weather or being stuck at the hospital a lot, I can cut back on calories and keep my weight balanced. It's simple! And, even better, it works. This ability to trade calories in for calories expended in exercise allows you to find the right balance of calorie restriction and exercise to develop an effective approach to long-term weight management that you can live with forever. Remember, it's a ''forever'' problem that requires a ''forever'' solution. I must add at this point that it is a little too simple to say that the only effect of exercise on weight is the calculated calories burned. The calories burned up running a marathon, twenty-six miles, are only equal to the calories in a twelve-ounce steak and a baked potato. Whoa! That's all you get for running twenty-six miles—one dinner at the Outback? It sounds pretty discouraging when you look at it this way. But there is obviously more to exercise than simply counting the calories expended and balancing them against the food you eat—take a look at most marathon runners and you'll see that they have very low levels of body fat. They are lean, mean running machines! Exercise reprograms your metabolism to discourage fat storage and accelerate fat burning in a way that is much more powerful than simply ''burning calories.'' Did you know how they actually determined the amount of calories in food? The original experiments were done with a device called a bomb calorimeter. It is simply a pot immersed in a water bath. The food in the pot is incinerated, and the resulting rise in the temperature of the surrounding water is measured in calories. Simple, huh? Of course, unless you're passing ashes in the toilet, your body with its immensely complicated metabolic systems is not an incinerator. Therefore, this model does not adequately explain the complex relationship between the food we eat, exercise, and weight control. The calorie-balancing method gives us a way to rate one exercise against another and a rough estimate of the effect of exercise and food on daily calorie balance, but it is only an approximation. The overall impact of exercise on weight maintenance is much more powerful than a simple exchange of calories in and calories out, but understanding it at this level is a start.

5. Regular exercise makes you feel better about yourself and improves energy levels.

Getting in shape makes people feel better about themselves. Improving your strength and endurance, shedding flab, and seeing your muscles toning up from working out gives you a sense of accomplishment. Knowing you look better makes you feel better about yourself. It improves your self-confidence in just about everything you do, including your love life. It makes a woman feel sexy to know that she looks good. Doesn't getting a new hairstyle or a new dress that you *know* looks good on you make you feel better? Absolutely! Exercising regularly and getting in shape will do the same thing for you. Exercise itself makes us feel better. When you exercise, your brain releases chemicals called endorphins. Endorphins chemically look a lot like morphine, specifically the part of the morphine molecule that causes the sense of euphoria, or "high," that drug users look for. Regular exercise improves the brain's ability to produce endorphins. This is one reason that exercise can help you feel better and less fatigued.

9

Diet—What Really Works and Why

Dieting is a very popular "sport" in America today. In fact, over 50 percent of American women have been on a diet this year. Of course, most of them have not *stayed* on their diet, but at least half of the women in the United States have attempted to diet at least once this year. However, only 5 percent of these women actually reached their goal weight. But even more telling is that of those that lost weight, *over 90 percent gained it all back within twelve months.* More proof that being overweight is a "forever" problem.

Fad Diets Don't Work—Period!

A quick stroll through the health section of your local bookstore will reveal literally hundreds of diet books and different diet methods, all touted to be "the best." Whether it's one of the high-protein, carbohydrate-starvation ketosis diets, Sugar Blasters, Butt Busters, or the Diet-of-the Month Club diet, they all pitch their "unique" approach, along with some testimonials from satisfied customers and with some scientifically feasible but nonetheless unproven arguments for why their method is superior to the other gimmick diets available.

I am not a biochemist, exercise physiologist, or a nutritionist. And even though there are some very smart experts out there with these fancy titles writing too-numerous-to-count books on dieting, I think it is clear from reading what they say that there is no agreement among them as to the absolute best method to achieve long-term weight control. In fact, I really don't think any of them are that interested in the long-term picture anyway. Most fad diet books stress short-term weight loss and, sadly, often miss the important role that exercise plays in successful long-term weight control. If you are trying to drop a dress size in two months for your best friend's wedding and really don't care what happens after that, then by all means feel free to choose a fad diet. But if you'd like to take a more long-term approach and *keep the weight off* afterward, you need to keep reading.

In addition to missing the boat on exercise, fad diets don't work in the long run for three important reasons: (1) fad diets are usually "unbalanced" diets and will often turn on survival genes, which make the diet become less effective over time: you reach the "plateau phase" and stop losing weight; (2) the weight loss gimmick doesn't allow for diet flexibility in food selection or match the way you normally eat; and (3) once the weight is off, you must change your eating habits again to another diet method for long-term weight control or the weight will come back—you have a "forever" problem that requires a "forever" solution.

Keeping Your Balance

Most nutrition experts agree that a healthy diet should distribute its calories among the various energy sources as follows:

Protein	40%
Fat	30
Carbohydrates	30
Total=	100%

When these ratios become distorted, as is the case with most fad diets, the imbalance causes complex changes in the body's metabolic systems to "fight" the starvation it's experiencing. If the starvation is harsh enough or lasts long enough it can cause malnutrition. In fact, Dr. Sears says that malnutrition, particularly protein malnutrition, is quite common among people on a diet. However, more important for the success of the diet, starvation can turn on the survival genes we discussed earlier, which makes the diet lose its effectiveness over time. Ultimately, most women hit the "plateau phase," where the weight loss comes to a screeching halt, and decide to bail out.

Rather than trying to begin a lifelong commitment to weight management with some oddball diet scheme and then shifting out of it later, doesn't it make more sense to start a diet and exercise program that uses these optimal ratios in the first place? Fad diets manipulate these ratios to achieve faster short-term weight loss, hoping to encourage the new dieter. But remember, you must be committed to the long term and fad diets are not healthy in the long run. They are not friendly to your system over the long haul and can cause metabolic disturbances. My advice is to get on the right program—one you can stick with forever—right now and stay on it.

Gimmick Diets Aren't Flexible

For a fad diet to sell, it must be unique. In fact, the more unusual, the better. Most dieters have already tried several diets through the years, and since dieting is incredibly tedious and rapidly leads to frustration, any diet that is perceived as brand-new or glamorous or clever in how it "tricks the body into giving up its stored fat calories" (yeah, right!) gets a lot of attention—sells books. Of course, the gimmick used—for example, high-protein, super low-carbohydrate, or special food you can only purchase from the chain of diet centers—ain't no "natchal" (natural) way to eat, and therefore, to paraphrase Jerry Lee Lewis "there's a whole lotta cheatin' goin' on!"

When you cheat on one of these fad diets, you lose a lot of ground on the diet because your cheating reverses the metabolic gimmick quickly, since your body is ready and willing to save you from the death grip of the famine you've placed yourself in, and it takes a couple of days of "being good" to get the gimmick back working again. Fad diets don't allow you to do much manipulation to fit the diet to your individual needs—you just can't "personalize" them.

Most Fad Diets Don't Have a Follow-up Plan

If you beat the odds and are successful at losing your weight with a fad diet, what do you do next? Most fad diet books don't give you a viable follow-up plan. They focus on the short term but fail to provide a long-term solution. You have to do that.

And what about the diet programs that require you to purchase special food? How long do you think most people stay with those programs and how much do they cost? The answers are "not very long" and "too much" to be practical for most normal humans anyway. No one is going to pick up seven to ten brown bag lunches each week for the rest of their lives at $200 per month. Get real!

Again, my advice is to get on a program of diet and exercise that is inexpensive, allows for flexibility in food choice and timing, has been proven to be effective, and can adapt to fit your lifestyle—which includes not having to prepare two or more different meals for each mealtime to meet the needs of everyone in the family.

So, by now, you've got to be asking yourself, *When is he going to tell me what is the best diet method to lose weight and keep it off for the long haul?* Well, I have to admit that it isn't particularly glamorous, sexy, or fun. Are you sure you're ready for it? (You might be shocked, you know.) OK, I'll tell you. *Lean a little closer; it's a secret*—I want to be sure to sell a bunch of books before the word gets out! The most effective diet for long-term weight management is: counting calories.

I know, you're thinking, *I hope I saved my receipt for this stupid book so I can get my money back! I can't believe this toad is recommending counting calories. There's nothing new or glamorous about that method. It's been around for years, it's boring as hell, and you have to be an accountant to be able to keep track of all those numbers.* I admit that a lot of patients look at me as if I had just walked out of a storm drain when I tell them that balancing calories is the most effective long-term method to manage their weight. But after years of counseling patients on the subject of weight loss and watching their progress on all kinds of diets, I assure you that calorie counting done properly works and works well, compared to any other diet method I've seen.

Balancing calories is:

Simple: Once you learn some simple rules and conversions, you will be able to accurately estimate the calories you eat.

Flexible: As long as you maintain the proper ratio of carbohydrates, fats, and proteins, you can chose to eat reasonable portions of what you want at mealtime. You don't have to make or buy special foods unless you want to. This lets you eat the same food as your family and also allows you to eat out without the embarrassment of bringing a doggie bag into the restaurant.

Adaptable: You can learn to "cheat" by overeating one day and then making up the difference by undereating the next day. You can trade exercise calories out for more calories in. These two facts allow you to individualize your weight management system of diet and exercise to fit your personal needs for the long haul.

Effective: In fifteen years of practice as an obstetrician/gynecologist, this system of calorie balancing and exercise is the most effective method I've seen to get the weight off and, most important, to keep it off. And it works for everyone. You don't have to become a ''diet guru'' or get your Ph.D. in molecular physics to monitor your progress and make the adjustments described in the next chapter to make it fit your individual needs.

Fun: Right! I threw this in just to be sure you are still awake. Of course, if you read past this silly comment and didn't catch it the first time, you obviously *are* a Hurried Woman! Slow down, and read more carefully. You'll get more out of this *(and life)* that way.

10

Getting Started

"Ready, set . . . Now wait a minute!"

I know you have read a lot and thought about it for a good long while and are now charged up and ready to begin your new life as a calorie-balanced, physically fit woman. Actually, if you're like most women faced with the prospect of another diet, you're probably moping around the house, kicking the cat, and feeling like you'd just lost your last friend—the key lime pie, to be exact! But you need to think of this as a fresh start on an almost guaranteed method to lose weight, improve your energy levels, and live healthier that will last you the rest of your life. Besides, once you learn the method and how to adjust for fluctuations in calories in and exercise calories out, you can pretty much eat what you want within reason and maintain your weight where you want it.

There are a few preparatory steps I think you should take during the first week of your new weight management program, before you start the diet, that will pay big dividends if you invest time in them now:

1. Keep a food diary (Appendix D).

During this week of preparation before the diet begins, start keeping a food diary. A form for your use with explanations is in Appendix D. Record the date, time, amount of food eaten by weight or volume, and the estimated calories in immediately after you eat anything, and I mean *anything!* Even a half of a cracker or a taste of your child's Dr. Pepper goes on the form. The vast majority of my patients are shocked to see how much they actually do eat in a given week. In fact, a majority of patients will lose weight simply by using a food diary. In other words, when they begin to pay attention to what they eat, they will begin to eat less and make better choices about what they do eat. Besides, to keep track of your calorie balance you must learn how to estimate the calories in your food and get in the habit of writing them down, so it's good practice to start now. For a food diary to be accurate and therefore helpful, you must write down what you eat as soon as you eat it. If you wait until bedtime to record your calories in, you will invariably miss things that you ate during the day, simply because you forgot. You can total up the calories later if it's more convenient for you, but you must record the food that you eat, *when you eat it*—otherwise the diary will lose its effectiveness for the weight management program.

2. Get a good calorie-counting book and study it before you begin the weight management program.

There are several excellent calorie-counting books available to you, most at a very low price. I leafed through several of them just the other day at one of the big chain bookstores. Some of the better ones are: *The Nutribase Complete Book of Food Counts,* by Dr. Art Ulene (Avery, 1996); *The Nutrition Doctor's A-to-Z Food Counter,* by Dr. Ed Blonz (Penguin, 1999); *Convenience Food Facts,* 4th ed. by A. Monk and N. Cooper (IDC, 1997); and *The Most Complete Food Counter,* by A. Natow and J. Heslin (Pocket, 1999). Learn what your favorite foods are made of—carbohydrates, protein, and fat—and the calories associated with each of these components:

1 gram carbohydrates	=	4 calories
1 gram protein	=	4 calories
1 gram fat	=	9 calories

You will need to pick up a small food scale to help you learn to estimate the size of your portions so that you will be able to accurately account for your calories. Even though you may already be a "pro" at weighing and estimating food portions, verify that you are doing it correctly during the first two weeks of this program. This will simply make sure that you're "on the mark" in your calorie counting. Be sure your book lists total calories as well as the portion from carbohydrates, protein, and fats. Dr. Sears suggests a "quick and dirty" way to estimate portions when you are eating out at nice restaurants and don't feel like whipping out the old scale in front of God and everybody. He says that four ounces of protein (or twenty-eight grams of protein) will cover the palm of your hand. To maintain the proper ratio of protein to carbohydrate (3:4), you will want to have a slightly smaller portion of carbohydrates on your plate than the portion of protein. This method appears to be a valid rough estimate, but I still think the best way to get good at estimating portions is to measure them out at home over and over again until you feel confident that you're doing it right. It is very important that you give your best effort to be accurate. If you are off by only 10 percent on 1,500 calories per day, you will take in an extra 150 calories each day. That becomes 1,050 extra calories per week and 4,725 calories per month. Since there are 3,500 calories in a pound of fat, being off just 10 percent each day in your calorie estimation will give you an extra one and one-third pounds to deal with each month, or sixteen pounds in a year—ouch!

3. "Do the math"—determine your maintenance calorie level and desired weight goal calorie level.

To fully understand the calorie-balancing system, it's important to make a few key calculations:

Maintenance calories—this is the number of calories necessary to maintain any given body weight. This level varies from woman to woman, but a rough approximation can be found by multiplying your weight by 11. For a 170-pound woman, the maintenance calorie level would be 1,870 calories (170 lb. × 11 cal. /lb. = 1,870 calories). If the 170-pound woman wants to lose weight, she must drop below 1,870 calories per day by either decreasing her calories in or increasing her calories out through more exercise. Making this calculation can be an eye-opener for a lot of women, particularly those who are still in denial: "I don't really eat that much." If you weight 200 pounds, you must be consuming at least 2,200 calories per day to maintain your present weight! To calculate your *present weight maintenance calories* below:

Present weight	_____	lbs.
multiply	× 11	cal./lb.
Maintenance calories	_____	calories

Target or goal weight—this is the weight you hope to achieve and stay at the rest of your natural life. One problem a lot of patients have is setting this weight too low. In other words, they set an unrealistic goal for themselves, ensuring a sense of failure when they don't reach it. This disappointment is followed by guilt, which then quickly turns to anger, frustration, and ultimately diet failure. Remember that 90 percent of the people who get on a diet and actually lose weight gain it all back within one year. Setting both long-term and short-term goals that are achievable will encourage your success. It is a rare woman who can get her weight down to what it was when she graduated from high school, particularly after one or more pregnancies, but it is amazing how many women set that particular goal for themselves. It is an unreachable goal for most women over thirty. In fact, most women tend to gain a pound each year after thirty, so you should allow your goal weight level to go up some if you're over thirty—not necessarily a pound each year, but maybe a half or a third of a pound for each year after thirty. To calculate you *target weight maintenance calories:*

Target weight	_____	lbs.
multiply	× 11	cal./lb.
Maintenance calories	_____	calories to stay at your target weight.

A much more reasonable target weight might be your weight before your last baby. That weight may be too high, but you can still use it as a short-term goal and celebrate when you get there. Then add your age adjustment (a half-pound per year over thirty) to come up with your realistic target weight. In our previous example, let's say that the 170-pound woman determines that her ideal goal weight is 140 pounds. Using the formula, we find that when she gets down to 140 pounds, she will need to take in only 1,540 calories each day (140 lbs. × 11 cal./lb. = 1,540 calories) to stabilize her weight at 140 pounds. Looking at it from a slightly different angle; when she achieves her ideal weight she will need to keep her daily calorie intake at or below 1,540 calories or she will gain weight. She can do this by decreasing her calories in or by increasing the calories expended or trying some combination of diet and exercise—that's the flexibility of the calorie-balancing system. What calorie level should you start with to lose weight effectively? For this hypothetical patient, I would recommend going to the 1,540 calories per-day level (a decrease of 330 calories per day) and get started now on the new calories in that she will need to maintain her ideal body weight in the future. If she wants to start out a little lower (at, say, 1,400 calories) to lose weight faster that's OK, but remember that this is a lifetime commitment to weight management, not a "lose the weight and then go back to eating like you want" diet, i.e., *unsuccessful!* Why not go ahead and get conditioned now for this new calorie level? You are going to need to maintain it for a good while—like the rest of your life! I do not recommend initially dropping your calories in below 1,100 to 1,200 calories per day regardless of your target weight calculation or desire to lose weight quickly. This is the maintenance calorie level for a 100-to-109 pound woman. Such a harsh program is unnecessary for success, psychologically looks like a fad diet (deprivation), and may turn on your "survival genes," which will work against you. Besides, you have a built-in "calorie cushion"—we haven't accounted for your exercise calories expended. To summarize the calculations: (a) calculate your *current weight maintenance calories* (current weight $\times$ 11 cals.=lb.) (this shows you where you are now); and (b) calculate your *target weight maintenance calories* (target weight $\times$ 11 cals./lb.) (this is where you need to be). Use you calculated target weight maintenance calories as your new daily calories in when you begin the second week of your weight management program and then monitor your progress.

Congratulations! You've decided on your ultimate weight goal! But also take a moment now to set some short-term goals. These will give you a reason to celebrate along the way to your final goal. Calculate 5 percent and 10 percent of your current body weight by multiplying your present weight by .05 and .10, respectively, then subtract these from your present weight. When you lose 5 percent of your current weight and again when you reach 10 percent, you should celebrate because you have significantly lowered your risk of death from cardiovascular disease as well as other troubles by reaching each of these goals. Humans are goal-oriented and we all seek approval or praise for what we do. Set some intermediate goals to make the journey to your final destination not seem so long. I admit that this is a "mind game," but it works! Besides, when you reach these goals you will have done something you have not been able to do before—lose weight and keep it off. And you will be able to keep it off this time because you are now on a lifetime weight management program, not a diet.

4. Start your exercise program now.

I cannot over-emphasize the importance of exercise to successful weight management—it is critical! Remember that there is a minimum amount of exercise required for successful weight control, particularly for women over thirty. You have to turn in at least three half-hour sessions of uninterrupted exercise each week. This is a starting point. Some women require more activity than this to maintain their weight at any given level. Also, remember that you can trade exercise for food. If you exercise above your minimum, you can get "calorie credits," which you can exchange for (a) faster weight loss (the more calories you burn, the more weight you lose), or (b) more calories in—the more you exercise, the less you have to diet or the more you can eat. Start at three half-hour sessions each week. If you walk, that's two miles at a time or about 200 calories each session, for a total of 600 calories per week. If you have been a certified couch potato and are not used to any real exercise, you will have to start out slowly and work up to this level of exercise. Be patient with yourself and use your head. It's important to be careful to avoid an injury that might prevent you from exercising now, or worse, give you trouble in the future. Being overweight puts you at risk for ankle, foot, and knee problems anyway. Also, be sure you have the right shoes for your activity. Spend a little money and get the best shoes you can afford, particularly if you are more than sixty to seventy pounds overweight. Believe me, they are worth the money. One word of warning: A lot of women begin an exercise program and actually *gain* weight. Why? When you go from a sedentary lifestyle to one that is more active, you build new muscle tissue, often at the expense of fat tissue. Now that's a real heartbreaker, isn't it? But muscle tissue weighs more than fat. So, when you replace fat with muscle, you may gain weight initially but will be losing inches. Don't get hung up on your weight. Be more aware of how well your clothes fit. If your pants get loose, but you haven't shed any pounds yet, you're probably doing the right thing. Keep it up and the weight will begin to drop later. Also, remember that sore muscles are actually injured. Although this is generally nothing to worry about, these injured muscles tend to swell a bit with water and other nutrients that help heal and build new and better muscles. But they may weigh a little more during the "sore" phase than they will when the soreness and the extra fluid leaves. Common sense tells you that exercise is good for you and will ultimately help you lose weight or, more important, *inches.* Be persistent!

5. Get your mind and heart focused on the goal.

This is probably the most important single step toward a successful lifelong commitment to weight management. You have to want to succeed to be successful. Sounds trite, but it's true. If you make up your mind that you can do this, you will make it. If you decide now that you won't be successful, I can almost guarantee that you won't be able to do it. Many women already feel defeated by their weight, so it is sometimes hard to rekindle that winning spirit, particularly in an area where they've not tasted success in a while. But if you understand what I've shown you here and believe that, contrary to the fad diet culture, long-term success is the only success worth having, I think you can do it! If you have a relationship with God, you need to ask Him for help now. Ask Him to provide His strength where you are weak and help you realize that no one else can fix this problem but the two of you working together. Ask Him to help you stop craving foods that are packed with calories, to realize the hidden snacking that you do (a taste of this, a nibble of that) and cut it out or at least be honest with yourself and account for it, and to not make excuses about eating too much but actually stop eating before you're uncomfortable. Pray for a better attitude about yourself—that you are a person who has value—and decide that you are worth "fixing." If you don't have a relationship with God, I encourage you to get one. Ask for help from a minister or priest you know or ask a friend where he or she goes to church and when they meet for worship. It's a small step but a very important one—not just for your weight troubles but for the other troubles in your life as well. We all have them, you know. Having a personal relationship with God gives you a better perspective on what's really important in life and what's not—in other words, the "Big Picture." Just as a good soldier prepares to go into battle, be sure you prepare yourself mentally before you start the program and continually work on staying focused on the goal—lifelong weight management.

6. Start the diet phase of the program.

Cut your calories down to the target weight maintenance level you calculated earlier. Try to keep a balance between the different nutritional elements:

Protein	40%
Fat	30
Carbohydrates	30
Total =	100%

This is the healthy balance that many nutritionists recommend, and deviating from it may encourage your survival genes to kick in. They will continually fight your efforts at weight control. Continue to keep your food diary, marking down exactly what you eat at the time you eat it, and total your calories each day to watch your progress. I recommend writing down your exercise calories, too. This will help you keep track of your exercise frequency and duration and assist with adjustments to the program if you don't lose weight as expected. Remember that everyone's minimum exercise level and response to exercise is different, so knowing what has not worked in the past can be helpful in making adjustments to improve future results.

7. Keep track of your progress.

Write down your calories in and your exercise calories expended in your food diary. Always write down the food you eat as soon as you eat it. If you wait until the end of the day and try to remember what you've eaten, you'll blow it! You must write down the food you eat *when you eat it,* even when you are away from home—*especially when you are away from home!* It's OK to wait and total up your calories when you get home or at the end of the day, but write down what you eat *right away.* Weigh in weekly, preferably the same day and time of day each time; e.g., weigh in every Sunday evening. Weighing more frequently tends to drive women crazy. Besides, daily weight fluctuations are quite common, particularly around your menstrual cycle. Record your weekly weight in your food diary. It is also important not to get too hung up on your weight as a number. A lot of women who have been sedentary and begin a program of physical conditioning will notice an initial weight gain, probably due to an increase in muscle mass over fat, since muscle weighs more than fat. So as you develop better muscle you may weigh more but find you fit into your clothes better. I assure you that the latter is more important than the former in how you feel about the program.

Stick with it; the weight number will start down soon. If it doesn't within two or three weeks, you may need to reassess your calories in or exercise level. You should expect to lose about one to one and one-half pounds each week. Trying to shed weight faster doesn't seem to work well for very long—those damned "survival genes to the rescue" again. Women who lose weight rapidly tend to put it back on more quickly once the diet is over. Slow, steady weight is associated with the highest success rate. Realize that if you have fifty or sixty pounds to lose it will take almost a year to achieve this goal. Again, you have to be patient. This program of weight management will need to be a lifelong project to enjoy long-term success. If you don't lose weight as planned or you feel that you've reached a "plateau" weight you just can't seem to get below (two weeks with no progress), consider one of two actions: (a) decrease your food intake or calories in, or (b) increase your aerobic exercise levels (calories out). To adjust your calories, I recommend cutting out 100 calories per day to start with. (Drop down from 1,800 to 1,700 calories each day.) Remember to keep your overall carbohydrate: protein: fat ratios at the recommended levels. If you hit another plateau later or your initial adjustment didn't work after two weeks, drop another 100 calories from your daily intake (down to 1,600 calories) or increase your exercise level as described here. To adjust your exercise calories expended, consider adding a session each week or pushing to go an additional ten minutes in each session. Give this new level of exercise two weeks. If you don't start to see progress again, then add another session each week or ten more minutes of exercise per session, up to a maximum of one hour per session. Continue to monitor your progress, and whenever you encounter a plateau adjust your exercise level up by the same method—either add ten minutes to each session or add another session per week. If you add a session, it can be a thirty-minute session even if the original three are now each an hour long. The key is to burn more calories each week. Also, be sure that your rate of exercise is strong enough to get your heart rate up to between 130 and 155 beats per minute. This is the aerobic level needed to affect the body's metabolism and get the weight control benefits of exercise. If you have heart disease or diabetes or take blood pressure medication, you should consult with your doctor before beginning an exercise program. Also, don't ignore pain when you exercise. If you suspect you've incurred an injury, let your doctor know immediately. Injuries are the most common (legitimate) reason women stop exercising.

8. Start on a good multi-vitamin and calcium.

I recommend over-the-counter vitamins such as Centrum, Thera-gran-M, and One-a-Day with Iron. I am sure that there are many other vitamins that are equally as good, but I do not recommend going to the health food store and asking some "Valley Kid" what he or she recommends as a vitamin supplement. Use one that has been evaluated by the FDA for safety and effectiveness and is known to work. It is also currently recommended that women over thirty begin calcium supplements. The current recommendation is 1,500 to 2,000 milligrams of calcium each day. Contrary to the marketing attempts of calcium manufacturers, all of the supplements are pretty much the same. Watch for the right number of milligrams of calcium. Vitamin D is essential for calcium absorption, but unless you are a cave dweller or are stationed at Ice Station Zebra in the dead of winter (there's only four hours of sunlight each day there) you probably get a reasonable amount of vitamin D from sunlight, regular multi-vitamins, and "fortified" foods like bread and milk. But if you want to take a calcium supplement with added vitamin D, I won't sick the Vitamin Police on you.

9. Drink lots of water!

I probably should have listed this first to be sure you read it and realize how important it is to your general health and to your dieting efforts. Water is the essential element for all of the body's metabolic systems. You can fast for several weeks and do quite well (some of us can go a lot further than others!), but without water you will die in a matter of a few days. Water helps flush out metabolic poisons and ketones and draws edema fluid out of your legs and hands. Besides, when you're drinking water you are *not* drinking sodas. (A twelve-ounce can of your favorite carbonated drink contains about 150 calories—three of these a day is about the same number of calories as a Big Mac sandwich.) On the whole, I think water encourages more efficient weight loss.

10. Cut down on eating meals out and particularly fast food.

This is a big problem for the Hurried Woman. When she gets home from work, she is constantly on the go shuttling kids to karate, soccer, gymnastics, etc. When is she going to find time to cook a nutritious and delicious low-fat meal, and if she did have time to prepare it, when and where would she serve it? Prime choices include: the ballpark, the school PTA meeting, or in the car. Eating out is a logical conclusion to this dilemma, and fast food, as its name implies, is the only food that can fit into a hurried schedule. Unfortunately, there are no really low-fat alternatives at any restaurant with a drive-through window. Almost everything on the menu is fried in fat or wrapped in flour or bread. Look at the list of fast foods in any of the calorie-counting books recommended in chapter 10 and marvel at the number of calories in most of the foods on the list. You don't have to eat like a hog at a fast-food restaurant to consume a lot of calories. If you are going to eat out, you'll find better food choices at the sit-down restaurant. However, you're not totally safe there, either, because as any good cook knows, the last thing you want to do is have someone leave your table hungry. This is bad for business. When people pay money for a meal out, they want to get full value for their money. So restaurant owners cook food that is rich in flavor (and calories) and give you a lot to eat. This is a bad combination for someone on a diet. We were all taught as children to clean our plates, and besides, you paid good money for that meal so, by golly, you're going to eat it; all of it—every last overstuffed plate full of calorie-dripping food they gave you. And God help you if you're at a Mexican food place *with chips and hot sauce!* There's no way I can go into a Mexican restaurant and not consume half my weight in chips and hot sauce, and then . . . I have to eat all of my entreé, too—remember, "clean your plate, young man!" This adds up to failure for most diets and is one of the main reasons the Hurried Woman can't seem to lose weight—her schedule just doesn't allow her to control her meals out without Herculean effort.

11

Other Considerations

Medications

I am not an advocate of diet pills. They are the ultimate in short-term strategies. Diet pills that are a combination of caffeine and ephedrine are available over-the-counter as Dexatrim or Metabo-*whatever*. Amphetamines can suppress appetite and help you get a "jump start" toward successful weight loss but are absolutely forbidden for long-term use. They are actually unsafe when taken for an extended period of time. I have on occasion given selected patient diet pills, but for only thirty days *and not a day longer*. They are strictly short-term—basically a "crutch" to help you begin a diet. I much prefer to stress the long-term approach to weight management through decreasing calories in and increasing calories expended through exercise. It's natural and it works for the long run.

Meridia *(isbutramine)*, manufactured by Knoll Pharmaceutical, is claimed to be an appetite suppressant that works through the dopamine/serotonin system, rather than as a central nervous system stimulant (speed). Some patients can experience a significant rise in blood pressure or a rapid pulse rate on the medication, and blood pressure should be monitored regularly. It appears that between 20 and 50 percent of patients respond to treatment with at least a 10 percent loss in weight. Unfortunately, no information is available concerning long-term success with Meridia, as no one has data beyond one year of use. Women with a history of heart disease, stroke, high blood pressure, glaucoma, or seizures should not take the medicine.

Xenical, a new fat-blocking drug from Roche, holds some promise in helping patients effectively achieve a low-fat diet through stopping the intestine from absorbing about 30 percent of dietary fats. It causes loose stools and even explosive diarrhea in some patients. Unfortunately, it has not been available on the market very long, so it hasn't been fully studied yet. You may want to ask your doctor about it in the near future. Most experts believe a 10 to 15 percent sustained weight loss will be possible with this medication. However, women must take a good multi-vitamin while on Xenical to prevent certain vitamin deficiencies caused by blocking the absorption of about 30 percent of the fat.

Welbutrin, Prozac, and Paxil have all been shown to help depressed patients lose weight. Since many women with Hurried Woman Syndrome complaining of fatigue respond to these newer antidepressants (probably because they are pre-depressed—which is the same type of chemical imbalance in the brain that occurs in depression, just less severe), starting one of these medicines may have the spill-over benefit of decreasing appetite and encouraging weight loss. About 15 to 20 percent of women who take them lose weight.

Environment

A lot of us eat when we are bored or stressed out—it's something to do, or maybe eating helps us relax. Many people eat when they feel blah or down, probably because many of us have been programmed from childhood to view food as a reward: "If you'll bathe the cat, I'll give you some chocolate cake" . . . well, probably not this exact statement, but something similar was used on all of us as children. Also, many women are impulsive eaters: "I went into the pantry for a lightbulb when my gaze fell upon the double-stuffed Oreos. I turned to run before they saw me, but alas, I was too late. 'Eat us!' they cried compellingly. Since I was outnumbered, I had no choice but to capitulate and downed the entire package, plastic and all." You see something you know will fit comfortably in your mouth, and suddenly, even though you aren't really hungry, you want to eat it *right then.* The items that line the checkout stand at the grocery store are specially selected for that location because they are known to be "impulse items"—when we see them they stir something in us that wants to pick them up. Even more so because they are relatively inexpensive. We see our favorite candy bar or a horoscope or the silly magazines with headlines like "Elvis's Alien Love Child Found in the Vatican!" and we (some people, anyway) are tempted to pick them up, simply because they are available and not too expensive and we don't really think about it; we just do it—an impulse causes us to buy them. We do the same thing with food, particularly treats and sweets, which are also "reward" food. They make us feel good.

For all of the preceding reasons, it's very sensible to stock the kitchen cupboard with snacks that are low-fat, with moderate calories and get rid of the stuff that you have trouble saying "no" to. If you have a real weakness for Blue Bell Homemade Vanilla Ice Cream—like me!—then you might want to consider getting it out of the house so that you won't be tempted to cheat. Instead, stock up on fruit, like cantaloupe, and low-fat snack bars. (I suspect some of these energy snacks they say are "high-fiber" are actually pieces of cardboard with synthetic chocolate coatings, but I have not yet been able to verify my suspicions.) Most fruits are moderate in calories (an orange has 80 to 100 calories, while an apple has 60 calories); however, grapes and watermelon are very high in sugar content, so you have to eat these in moderation—of course, my two favorite fruits would have the highest calories!

Snacks

Snacks are an inevitable part of everyone's diet. It is *absolutely inevitable* if you are stuck at home with kids and enough food to feed the Russian army for two weeks. However, snacks can actually be good for you. Women with true hypoglycemia and even those who don't have it notice that they often slump about one or two hours after a meal. A well-timed snack, like cheese and peanut butter crackers, an hour and a half after a meal will often keep these symptoms under control. Since you know you are going to snack, have reasonable snacks on hand so you won't use up all of your calories in on junk or, worse, chronically overeat.

Also, watch out for what I call hidden snacks. These are the little bites and tastes of food that we eat almost subconsciously. Sampling the food as you cook so often that you are not even hungry when it hits the table and always taking a few bites of the children's food just to be sure someone didn't sneak in and poison it are common examples of eating that often go unnoticed by the patient until she keeps a food diary. If you start writing these down, you will either become aware that they exist and start to account for them accurately or stop snacking as much because you now "see them before you eat them" and choose to not do it anymore. A lot of people on diets don't count a "taste" of things that they eat or the assorted pieces of broken cookies at the bottom of the package because they weren't a whole cookie—don't lie to yourself; be honest and count it all. The only person you cheat by "looking the other way" is yourself. Do I sound like your mother?

If you like an afternoon or bedtime snack, you don't have to deny yourself; you just have to plan for it in advance. Save some calories for the end of the day if you want to have a bedtime snack. Also, you might be surprised to know that if you have sex right before a snack, the calories don't count. (Of course this isn't true, but I put it in here to make your husband happy!)

Summary

Weight gain is one of the three major symptoms of the Hurried Woman Syndrome. Being overweight affects your physical health (heart disease, high blood pressure, diabetes, and bone and joint problems) as well as your emotional health. When you feel fat you're more fatigued because you've been lugging the extra weight around. And if you're like most women who are struggling with their weight, you're down on yourself, and that drop in mood makes you feel more tired. Being tired most, if not all, of the time makes it hard to get up the gumption to go exercise, and this decreased level of activity drops your calories expended, making your weight go up further or at least makes weight loss harder. This is a vicious cycle that has many women feeling hopelessly trapped.

When you're down about your weight, you aren't going to be happy with yourself or the people around you. You'll be grouchier and grumpier and have less tolerance for the things in your life that stress or annoy you. (Gee, who or what might those things be?). There's a sign in our kitchen that says: "If Momma ain't happy, ain't nobody happy." No truer words have been spoken. And if Momma ain't happy with Papa, she won't want to "punch his ticket" anytime soon, either. When women put on weight, they often say that they don't look or feel sexy. Looking sexy and feeling sexy are very important to a woman. If she doesn't feel sexy, she won't want to make love, because she's self-conscious about how she looks, particularly *naked!* Being overweight or, at least, perceiving that she's overweight kills sex drive for most women. I hope that you are now beginning to see the relationship among fatigue, weight gain, and sex drive—the Hurried Woman Syndrome.

12

FAQS and Statements

"I don't eat that much and I'm exercising more. Why am I not losing weight?"
When patients ask me this question, I immediately ask them two questions: "What diet are you on?" and "How much exercise are you doing?" Almost invariably, the answer to the first question is one of the following:

"I'm cutting back," or, a variation on the same theme, "I'm doing better."

"Well, I'm taking Metabo*whatever* and cutting back on sweets."

"I've cut my fats down to twenty percent."

"I've stopped eating beef and switched to chicken."

"No more fried foods!"

Certainly these are all good ideas (except, perhaps the Metabo*whatever*) and many of them are incorporated into most diets; however, none of these strategies is an organized plan. None of them really restrict the amount of food eaten—yes, "20 percent fat" is a limit, but if you eat 3,000 calories a day, keeping the fat below 20 percent won't really do much to help you lose weight. You have to have a diet plan that is: (1) organized (has a defined set of rules and is balanced); (2) doesn't stray too far away from the 40 percent protein, 30 percent carbohydrates, and 30 percent fat ratio described earlier or you'll turn on those survival genes; and (3) works—don't just "play" at dieting; get a program that works and do it! If you diet off and on again, you'll become a victim of the diet "yo-yo" and actually gain more weight.

Answers to the second question usually require a lot more clarification:

"I'm working out at the gym [or spa] three days a week."

"I'm walking every evening with my mother."
"I do ten minutes on my exercise bike every morning."

By now, you've probably figured out what's wrong with each of these exercise strategies. First, "working out" means a lot of different things to a lot of people. Weightlifting is not really aerobic exercise unless you are really humpin' and pumpin' those machines. If you do your repetitions (or "reps" as Hans and Franz say) very quickly *and* don't rest between stations *and* do this for 30 minutes without interruption, *then* you're doing aerobic exercise. Anything less than that is "toning," not aerobic exercise, and it will not have the impact on your metabolism that you are looking for. (However, I think toning exercises are still good for you—they make you feel better and help you firm up some of the flab you don't like; such as the dreaded underarm dingle-dangle. You know, that's the stuff on your sixth-grade English teacher's arm that would hang down and flap around when she wrote on the chalkboard.)

To get the proper weight loss benefit from exercise requires a minimum of three thirty-minute sessions of uninterrupted aerobic exercise each week. This is a *minimum* and should be viewed as a "maintenance dose" of exercise. To really impact weight loss, you'll need to do more. Also, remember that this may not be enough exercise for you to be successful because everyone is built differently. You will need to experiment to find your maintenance level, but three half-hours per week is a good start.

Walking with your mother is good for your relationship, and I think it's a great thing to do. But if you're forty and she's seventy-five, you may not be walking fast enough to get the aerobic benefit from it. You might try carrying your mother while you walk—now *that's* aerobic exercise! Actually, I ask patients how far they are walking and how fast. Patients often tell me, "I walk two miles every day," only for me to find out that it takes them an hour to do it—that's walking at half the recommended pace to get your exercise benefit. No wonder they aren't losing weight! Certainly for some of my patients this is as fast as they can walk, since they are starting in the couch potato league. But that's OK because at least *they are starting!* Even ten minutes on an exercise bike is a good start, but you'll have to go further to see your investment in exercise really pay off. Don't be impatient that you have to start low and build up slowly to even the minimal exercise level. You have the rest of your life to get there. The key is to start something and start it now.

What has really happened for many of my patients is that the rules of the weight game have changed, but they just haven't realized it yet. What worked in the past to keep their weight where they wanted it just doesn't work anymore, and it frustrates them. Previously, if they gained a few pounds they could start skipping lunches or perhaps cut our breads and desserts at meals or maybe walk two miles a couple of mornings each week and the weight would come off—but not anymore! What happened? Their metabolism changed in some currently unexplained way. It's usually not thyroid disease or some other easily understood mechanism, but the way their body handles calories has changed and it makes them angry—and understandably so. I wish I could give them a more scientific explanation, but it appears age has something to do with it, being a woman *has a lot to do with it,* and having children seems to make it much worse. Perhaps medical science will unlock this mystery in a few more years. I certainly hope so. But in the meantime, they've got to do what their grandma would have told them to do—eat less and exercise more. It will work. But, unfortunately, it's the *only thing* that works.

"But I hate exercise!"

I understand the sentiment, but you must learn to hate being overweight more. I almost guarantee that until you get committed to a weight management program that includes regular exercise, you will not be successful in the long run. I don't give a hoot in hell for short-term weight loss—I could lock you in a room for a week with only a bucket of water and you'd probably lose ten pounds, no problem. But as soon as you got out (and called your lawyer!), you'd start gaining the weight right back again. Fad diets can make you lose ten pounds, mostly water, in the first week or two, but what really counts is losing the weight *and keeping it off.* That's the only success worth having. Besides, exercise is healthy for you. It improves your energy levels and makes you feel better about yourself. And the last two benefits will help you in your relationships with the people closest to you, particularly your husband.

Although I personally find most types of exercise boring, it doesn't have to be that way. If you enjoy tennis or racquetball, this can be a good way to get your exercise calories in while enjoying a sport. Aerobics classes are a popular way for women to exercise and enjoy time off-call from work and family. You can still love your family yet need time away from them. It especially helps women with small children to interact with people who have a vocabulary of more than twenty words and don't routinely have food or snot smeared on their faces. I run between eight and twelve miles each week. And when I run, I like to use it as a time to pray, think through tough problems, and sometimes just get away and be by myself for a little while. For me, running is cheap therapy, and it helps me stay focused on the Big Picture.

It sometimes helps to exercise with a friend. If you can establish a routine time and place for exercise, your friend may help you be more faithful in your exercise by encouraging you to go when you don't feel like it, and vice versa. You know that if you don't go, you'll feel guilty about letting your friend down, and sometimes that is the difference between going and not going. Staying on a regular exercise program is difficult for most of us, so take advantage of any help you can get. Stress the positives and try to ignore or work around the negatives. The payoff from regular exercise is significant.

"I don't have time to exercise."

Either this statement is a politically correct way of saying, "I am not going to exercise," or you could be the poster child for the Hurried Woman Syndrome. I don't care how busy you are; if it's really important to you, you can work a half hour of exercise into your schedule three days each week. You've done harder things before, right? Make the commitment to long-term weight control now, and with it comes the necessity for exercise. If you keep denying this fact, you will continue to fail at weight control.

If your schedule really is so busy that you cannot work in an hour and a half of exercise in each week, then I suggest you give up on weight loss until you can make the time to exercise or take a long hard look at your priorities and try to reorder them to incorporate routine exercise into your schedule. Until you do, I predict you will be unsuccessful at controlling your weight.

"What is the best exercise for weight loss?"

The one that you'll do! That's always my quick answer to this question. (Do you get the feeling that I can be a smart-aleck at times?) I do think that walking (or swimming, if you have ready access to a pool) is probably the best exercise because it requires no special equipment except good shoes, which are very important (I will talk more about this later), can be done almost anywhere (inside, at the mall or on a treadmill

81

if the weather's bad, or outside), and it works with relatively few injuries when compared to running or other aerobic activities.

Walking a mile and running a mile burn about the same number of calories (about one hundred), but most people can run about twice as fast as they can walk, so running burns off calories in about half the time. Therefore, if you're pressed for time—the typical Hurried Woman—then you may prefer running over walking from a time efficiency standpoint. Thirty minutes of running will burn off about 350 to 400 calories. The same time walking will burn off 200 calories). The main thing is to get your heart rate up above 120–130 for at least thirty minutes each exercise session without interruption. (You couch potatoes may have to work up to this level, but that's OK. Be patient. You have the rest of your life to get there.) If you exercise for a shorter period of time, you will not get the full benefit of aerobic training for weight control. Three thirty-minute sessions per week is the minimum level of exercise, and some people will need more to achieve their weight goals.

Good shoes, matched to your choice of activities, are critical to help avoid discomfort and even injuries that could keep you from exercising appropriately. When I started running twelve years ago, I just wore my good ol' tennis shoes. I thought to myself, *Self, these shoes are what I wore in high school and I didn't have any problems back then. Why do I need to spend all that money on jogging shoes? I can do this!* So I took off running—about one hundred yards, as I remember—and fell down in a heap, my rib muscles in spasm and gasping for air like a carp out of water. (Lesson no. 1: Warm up first and build up your level of exercise *slowly*, particularly if you are starting from scratch.) I decided I'd better *walk* a few trips after that, going a little farther each time. Then I picked up my pace so that I was walking two miles in thirty minutes. After that, I began to jog a quarter-mile, then walk a quarter-mile, alternating them to not get too worn out. Eventually, after about two or three months, I was running between two and three miles three times a week. That was great; I really felt I had come a long way with my wind and endurance. I also noticed I had more energy and just a better attitude in general. But I kept having sore feet, my ankles hurt, and sometimes my legs hurt at night and I'd wake up with calf muscle spasms. At first, I thought it was just age—my thirty-year-old joints were just not recovering like they did when they (and the rest of me) were younger. Then I asked my brother-in-law's wife (that would be the woman who married my wife's brother—confused yet?), who was an avid runner, if she ever had that kind of trouble. She told me I needed to get some good running shoes. I went and priced them at the mall: $100. Ouch! I decided that she was crazy and that I, being a doctor and having descended from Mount Olympus to live among mortals, would eventually work out the soreness and get better. Well, you guessed it: I kept getting worse. In fact, the more I ran, the worse it got. I finally broke down and bought the $100 air-sole running shoes, not admitting I was wrong of course but thinking, rather, that I could afford to have the best equipment so I might as well try them. I strapped them on, still not believing they would help much, and took off running—it felt as if I were floating above the pavement! I couldn't even feel my sore feet hitting the road. The pain was gone! Lesson no. 2: Get the right equipment from the start. It's worth it. My wife's sister-in-law insists that this is actually Lesson no. 3. Lesson no. 2 should be: your brother-in-law's wife is always right! (Who *are* these people?)

"I'm on my feet all day at work. Isn't that enough exercise?"

I wish it were. When I have a patient in labor at the hospital, I walk over from my office to check her anywhere from eight to ten times a day. It's about 0.4 mile round-trip from my office to the hospital and back, so that's about 3.2 to 4.0 miles of walking each day, not counting the walking I do in the office seeing patients. But it doesn't count as aerobic exercise. Why? Because *I don't do it all at one time.* If I went back and forth to the hospital eight times without interruption, it would be aerobic exercise. But since I go back and forth piecemeal over several hours, all it does is make my feet and ankles sore at the end of the day. It won't help me control my weight.

"I'm too tired to exercise, particularly after a busy day."

I can really sympathize with this statement. Some days I come home, as my mother would say just "bone tired." The last thing I want to do after one of those days is hop up on the treadmill and go thirty minutes "for the Gipper." I am "just too beat to slap the feet," if you know what I mean. **But** (and this is a big but!) when I do go ahead and work out, I feel much better. It reenergizes me to exercise. I guess those endorphins that are released with exercise make me feel good, or perhaps it's the sense of accomplishment that I'm still on track with my exercise routine. Either way, I feel much better after I exercise, even when I feel too tired to do it. Besides, when do you *not* have a busy day? I should clarify that if I am exhausted (perhaps I've been up all night with someone in labor), I don't go hit the track the next day until I've had a chance to rest. I think if you are absolutely "wasted," you should skip exercise that day and try to make it up the next day after you've rested. Remember, you only need to exercise three times a week, so you have a lot of flexibility about when you go. My point is simply that you need to exercise three times a week, and some days when you feel too tired to go if you'll just go and do it you will feel better. I've proven this to myself over and over again. I admit it's awful hard sometimes to push myself out the door when I've had a hard day, but it will pay off in the long run. And that's where it counts.

"What is the 'diet yo-yo' again and how does it cause me to gain weight?"

The so-called diet yo-yo describes the phenomenon that a lot of women see when they try a new diet, lose a few pounds, then fall off the diet only to gain the weight back, plus a few extra pounds. Each time they try a new diet and fail, they end up weighing a few pounds more than they did when they started. This is a big source of frustration for the woman who diets frequently and is a good reason not to start a diet if you're not really committed to losing weight.

When you diet, you send a signal to your body that you've fallen on hard times—food is scarce, it's a bad winter, etc. Because, the body thinks it's starving, it becomes much more efficient at holding onto the calories that you do take in and stingier at giving them up for exercise. You may lose some weight, but when you stop dieting and increase your calorie intake back to your previous level, you begin to put the weight back on. But now, since your body has been "reprogrammed" by by starvation to be more efficient with the same calorie load you had before starting the diet, you will gain your weight back faster and eventually go up to a higher weight than before. If you keep starting and stopping diets, you will see a weight chart that looks like the following:

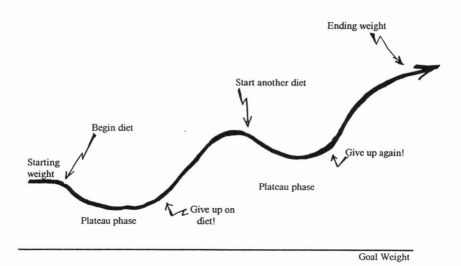

The diet yo-yo phenomenon is why women who keep dieting off-and-on again see their weight gradually rise over time and find it harder to lose weight each time they try to diet. To be successful in the long run, you must find a diet you can live with *forever* and stick with it.

"What about using sugar substitutes, particularly NutraSweet?"

I think sugar substitutes can ease the pain of dieting by allowing food that is low-calorie to taste better. This makes giving up sugar less painful. But I think they should be used in moderation. Saccharine works well for most dieters, particularly in hot drinks like coffee and hot tea, since NutraSweet is not supposed to be heated. Most people sweeten iced tea while it's still hot, so saccharine works best here, too. However, evidence continues to link saccharine to bladder cancer in animals, so I think limiting yourself to six or eight packets of saccharine sweetener per day makes sense.

Similarly, aspartame and NutraSweet may cause problems if used excessively. I have heard many patients complain that they have swelling and fluid retention if they drink a lot of diet drinks. One time I tried to lose some weight by drinking only a diet drink for breakfast and lunch and eating supper as I pleased. It didn't work and I noticed edema in my ankles at the end of the day and stiff, swollen hands in the morning. When I changed over to a Dr. Pepper for breakfast and lunch instead, I actually began to lose weight. Looking strictly at the calories, I swapped two ten-ounce Dr. Peppers—a total of 300 calories—for two diet drinks that had a total of two calories and *lost* weight. To tell the whole story, I was also drinking five or six additional diet drinks at various times during the day and I cut back to two diet drinks per day and began drinking water during the day. I have tried this experiment again with similar results and have discussed my suspicious about excessive aspartame with patients who were having trouble losing weight on a reasonable diet but drinking a lot of diet drinks. When they go home and cut back on diet drinks like I did, many, if not most, have similar results. This revelation came as a shock to me.

I used to drink a Diet Coke and eat a thickly glazed doughnut each morning, somehow deluding myself that the aspartame nixed out the calories in the doughnut—perhaps, the diet drink was some kind of caloric "black hole" that sucked the calories out of the doughnut! Yeah, that's how it works! (Weird, huh?) More like wishful thinking actually. But I am convinced that too much aspartame is not good for dieters because it may cause fluid retention and, in some unusual way, may slow down weight loss. In addition, if I drink too many diet drinks I get a great deal of abdominal gas and bloating, which really hurts and also makes my clothes fit poorly. Moreover, if I eat sugar with a diet drink, it produces a huge amount of gas bloating and abdominal distension. If you don't believe me, try this little experiment yourself: Take a handful of candy corn and chew it up, but leave it in your mouth. Then put some Diet Coke or other NutraSweet diet cola in your mouth and check out what happens next. I advise you to lean forward, because when the diet drink hits your mouth the foam will literally pour out! There must be some kind of reaction between the sugar and the aspartame that produces the gas, but it is simply amazing. Think about swallowing the two together. They will produce this kind of gas in your stomach or upper intestine, and once the gas is in your GI tract it has to travel all the way through your intestine and then out rectally, with a lot of bloating, cramping, and embarrassing flatus (that's toots, if you haven't guessed by now) before you get relief. Beware of this combination if you have a spastic colon or irritable bowel syndrome.

"Do I have to follow my calculated daily calories in rigidly or can I cheat a little?"

You haven't even started the program yet, and you are already asking about how to cheat! Of course, everybody cheats on a diet. That's what a diet's for, right? I sincerely recommend, though, that for the first two weeks you exercise the minimum three half-hour sessions each week and stick to your daily calories in until you get the hang of it and see what this level of exercise and calories will do for you. Remember, each woman is different and must find the calories in and exercise calories out level that controls her body weight.

However, once you establish a daily calorie level at which you will consistently lose weight, I think it's OK to stretch the program out a bit and get the full benefits of its flexibility. Most people don't eat the same amount of food every day; they have big-calorie days and medium-calorie days (I never seem to let myself have a low-calorie day!) In other words, we eat more some days and less on others. Since a diet must fit your lifestyle to be successful, it's important to know that you can let your daily calorie levels fluctuate somewhat from day to day, as long as you keep track of the overall calorie balance. For example, if you calculated your maintenance calories to be 1,800 but only eat 1,600 calories one day, you can carry 200 calories over to the next day and eat a little more without affecting your overall weight management program. Similarly, if you overeat 300 calories today because you just had to have the cherry cheesecake at supper, you need to cut back by 300 calories the next day to not affect your overall calorie balance. This flexibility helps a lot when an occasion is coming up where you know you're going to eat a lot—say the office Christmas party. You can cut your calories down below your maintenance level one or two days in advance to get a "calorie credit," which you can use to cover the extra calories you want for the office party. Most fad diets can't do this. However, be careful—you can get carried away with trying to stretch this too far and hurt your overall weight control efforts. For example, if you are on 1,800 calories a day and decide to eat only 500 calories one day to get a 1,300 calorie credit and then "cash it in" three days later on an eating binge (for a total daily intake of 3,300 calories), you will see your weight start to do some crazy things—and you won't feel very good, either. I wouldn't recommend trying to carry a "calorie credit" of more than 500 calories, and I wouldn't try to carry it forward more than two days. As in most things, moderation is the key.

The other way you can create a "calorie credit" is through additional exercise. Once you have turned in your exercise minimum of three half-hours per week, any additional exercise calories you burn make room for more food in your daily diet (or help you lose weight faster if you chose not to eat them). So if you've already met your exercise minimum by walking two miles three times this week (600 calories) and you walk an additional three miles, you can eat an extra 300 calories this week if you want them without affecting your weight program. Pretty neat, huh? If you want more food, you can "pay" for it through additional exercise.

Unfortunately, it also works the other way. If you fail to exercise one of your required sessions in a week, you should withhold 200 calories from your diet. However, don't routinely cut an extra 200 calories out of your diet so you only have to exercise two times each week—it doesn't work that way. You need to turn in at least the minimum amount of exercise for the program to be successful. Adults just can't seem to maintain their weight without regular exercise. But it is nice to have the flexibility that the calorie-balancing method gives you to trade more exercise for less dieting and vice versa. This feature lets you tailor the program to fit your eating "personality."

"My family won't eat 'diet food' and I really don't have time to make two different menus for each meal."
This is a big problem confronting a woman trying to diet: her husband and/or kids just don't want to eat those oddball diet dinners or stick to a high-protein, low-carbohydrate food selection fad diet. Can you blame them? You don't want to do it, either! Plus, it's hard for you not to want to taste their "real" food if you are forced to cook it. (Besides, someone could have slipped into the house and poisoned it, so you have to sacrifice and taste it, don't you?) This is one of the main reasons fad diets fail, because no one wants to eat Mom's crazy food (including Mom, for that matter!) and Mom is tempted to the brink of insanity fixing her favorite foods for everyone else to eat while she eats her brown bag cuisine from the Jimminy Craig Diet Center or wolfs down a nutritious fiber energy bar or rice cake—yum!

The calorie-balancing program doesn't require you to purchase special food or prepare oddball meals your family won't eat. You do have to eat less of what you serve, particularly if you prepare high-fat, high-carbohydrate meals. But you do need to maintain the proper protein:carbohydrate:fat ratios mentioned earlier and stay within your calorie limits. If you opt to make healthier food choices (more vegetables, less red meat and fatty fried foods), you can get more food to eat and feel less hungry after mealtime.

However, your family often balks at those healthier food choices, don't they? The kids especially want the french fries, chicken-fried steak, mashed potatoes with gravy, and buttered bread at every meal. Oh, yes . . . and the cherry cobbler, too. Besides, they don't have a weight problem, right? Think again! Humans aren't born knowing the proper food choices to make any more than they are born knowing how to drive a car or balance a checkbook (a lot of adults still can't do this). They've got to be taught, and not just in the classroom format but in the "classroom of life" format. They need to be shown day in and day out what makes a balanced diet and the importance of maintaining it—forever. If you can help them get used to it now, they'll be more likely to continue these good diet habits when they leave your loving guidance and take off on their own. And don't forget; they are genetically programmed to become just like their parents—namely, *you!* It's very probably that they also have your predisposition to gain weight. I know what you're thinking: *They don't have a weight problem now, so why should they be forced to be on a diet?* I'll bet you didn't have a weight problem when you were their age, either. But you've got one now, don't you? And you got where you are now by continuing to make the same wrong food choices you were taught as a kid, not realizing the consequences they would have on you later in life when your metabolism changed due to your age and the reprogramming that pregnancy causes. If you had been taught as a child how to eat properly and balance exercise with diet to maintain your weight, you might not be in your current predicament. Teach your children how to eat properly and exercise now, but more important, *show* them by your example how important it is to eat healthy and stay fit. Unfortunately, our children are far more likely to do what they see us do than what we tell them to do. Did "do as I say and not as I do" motivate you as a kid? Not me, either. (Unless they were beating me senseless at the time!) No, you've got to set the example by showing them how to do it the right way—now. You owe it to yourself first, but also to them.

"I diet and exercise as hard as anyone else and I still have to always struggle with my weight. It isn't fair!"

You're right. It isn't fair. But *fair* is a four-letter word that starts with *f* and you aren't supposed to use them. You were dealt a set of genes that, albeit great for survival in bad conditions, make you have to diet more and exercise harder than other people to effectively manage your weight. Well, as I see it, you have two choices. You can either (1) continue to feel sorry for yourself and complain about it, looking for shortcuts to weight loss through fad diets, or (2) recognize that you can't change your genes, but you can change your attitude about them and learn how to cope with them to achieve the long-term weight control you want through sensible diet and exercise. Yes, you will probably have to work harder at it than others, but no one promised us that anything in this life would be easy or "fair." Decide that you are going to be a winner, not a whiner, and go after it!

"Are there any other diet programs that you do recommend?"

I think Weight Watchers packages an excellent diet program that is reasonably affordable. They use a "credit" system to regulate calories in rather than actually counting them, but it is essentially the same method. In addition, Weight Watchers provides a support group that meets weekly to encourage compliance and these meetings are very help-ful for some women. Let's face it: we all need support when things get tough and recognition when we succeed. The Weight Watchers program provides both. Through my fifteen years in practice, this program has been the most successful at achieving long-term weight loss and I have no reservations about recommending it to anyone.

You can also consult a dietician. Your doctor probably knows where to refer you should you choose this route. Sometimes one-on-one discus-sion and personal attention help patients get a better handle on their unique situation. Certainly if you are a diabetic or have other special diet restrictions or if you have tried calorie counting several times before and never been successful with it, you should consider a consultation with a registered dietician. Your individual circumstances may be unusual and not allow a simple "cookbook" approach to weight loss. Consulting an expert should help.

"Are some people literally 'addicted' to food?"

Well, since none of us can live without it, I guess we are all addicted to food to some extent. However, there are people who think about food all day. These people spend virtually every waking moment planning the next thing they are going to eat. They crave foods almost all the time. Food is an obsession for them. I would say that these poor souls are addicted to food, or at least, they are addicted to *eating*. Overeaters Anonymous has been helpful for some of my patients who felt that they had this type of addiction. You can get their number from the toll-free directory. Give them a call if you think that this applies to you.

However, unlike, other addictions—to cigarettes, alcohol, and other drugs—you can't quit food "cold turkey" or totally abstain from "the habit." Alcoholics Anonymous and most other drug rehab programs preach abstinence as the *only way* to kick the habit, and rightly so, yet food addicts can't use this technique for obvious reasons! This is one of the main reasons that dieting is so hard. We must change a bad habit but can do it only by degrees, not by completely eliminating it. Since success is only a few bites away from failure, it is very easy to veer off-course, even just a little bit, and soon be back on the wrong side of the line—right where we started. When someone gets lost in the desert or a dense forest, unless he or she has a compass to guide him or her, he or she will typically start walking in a big circle. (Interestingly enough, this happens because one leg is usually longer than the other, but that's not the point of this example!) Without a "compass"—a plan of diet and exercise to guide us—we will find ourselves going in circles when it comes to weight management.

Staying-on-track with diet is even tougher, because the bad effects of our overeating come on us very slowly, which makes the link between misbehaving and the subsequent punishment hard to see. If the effects of eating excess calories were felt immediately, we would all have a much easier time not overeating. Imagine how much easier it would be to eat appropriately if after my nightly bowl of Blue Bell Ice Cream, when I got up to put the empty bowl in the sink, **POW** a *four-by-five inch ball of fat appeared on my left hip!* I finish my reasonable plate of victuals at dinner but then sneak past the stove to eat an extra roll—**ZAP!**—another chunk of lard pops out by my belly button! I guarantee you one thing: it sure wouldn't take me long to figure out what was causing all that fat to pop out and I would be a lot less likely to cheat and overeat. In fact, I predict that if food worked on us like that, there would be very few overweight people anymore. My constant prayer for people with weight problems is that God will show them more clearly the link between what they eat and how it affects their bodies.

"I have so much weight to lose, I just don't know where to begin."

Confucius said (or maybe it was Elvis), "A journey of a thousand miles begins with one step." Although it looks like a long way to your goal, you can get there if you will just get started. Take the first step and become committed—not to a diet but to a lifetime weight management program. When you think about it, the rest of your life is a long time, and you've got all that time to work on this problem. Don't be in a hurry. Take it slow and do it right the first time. Remember, the tortoise won the race, not the hare.

It can be very discouraging when you've got a hundred pounds to lose and you remember that you should only expect to lose one to one and one-half pound each week. When you do the math you realize that it may take a year to lose your weight. A whole year! But if you think about it, a year, compared to the rest of your life, is not very long. If you are thirty-five now, and we all hope you make it to at least seventy-five, you've got forty years left. Investing one year, or one-fortieth of the rest of your life, in getting the weight down and keeping it off looks like a pretty good investment to me. Also, this is not a year in "calorie prison" on a starvation fad diet; it is merely the first year that you have begun to eat properly and exercise to begin to maintain your ideal body weight, or at least your target weight. That's why it takes so long for the weight to come off. This is not starvation or total food deprivation but simply a change in your eating habits and level of physical activity to fit the weight you want and allowing your body to slowly but surely correct down to it. There is no gentler way to do it, and besides, this is the way you will need to eat and exercise to stay at your target weight once you get there. These are the facts. If you understand and believe them, the only logical conclusion is to get started now and be patient.

"What do you think about the Atkins diet and the Zone diet?"

The Atkins diet is the typical fad diet that I don't believe leads to successful long-term weight loss. Remember, unless you're trying to drop a dress size for your sister's wedding in two months and don't care what happens afterward, long-term success is the only success worth having. The Atkins diet is a high-protein, low-carbohydrate starvation diet that does work for short-term weight loss (mostly water) but is a failure for sustained weight loss efforts. It remains popular because it gives quick gratification, as most people lose several pounds of water weight in the first two weeks. However, it isn't worth a hoot for long-term weight control, and in my opinion, it perpetuates the diet yo-yo that plagues many women trying to lose weight. In fact, most nutritionists criticize the diet for these same reasons. I guess the Atkins diet is much like a bad case of hemorrhoids: it just keeps coming back.

The Zone, however, does offer a long-term program for weight management that should prove quite successful. Dr. Barry Sears is a well-respected molecular biologist and bases his recommendation on several scientifically based nutritional studies that are, of course, unfortunately flawed by the inherent limitations on all nutritional studies that were discussed earlier, in chapter 6. Much of what he says makes sense, though, and I have incorporated that information into this book. However, I do have two areas of concern with Dr. Sears's concepts. First, he feels that staying in "the Zone" will prevent heart disease, cancer, arthritis, lupus, depression, alcoholism, AIDS, jet lag, PMS, impotence, chronic pain, eczema, psoriasis and—oh, yes, aging. (He left out under arm dingle-dangle).

It is clear, from an abundance of research, that eating a balanced diet and following a program of regular exercise will lower one's risk of death from heart disease, and *The Zone* certainly offers an acceptable approach to this problem. However, the body of available scientific evidence becomes quite thin in support of Dr. Sears's assertions that his program can ward off the other diseases mentioned earlier. In this area, *the Zone* becomes more like the *Twilight Zone*. Although he may be proved right one day "in a galaxy far, far away . . . " Dr. Sears's evidence to support the other reported benefits of "life in *the Zone*" is really from *The Outer Limits* instead.

Staying within the Zone requires an excessive restriction in calories compared to other successful diet programs, including the one I have proposed here. For example, Dr. Sears calculates that Bubba, a 220-pound man (strangely, like me) who is moderately active (three half-hours of exercise per week) should have a maintenance calorie intake of 1,680 calories per day, balanced in a ratio of 2:2:3 protein:fat:carbohydrates. This will keep Bubba in the Zone and reaping all of the benefits(?) described in his book. However, the maintenance calorie level calculated by the calorie-balancing method I've show you in *The Hurried Woman* is 2,640 calories per day! (220 lbs. × 12 cals. = 2,604 cals. Sorry, but men get to use a factor of 12 instead of 11. It really is a man's world, isn't it?) Now, which diet would you rather be on to achieve the same weight goals? I don't know about you, but I can find a whole lot of creative ways to spend the additional 960 calories allowed me by the calorie-balancing method and should still be able to keep my weight where I want it in spite of being "outta 'da Zone.' "

Besides that, I have degrees in biology, chemistry, economics, and accounting, an M.D. degree, and an M.B.A. Nonetheless, in spite of all that "learnin'," it took me about thirty minutes to calculate my maintenance calories based on Dr. Sears's method. In fact he doesn't give his diet recommendations in calories at all; I had to convert the results from his "blocks" of protein and fat into calories to make the comparison. *The Zone* isn't really rocket science, but it isn't too far from it. I'm afraid that most normal humans will have trouble walking the narrow nutritional path outlined in *The Zone,* much less being able to locate and land on it (or in it?) in the first place.

"I am thirty-seven years old, five-feet six inches and weigh 180 pounds. I want to lose weight. How do I get started?"

First, let's establish your ideal or target weight. Looking at the BMI table in Appendix B, your current BMI is 29, or "overweight" to any government employee. A "high normal" weight for you would be 148 (BMI = 24), so let's make 148 pounds your target weight. Therefore, your target maintenance calories would be calculated by taking your target weight of 148 and multiplying by 11 to find the number of maintenance calories needed to sustain you at your target weight.

148 lbs. $\times$ 11 cals./lb. = 1,628 calories in per day

We have also calculated that you wish to lose 32 pounds. You should begin a food diary to track your food intake and your exercise calories expended, start a balanced diet with 1,620 calories in each day, and exercise for three half-hour sessions per week. Although you may experience more rapid weight loss at first, you should routinely expect to lose between 1 and 1.5 pounds each week until you reach your goal weight of 148 pounds.

Remember, this is a lifelong commitment to weight management, not a fad diet. Your weight loss will go *very slowly* at first, but in the long run this program will give you the very best chance of getting the weight off *and keeping it off.*

"I did what you suggested and lost about seven pounds in a month, but now I can't seem to lose any more weight. What should I do now?" (This is the same woman who asked the previous question. *Four weeks went by so quickly. Doesn't time fly when you're having fun?*)

Congratulations! You've successfully lost seven pounds, a feat not every woman can accomplish. However, it appears that the remaining weight isn't going to be as easy to ditch, which should come as no surprise. Some organized trial and error will pay off here.

You can approach this "plateau" in one of two ways. You can either (1) decrease your calories in by 100 per day, down to 1,520 calories per day, or (2) add ten minutes to each of the three exercise sessions each week. (If you prefer, you may add one additional half-hour session each week. Whichever way you choose should work out about the same.) Either approach will effectively decrease the overall net calories in from the original calorie-balancing equation.

Decreasing your daily food intake by 100 calories will decrease your calories in each week by 700 calories, whereas adding ten minutes to each exercise session will increase calories expended by about 200 to 400 calories each week, depending on what type of exercise you choose. If, after two weeks, your weight is still holding steady and you want to continue to lose weight, then make a similar adjustment again—decrease calories in by another 100 calories each day (down to 1,420 calories per day) or increase calories expended in exercise by going ten more minutes each session or add that fourth session each week. Continue to reassess your progress every two weeks and step up the dieting or exercise regularly until the weight loss resumes—which it will. Be patient, but also be persistent.

"I've never needed (or wanted!) to exercise before. What's the best way to start?"

This is a very common problem for us forty-something people. We can't just hop up one Saturday morning, slap on some tennis shoes, and boogie two miles down the street simply because we feel like it. We have to approach exercise more carefully now, as our bones and joints aren't as limber or resilient as they once were. It's best to make a few necessary preparations before taking on a new exercise program:

1. *Check with your doctor before you begin:*

Most health clubs and workout facilities will require a note from your doctor anyway before they let you die on their equipment—it makes them look bad, you know! Seriously, discuss your workout plans with your physician before you hit the track. He or she will probably want to check your blood pressure and get an EKG if you have any symptoms suggestive of heart disease or significant risk factors. Once you get the "all-clear," then get started.

2. Get the right equipment:

Older ankles, legs, and feet need help getting started with exercise. I recommend walking to begin with, and do it on a track rather than the street. Many school or workout tracks are actually padded to help decrease the chance of injuries. You also need to invest in the right type of shoes for your chosen activity. If you aren't sure what shoes to get, start with "cross-trainers." These shoes are designed for moderate use in almost any activity.

3. Pick the right exercise for you.

I wish channel surfing, or even sex for that matter, was aerobic exercise, but alas, it isn't. Walking is absolutely the best exercise for most people, as it requires little equipment and can be done almost anywhere and in any weather. (There are lots of *used* treadmills available, and most malls welcome walkers). However, some people have leg, ankle, or hip problems that prevent them from walking. Even worse, the extra weight they would like to get off makes the leg, ankle, and hip problems worse. It's a vicious circle for these folks. Consider swimming or riding a stationary bicycle as an alternative, at least until you can get some of the extra weight off your joints so that walking or jogging might then be possible. The absolute key to success at this juncture is to not get injured, which will kill your exercise efforts. If you aren't sure what to do, consult with your doctor or ask to be referred to an orthopedic surgeon or physiatrist (physical medicine and rehabilitation specialist), who can prescribe physical therapy and/or alternative exercise options for you. Remember, for people over thirty, exercise is a critical part of successful weight management. If you can't exercise, you're going to have to diet a whole lot more, so try hard to incorporate some type of calorie-burning activity into your program to help ensure your success. It'll be worth the trouble.

4. Build up your exercise stamina slowly:

It's critical that you build up your exercise tolerance slowly to avoid injuries. The sad fact is that overweight people suffer a lot more leg, knee, ankle, and foot injuries when they begin an exercise program, because the extra weight they are carrying puts too much strain on their legs and associated parts (not to be confused with the "parts" or "lower unit" in the section of chapter 15 on male anatomy). These poor women are in a Catch-22 situation, because exercise will help them lose weight, but their weight prevents them from exercising effectively. Ask your doctor or health club adviser to help you find a suitable aerobic exercise, given your current limitations. As you lose weight, you will begin to have more options for safe and effective aerobic activity.

Part III
Sex Drive

"Not Tonight, I've Got a Pulse"

13

Low Sex Drive—Physical Factors

Women have complained about low sex drive since time began. Perhaps it's the constant whining, begging, and pouting of their *men* that upsets them most. I'm not certain. But whatever the reason, men and women have complained about their different sexual urges for centuries.

A women's sex drive is influenced by several factors. Let's divide them into three primary areas, and discuss each separately although there is some overlap between them: (1) physical, (2) situational, and (3) emotional or psychological.

Animal Instincts

Humans belong to the animal kingdom. And even though we don't like to think of ourselves as animals, it is quite apparent that there are many physical and behavioral similarities between animals and humans. Most female mammals will not accept the amorous advances of the male unless they are in estrus or "heat," which is the time of ovulation—the only time pregnancy can occur. Such an attitude encourages reproduction in a species and avoids "wasted" encounters. Interestingly, many women notice that they are more likely to fantasize and show a more positive attitude about sex around the time of ovulation and much less so when their period nears. A woman's sex drive appears to have an underlying basic rhythm, which peaks once a month when her eggs are ready for fertilization.

Similarly, a man's sexual rhythm also seems to run parallel to his ability to reproduce. The difference is that sperm production is a continuous process. Sperm are being produced every day, always keeping "the lower unit fully charged." No wonder men are ready for sex virtually all of the time. Of course, these underlying sexual "currents" flow very

101

differently in men and women and may provide an explanation for some of the differences in libido seen between the sexes.

Additional proof for at least some holdover influences from our animal ancestry is found in the seasonal nature of human births. More babies are born in July, August, and September than any other three consecutive months during the year (not the best timing, considering that most new doctors-in-training start in July). This seasonal concentration of births would imply at least some cyclic increase in fertility and perhaps sexual frequency as well among humans. Most women would argue, and rightfully so, that this animal nature isn't the primary factor in deciding whether or not they want to have sex on any give night, but it may provide an underlying rhythm of rising and falling sexual awareness.

Understanding your own sexual rhythms might help explain *why* you feel the way you do *when* you do. Helping your partner understand your sexual rhythm may lead to less frustration and more satisfaction in your love life. Many women notice that they are just not in the mood to make love immediately before and during a menstrual cycle. Sex is often more uncomfortable then, too. The pelvic organs are congested and swollen with blood, and many women suffer from PMS or other mood changes that may make them less approachable during the week or so prior to the menstrual cycle. Don't just bite his head off when he makes the mistake of approaching at these times. Tell him what's going on so he won't keep making the same mistake. Men *are* trainable, you know!

Also, remember that your partner's natural rhythm is not a couple of beats on a bass drum each month but more like a snare drum roll. Try to be more patient with him. Don't necessarily read his almost constant readiness as "pressure to perform" but rather as a natural consequence of his underlying physical rhythms.

Illness

Illness has a huge impact on sexual functioning in women. Women who are debilitated by chronic disease or in pain are likely to have a much lower sex drive. You wouldn't expect a woman in a body cast to set any records in the Pelvic Olympics now, would you? Patients worn down by advanced cancer, severe anemia, low thyroid, and chronic infections all report lower levels of sexual desire. In fact, fatigue from any cause seems to distract women from their normal interest in sex.

102

Women who suffer from chronic vaginitis (yeast infections, bacterial vaginosis, and trichomoniasis), endometriosis, or uterine prolapse will complain of painful intercourse and begin to have less desire for sex. (Uterine prolapse is a condition where the uterus drops down into the lower pelvis, making intercourse painful. It usually comes from delivering a baby.) Let's face it: if you have to fish your uterus out of your panty hose just to have a brief and unfulfilling rendezvous with "Homeboy," how excited are you going to be about the opportunity? It makes sense for these patients to shy away from sex, because it hurts. Trying to force the issue over time is not a good idea because it may lead to a condition called vaginismus as well as a lot of resentment. Vaginismus is an involuntary spasm of the powerful pelvic muscles that close off the vagina, making sex extremely difficult, if not impossible, to complete. This condition can absolutely wreck your sex life until it is treated. If you have painful intercourse or dyspareunia, it is almost always a sign of some type of illness. Don't let this condition go undiagnosed and untreated—see your gynecologist immediately.

If you suffer from a chronic medical condition, try to comply with treatment and get your medical problems under control as much as possible. This will make you feel better overall and maximize your chances for a happy sex life.

Testosterone

Testosterone has recently received a lot of attention in the popular press, as well as scientific journals. As you probably already know, testosterone is the most active male hormone in both men and women. It has some similar effects in both sexes but can also have the opposite effect in certain areas. Testosterone encourages sex drive, or libido, in both men and women. Perhaps it would be too simple to say, "He's got too much and I have too little!" But it may be the truth. Women who complain about a low sex drive should have their testosterone levels checked and take hormone replacement if the levels are low. We replace estrogen in menopause and should also replace testosterone if the levels are low. However, I don't recommend taking male hormone "just to see if it works." You might start singing bass in the choir or need to shave every morning if you take extra testosterone and don't need it. Nor do I recommend the homeopathic approach either—"a little dab'll do ya." If your levels are already normal, adding a little more won't help anything and may wind up leading to an overdose. Overdose symptoms include extra hair growth, acne, irritability, channel surfing, scratching private parts in public places, and declaring war for no apparent reason! Seriously though, if there's a documented deficiency, taking an appropriate dose of medicine that will bring you back into the normal range makes sense. Taking extra might be harmful.

Besides improving sex drive, testosterone is anabolic. In other words, it tends to build muscle and not fat by modifying your metabolism. It also appears to build bone and blood elements that prevent osteoporosis and anemia. Other areas of current testosterone research include hair loss, Alzheimer's disease, depression, and connective tissue diseases like lupus.

If your testosterone level is low you should receive replacement therapy. I usually recommend topical or trans-dermal testosterone preparations compounded by a pharmacist. The skin absorbs certain hormones and other medications very efficiently, and in my experience transdermal testosterone gives more dependable blood levels than the currently available oral preparations. You don't need to worry about growing a patch of hair where you rub it on—usually the forearm—and it's not much more expensive than pills. Once you begin hormone replacement, you should have your testosterone level checked in about four to six weeks. Remember, not too much and not too little. Take the medicine faithfully and get your level rechecked to be sure it is where you need it.

Estrogen

Testosterone is not the end of the hormone story. Your female hormones are important as well in supporting a normal sex drive. Women in menopause still report a desire for sexual activity but are much more satisfied with sex if they are on estrogen. In fact, I remember early in my medical practice talking to an eighty-six-year-old patient about surgery to fix her fallen bladder. During the discussion, she stopped me in mid-sentence to ask, "This surgery won't stop me from 'getting it,' will it?" In my ignorance (I was a lot younger then but still a man, so take my last thought with a grain of salt) I thought maybe she meant "getting" the paper. I'm sure I looked puzzled.

"You know, Doc, the 'horizontal dance' . . . 'going for the gold.' "

(I was still awestruck. Surely this sweet little grandma wasn't referring to s-e-x? No way!)

"You know, *sex!*"

"Oh," I said (or something equally as profound). "It should be OK after six to eight weeks."

"Six to eight weeks! I don't know if I can wait that long. What about oral sex?"

I'm sure I was starting to fidget by his point in the conversation, trying to appear professional and compassionate and not bust our laughing at the same time. Fortunately, my nurse rescued me.

"Dr. Bost, don't forget Dr. Green is holding on line two."

"Yes, thank God . . . I mean, thank God Dr. Green is patient. I'll be right there." Shheww!!

I tell this story not to embarrass my patient but to criticize my own previous prejudices regarding sex later in life. It's actually OK to have sex up to the time you die. Of course, the older I get, the better that sounds. In fact, dying of old age *during sex* sounds good to me! I guess perspective alters our opinions.

Well, I said all of this to stress that estrogen primes the female sex organs for intercourse. Estrogen allows for vaginal lubrication as well as making the vagina more elastic for sex. Menopausal women will often complain of vaginal dryness and even painful intercourse if estrogen levels are too low. Estrogen has also been shown to improve sexual sensitivity and heighten a woman's ability to achieve orgasm or climax. Women in menopause report more satisfaction with their sex lives if they receive estrogen replacement therapy. Moreover, the levels of satisfaction improve even further if testosterone replacement is given as well, but only in women whose hormone levels are low. Achieving the appropriate balance of estrogen and testosterone can allow most women to enjoy a healthy sex life far into menopause.

Estrogen and Cancer

There has been much written lately about estrogen and cancer risks. Unfortunately, much of what you've heard or read is emotionally charged misinformation, some of it coming from physicians. I feel obliged as a gynecologist to discuss estrogen replacement briefly in order to clarify some of the contradictory information floating around out there like a dead frog in a swimming pool, much of which comes off the Internet. By the way, no one filters what's on the Internet for accuracy. Just because some *idiot* took the time to publish an official-looking Web page with his or her harebrained opinions on it doesn't mean that what he or she has posted for your viewing pleasure is actually true. I have found many Internet publishers, even *doctors* (can you imagine?), suffer from osteocephaly. If you're going to "surf the Net" for information, be sure to take what you read with a grain of salt, particularly from sites like www.estrogenkillswomendead.com or obgyndoctorsstink.net.

If women take estrogen alone, they run a tenfold increase risk of developing uterine cancer. Sounds pretty bad at first, until you find out that if they take progesterone with their estrogen, *they have a **lower risk** of developing uterine cancer than women who take no hormones at all.* Of course, if you've had a hysterectomy, this potential risk no longer applies to you.

No doubt by now you've heard that estrogen causes breast cancer. In fact, several major medical journals have recently published papers showing a slightly higher risk of breast cancer in estrogen users, particularly those who have taken it for more than ten years. However, let me stress two points about the body of evidence regarding breast cancer risk and hormones. First, the majority of high-quality scientific evidence *does not* show any link between estrogen use and breast cancer. Only three of the approximately ten articles available on the subject propose any link between estrogen use and breast cancer while the majority of papers show that using estrogen does not increase breast cancer risks *at all.* Therefore, the weight of scientific evidence supports the use of estrogen in post-menopausal women. Second, those few studies that do report an association between estrogen use and breast cancer can only demonstrate a *very weak* association. In fact, many experts in the field don't agree with the statistical methods used by some of these authors to demonstrate their proposed link between breast cancer and estrogen. Like my Dad warned me, "figures don't lie, but liars can figure." I'm not saying that these researchers are unscrupulous and would lie to us on purpose, but perhaps they believe so strongly in their cause that they see what they want to see in their numbers—maybe something that isn't really there.

It is clear that some breast cancers are stimulated by estrogen and if a woman finds out that she has breast cancer she should stop taking estrogen immediately, because continuing it might encourage the cancer to grow faster. However—and this is important—*the estrogen most likely*

106

did not cause *the breast cancer to occur.* It stands to reason that normal breast tissue is different from breast cancer. One of the things that makes breast cancer tissue different from normal breast tissue is its appearance under the microscope. But another more important difference is that normal breast tissue will not respond to estrogen as an abnormal growth stimulant while some breast cancers will. That's another reason why most experts believe that estrogen does not cause breast cancer. Unfortunately, the final answer to this question will have to wait for the right type of evidence—randomized clinical trials—which will take twenty-plus years to complete. I predict this research will reveal that there is a small group of women who are predisposed to developing breast cancer and should not take estrogen, yet the vast majority of women will benefit greatly from estrogen replacement therapy and will be encouraged to do so.

Current research also shows that the benefits derived from estrogen are very important and far outweigh any associated risks for the average woman. Estrogen, along with calcium and exercise, is extremely effective in preventing osteoporosis. Osteoporosis is a leading cause of death in elderly women. Of course, the death certificate does not list osteoporosis as the cause. Things like "pneumonia" or "pulmonary embolism" (a blood clot that goes to the lungs from the leg or pelvis) are given as the official reason for death. But these problems are complications of being confined to bed for eight weeks from a fractured hip that was caused by, you guessed it, osteoporosis. Thank goodness most women are starting to hear this information and are taking steps to prevent osteoporosis. The biggest problem with osteoporosis prevention is that most women have no symptoms of trouble until the damage is already done. Studies show that if a woman waits more than three to five years after menopause begins before starting estrogen, she will have lost most of the benefits of the estrogen. In other words, estrogen *prevents* osteoporosis but it cannot *reverse* it.

Estrogen is clearly helpful in preventing heart disease in women. Interestingly, it may also have a similar effect in men. Cholesterol patterns are improved by estrogen—less LDL ("bad" cholesterol) and more HDL ("good" cholesterol)—even though estrogen may slightly increase cholesterol levels overall. Heart attack is still the leading cause of death in American women today. In fact, a woman is ten times more likely to die from a heart attack than breast cancer. Many women do not believe this statistic, but it is absolutely true. So even if estrogen is someday

107

shown to encourage breast cancer (which is doubtful), you are still much more likely to receive protection from estrogen than to die because of it. If I were a woman in menopause (God forbid!), I would take my estrogen, testosterone, and calcium, have my levels checked periodically as directed by my doctor, and add progesterone if my uterus was still present—no doubt about it. I would also get my mammograms done on schedule and perform breast self-examination every month.

Menopause

Menopause is the state (it might even be a country) in which the ovaries no longer produce estrogen and progesterone. Women in menopause will stop having periods, can no longer get pregnant, and immediately begin to slowly but surely develop osteoporosis and an increasing risk of heart disease if left alone. Most women will also complain of hot flushes, night sweats, mood swings, irritability, and low energy levels. In addition, as menopause progresses, many women will begin to notice dryness in the vagina, painful intercourse, a decreased ability to concentrate or focus their attention on certain tasks, and a decrease in libido or sex drive.

Presently, medical science cannot predict menopause; we can only tell if you have arrived there or not. A blood test called FSH is used to detect menopause. If your periods are becoming increasingly irregular, you are experiencing hot flushes (sometimes called flashes) and night sweats more than just a few nights each month, or you are complaining of worsening moodiness or vaginal dryness, you may be in menopause. Notify your doctor of your symptoms and suspicions and he or she will most likely offer you the test to see what's going on. If your FSH level indicates that you are in menopause, you should start estrogen replacement therapy as soon as you can, to receive the maximum benefits from the hormones. If your blood test shows you are not there yet, you may be there soon. Unfortunately, no one can accurately predict exactly when *you* will go into menopause, and for some women these symptoms may persist for many years until you ''arrive.'' This time of menopausal symptoms prior to the actual menopause is called **SLOW TORTURE!** No actually, it's officially called peri-menopause.

Peri-Menopause

In peri-menopause, estrogen levels are not absent, but they may fluctuate widely and produce many of the symptoms outlined in the previous section, particularly moodiness and irregular bleeding. It is often difficult to treat patients in peri-menopause with simple estrogen replacement therapy because the estrogen may help take out some of the hormone "lows" but will not suppress the underlying hormone cycle. Because of this, peri-menopausal women on estrogen supplements will often experience *more* irregular bleeding and worse moodiness. An alternative solution may be birth control pills. For women who feel good on it, the pill may provide a way of smoothing the transition between peri-menopause and menopause.

We previously felt it was unsafe for women over forty (thirty-five for smokers) to take the pill. However, research now shows that birth control pills are safe for non-smoking women up to menopause—around age fifty-one in this country. The estrogen-progesterone combination pill provides estrogen, to prevent osteoporosis and heart disease risks, contraception if needed, and regular cycles without the hormone ups and downs that cause mood swings and irritability. Unfortunately, birth control pills are not suitable for everyone, but for those who can take, they may be the difference between misery and happiness. Certainly for many women the pill can help avoid surgery. Women in peri-menopause often bleed irregularly. However, traditional estrogen replacement therapy will not usually control this type of bleeding. In addition, many women experience heavier and more painful periods as the years go by. Ten years ago when a woman reached forty, she had to be taken off the pill—remember, back then we thought pills were unsafe after forty—and that's when the trouble began. When menstrual cycles got heavier and more painful, many women had no viable options other than to continue to suffer or have a hysterectomy. Now that women know they can safely take birth control pills into menopause, many are choosing to stay on the pill and thus avoid suffering through bad cycles and peri-menopause without help or having a major operation to find relief. In the future, as the rate of hysterectomy comes down, managed care will claim that they "scored a big victory for women by not allowing 'unnecessary surgery' and forcing women and their doctors to try other alternatives." But the real reason hysterectomies will become less frequent is that women have become empowered by finally having a viable alternative to "biting the bullet" or resorting to major surgery when it comes to the problems of peri-menopause and the worsening menstrual cycles common after childbearing.

I've often wondered why this condition was called menopause. It only occurs in women, right? Shouldn't it be named *women*opause? I think this is just another example of hidden sexism in medicine. Let's face it, the first doctors were all men and, like Adam in the Garden of Eden, named things to suit themselves. There are lots of examples of this sexual bias in medicine: Why isn't a hysterectomy called a *her*sterec-tomy?'' Doesn't make sense, does it? Shouldn't hemorrhoids be called *her*orrhoids if a woman has them? (My wife says that since men are such a pain in the rear that . . . well . . .maybe we should leave it hemorrhoids, regardless of who has them.) But what about herpes? It should be hepes if a man has it, right? And "he-dies" if he gave it to you! And finally, what male chauvanist pig named the footholders at the end of the gyn exam table "stirrups?" I guess he thought that was *funny* somehow. I can just imagine a bunch of old dudes in powdered wigs sitting around the table at the club snickering about the "stirrups"! Ha, ha, ha. . . .

There are many other examples, but I suppose we should move on to other factors that shape a woman's sex drive. (Seriously though, shouldn't menstruation be *women*struation or perhaps *whoa*menstruation on a particularly bad cycle? It would make a lot more sense!)

14

Low Sex Drive—Situational Factors

Stress Affects Sex Drive

Situational factors have an important role in determining the level of libido in women. Women under pressure are much less likely to fantasize about sex than men. Big deadlines at work, hectic schedules at work and home, troubled teenagers, and money problems all produce stresses that decrease a women's desire for sex. Living at your mother-in-law's house for a month, preparing for your daughter's wedding, or bringing a new baby home are all examples of stressful situations than can decrease sex drive. Fortunately, most situations like these are temporary and their effects are easily recognized. But what about situations that are not so temporary—an extremely stressful job, a chronically sick parent or child, or precarious financial circumstances? These situations may last a lot longer. Sometimes when the immediate effects of the initial stress die down we forget that the chronic stress that is left behind can take its toll on our energy levels and our desire to enjoy many aspects of life that we once found pleasure in, including sex. After one of these situations has gone on for a long time, many patients claim that they are used to the stress and that it no longer affects them. At this point they are suffering from denial and perhaps even depression (or pre-depression) is setting in—unrecognized by the patient, but nonetheless having a significant impact on her life and her relationships.

Most people would eventually recognize the preceding situations as stressful. It might take a while to appreciate the full impact of the stress on their health and attitudes, but most people would agree that these situations at least *could* be stressful. But what about the little things that stress us, like Little League baseball, Little Dribblers (sounds like a bunch of midgets with prostate trouble but is actually Little League basketball), gymnastics, cheerleading, twirling (do girls still do this?), dance lessons, children's activities at church, or—dare I say it—**soccer?** Don't these events weight on your schedule and, therefore, your mind? Could the stress of all these "little things," when combined with the big things in your life like work, husband, family, church, school, etc., produce a very hectic schedule? Of course they can and *do* for most women. *Do not make the mistake of underestimating the stress that you are living under.* Trying to juggle your busy life and the busy lives of your children takes its toll on your mental as well as physical energy. Sure, no one of these things will "make or break you" by itself, but *do not underestimate the overall effect that combining each of these "little things" with your big things has on your stress levels.* It is very significant.

Even when a woman understands the situational stress she is under, she often feels that changing the circumstances is beyond her control. Sometimes it is, but sometimes there's another problem:

"My husband's work is too important" (. . . *and I'm not*)

"No one else can take care of my mother" (. . . *like I want it done, anyway*)

"My job is very demanding, but I can't cut back" (. . . *I like to feel important and needed—even though it's killing me*)

"My kids just can't give up soccer" (. . . *but I guess they can give up* my *happiness without too much trouble*)

Women have told me these things over and over again, and when I confront them with the message in parentheses they sometimes look at me as if I am from another planet: "You just don't understand, Doctor," meaning *they* are totally clueless. Occasionally, maybe in every third or fourth patient, I see a little light pop on in her head and she begins to understand that *she* may be part of the problem, too. She has put herself too low on her own priority list. Everyone else's needs get met first. Then, and only then, does Mom really take any time out for herself, time to unwind, give herself a break, think, relax, etc. As I have said before, women are very willing (too willing, in my opinion) to sacrifice themselves for the benefit of their families. It is this trait that makes my wife a hero in my eyes—she constantly denies herself to serve her family, in so very many ways—but at what cost? I see so many women suffer under a horrendous workload of trying to run the kids to gymnastics, swimming lessons, baseball practice, soccer games, music lessons, school programs, church programs, etc., etc., etc., etc.! All of these are "worthwhile" endeavors, surely. Who could argue that playing sports or taking music lessons is "bad" for your child? But what is it costing you in "physical capital" to meet all of their schedules, project deadlines, practices, and performances—much less, your budget!? Do you realize how much all of this stuff costs? Erma Bombeck said that raising kids was "like being pecked to death by chickens." Not that any one "peck" is going to kill you, but after dealing with this kind of stress over several years you're going to start looking like Suzanne Pleshette in *The Birds!* Not too pretty, eh? You can bet that after a long day in the "chicken coop," when your husband fans out his tail feathers to pique (peck?) your interest, you'll probably be thinking, *What does this bird want?* rather than responding in kind. The hurry in your life simply drains the sex drive out of you too.

Don't expect the people around you to fix the situation for you. They don't realize how much you are hurting, *because you won't tell them.* Remember, your kids are too young to realize what anything really costs and your husband is genetically defective, so he'll never figure it out by himself. No, Virginia, you are going to have to take the bull by the horns and change things to make your life, and your love life, better. Otherwise, they will continue to peck away at you until your melt down or the circumstances change by themselves. (Your kids move away or maybe your husband moves away, whatever!) It's not that your children, boss, husband, or friends hate you. On the contrary, they love you, *but* they don't realize (and maybe you don't, either) how much all the little things they ask of you (and you ask of yourself, for them) affect you and how you react to them. The first step to fixing the problem is recognizing the importance of "the little things" and how they affect you and your attitudes toward sex and life in general.

We discussed this in some detail in the first part of the book on fatigue. I bring it up again here because it is critical to your understanding of the Hurried Woman and why she feels the way she does. In the fourth and final part, we will discuss how to fix the problems of the Hurried Woman—"un-hurry her," so to speak. At this point, it is important for you to understand that situational stress lowers your sex drive. Indeed, it may be one of the major reasons that you are where you are—unhappy. The good news is that it is one of the major causes that you can exert some control over.

15

Men and Women are Different—Duh!

I'm sure that you've read or heard a lot about this subject lately. There are several interesting books out on the topic, including the popular *Men Are from Mars and Women Are from Venus: A Practical Guide for Improving Communication and Getting What You Want in Your Relationships,* by John Gray (Harper Collins, 1992), which also ranks second in the world on the list of books with the longest title. If you've read any of these books, some of what I say here will probably be repetitive for you, but you need to have at least a basic understanding of how the sexes differ or you will continually be frustrated in your marriage for one very important but simple reason—your husband will *never* be like you. It isn't going to happen! And if he did become like you, you probably wouldn't like him anymore! You would probably view him as "less manly" somehow and long for "the old caveman days" again. Oh, sure, he could become *more* like you and it would improve your marriage in some ways, but he will never think and act as you do (unless he's a gynecologist) because he is a man and you are a woman. This is a fact of life that cannot be changed, no matter how hard you try. Men and women are not only built differently; they also approach life and their relationships very differently. This is why they approach sex differently as well.

Much of the information in this chapter is based on observed behavior. In other words, scientists have studied the habits and opinions of men and women, both as children and adults, and observed differences in how the sexes act and say they feel. This type of information is pretty reliable because it is based on observation. However, the underlying reason that men and women behave differently is still a mystery in many areas. This type of information is speculative—in other words, we don't really know that much about it for sure—but reasonably intelligent people are giving us their best guess as to why men and women don't approach

114

certain tasks in the same way, act the same in certain situations, or express similar emotions when challenged in a given way. The other problem with this type of discussion is that it leads to stereotyping. Everybody knows that all men are not the same—some are more athletic, others more effeminate, some aggressive and others more passive, etc. Likewise, you can't cubby-hole all women into two or three tidy slots; most people are a blend of several stereotypes. So, don't be surprised when you find that some of the examples don't exactly fit you or your situation.

In this chapter, we'll explore some of the more important differences between men and women. It may be a review for you, but it will still help you focus your thoughts on the subject. In the next chapter, we'll see how these differences apply to your marriage and particularly to your physical relationship as husband and wife.

Relationships and Identity

Men relate to one another through activities such as sports or work. They will gather with their friends to go golfing, hunting, or fishing, watch a ball game, play poker, or swap stock market stories with one another. Men obtain their identities through competition and goal-oriented activities like work. How often do you see your husband "chatting" with his buddies? You know, "guy talk." Men are much more likely to gather for an event or activity than to simply talk. Is it a mystery why men find work and sports rewarding? It's the way they receive gratification. Competing and accumulating "prizes" (such as money, a good car, a nice house, a pretty wife and family, or a promotion at work) give a man his self-esteem. Unfortunately, losing the race can sometimes take it away, too.

Women, however, often call each other just to find out what's going on, how the kids are doing, or what happened over the weekend. Now don't think that men don't gossip, because they do. Yet gossip is not the primary reason for male interaction; the event is—gossip just occurs at the event. Women show affection for one another through "relating" or talking, sharing emotions, and touching. Establishing and nurturing relationships with the important people in their lives give women much of their identity and purpose. Certainly women entering the work force have blurred this male/female paradigm; however, studies of professional men and women demonstrate that these differences are still present. Male executives place more emphasis on achieving work-related goals than their female counterparts, while female executives stress relationship building at work as more important than their male colleagues do.

Perspectives and Priorities

These inter-sex differences can also be seen in how men and women view the same event from different perspectives. A few months ago, my wife and I were told by friends about a car accident they had been involved in over the weekend. I asked the husband about the particulars of the accident: "How much damage was done? What's it going to cost to fix it? How did the accident occur?" My wife, however, asked, "Was anybody hurt? Are you still shaken up?" I was more interested in the action and the "prizes-at-risk" in the accident, while my wife was more concerned about the people and "relationships-at-risk." Men and women approach life and view its events from different perspectives and with different priorities. Knowledge of these differences can help us understand each other's behavior and attitudes as well as help improve communication in our marriages.

Traditionally, the reasons for these differences have been explained by the "gender programming" that our parents and society at-large encourage. Little boys are given toy guns and baseballs to play with while little girls get tea sets and Barbie dolls. The theory proposes that the specific toys and the encouragement our parents and others give us in our play as children determine our gender identity and the traditional male and female roles are learned in this fashion. This theory seems a little too simple to me. Besides, it doesn't explain why my middle son sees anything including a Barbie doll, as some type of weapon. I have been repeatedly shot, stabbed, and clubbed senseless with a (.45-caliber, 10-inch long, five-pound, respectively) Barbie doll. He was never shown any of these alternative uses for a Barbie doll; he just dreamed them up all by himself. I think the real reason men and women are different is genetic. I'm not talking about the fact that women are 46, XX, and men are 46, XY; everybody knows that. No, there's more to it than that. I feel it's time to share with the world something that men have known and women have suspected for many years: men are genetically deficient.

The Missing Gene Theory

Oh, I know—it's been a horrible thing to keep quiet. I'm sure that a lot of men are going to hate me for letting this one out of the bag. But, alas, it's true. Men *are* genetically deficient. Let me explain why.

As I said before, women have two X chromosomes and men have one X and one Y chromosome. Obviously, X and Y chromosomes are not the same. Some genes are found on one chromosome and not on the other. In other words, men have some missing genes. The X chromosome is much bigger than the Y, as shown:

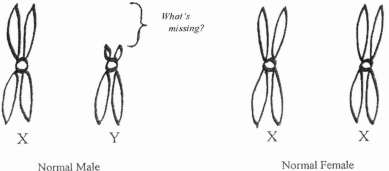

What's missing?

X   Y   X   X

Normal Male   Normal Female
(Is this an oxymoron?)

You can see from the diagram that men have fewer genes than women. Where they went and who took them is still a big mystery, but this paucity of genetic code leaves men with only one copy of some very important genes. These include:

The shopping gene
The gene that allows you to stop and ask for directions
The birthday/anniversary memory gene
The lost item locator gene (sometimes called the find your rear end with both hands gene, because if you don't have two copies of this one, you really *can't* find your rear end with both hands.)

Since men have only one copy of these genes, women can usually out-perform men at these "essential" tasks.

Although these are the major genes in which experts agree men are deficient, I have an alternate theory about why I can't seem to find anything around the house. When I use something, perhaps my left-handed

117

belly button lint remover, and set it down somewhere, my wife finds it and decides that she has a *better* place for it than where I left it, so she moves it. Now I intuitively go back to the general vicinity of where I left it (of course, I don't remember *exactly* where I left it), but somehow it isn't there anymore. After looking around for ten or fifteen minutes, mumbling and grunting unintelligible things as I wander aimlessly around the area, I sheepishly utter the dreaded phrase, "Honey, have you seen my . . . ?" at which my wife disdainfully but with a touch of bravado replies, "It's right where you left it," and goes straightway to the darn thing, brandishing it like a prize won in battle. Of course, if I had just a few more functioning brain cells, I would be able to remember I had *not* put it there, but since I can't muster them up on command, I must admit defeat and wear the "I can't find my rear end with both hands" badge for the rest of the day. It took me several years of painstaking research to finally sort out this enigma and realize exactly how she was pulling the wool over my eyes. I would have worked it out sooner, but I lost my notes somewhere, and . . . well . . . skip it! Let's get back to the matter at hand.

Men also have only one copy of some very important suppressor genes. Suppressor genes are those that turn off or turn down some bodily function, such as:

The gonadal scratch suppressor gene, sometimes called the crotch grabber gene (some pro baseball players don't have one working copy of this gene!)

The gene that stops remote control channel surfing

The flatulence inhibitor gene (referred to by many as "the ripper snipper"), that stops those little gaseous eruptions, which can be most embarrassing and usually get blamed on the dog.

As it turns out, there are only two genes that are unique to the Y chromosome. One of these genes is responsible for forming the external male genitalia (often referred to as "parts" or "the lower unit"). The other gene that is found only on the Y chromosome controls the digital-rectal reflex, or the old "pull my finger" trick your dad used to show you. I must say that women are better off without either of these genes. Well, I hope it is now clear to you, as well as the rest of the world, why men act the way they do—it's in their jeans. I mean *genes!*

These general differences between men and women lead to some very specific attitudes regarding sex. Although the stereotypes presented here don't apply universally to all men and women, they will, I hope, help you see the important differences that do exist between the sexes.

16

How the Sexes View Sex Differently

Arousal

Men are very physically oriented when it comes to sex. If you touch a man in the right spot, he'll probably be ready to have sex (sometimes with the wrong person, which can get him into serious trouble!). However, if a man touches a woman in the "right spot" without her permission, he'll probably get slapped. Same stimulus, but a very different response.

A woman is much more cerebral about sex. She must be properly courted—"in the mood." The proper mood includes being "happy" with her partner. If she's angry with him, she will probably not want to have sex with him. This anger could be from recent or even remote events. If she hasn't forgiven him for an affair he had five years ago or is upset by his not helping out with the kids enough or siding with his mother too often, she may not want to make love to him. Often these attitudes are not conscious efforts to punish him but travel just under the surface of her awareness—flaring up occasionally and then subsiding. In fact, when I have asked women complaining about decreased libido whether any of these situations applied to them they have vehemently denied it. Yet when I see them back in the office a few years later for their annual visit (a perennial favorite), suddenly their sex life has improved dramatically. What's different? They have a new husband! *Now* they will admit they were having trouble at home the last time I saw them. Their ex-husband was abusive or an alcoholic or had a girlfriend, or they were angry with him over some issue. So, if your sex drive is low it's important to ask yourself:

"Am I happy in my relationship with my husband?"
"Are there problem areas we need to work on (other than low sex drive)?"

120

"Do we need counseling?"

If you have asked yourself the last question more than once, you probably do need counseling. Virtually all marriages have room to improve, but if you and your spouse communicate well, then counseling may not be needed. However, if you find yourself butting your head up against the same wall over and over again, counseling may make the difference. I recommend starting with your pastor, rabbi, or priest. These people are sworn to secrecy and usually have experience in dealing with couples having problems. It is highly doubtful that they will help much with specific sexual problems, but they do usually understand the underlying problems in marriage. If your clergy doesn't seem to be the right person for counseling, then ask your doctor to recommend someone.

The most common areas for disagreement in marriage are (you probably already know what they are):

Raising the kids: Often one parent takes on the role of disciplinarian while the other parent disagrees with the first one's methods and doesn't help enforce the rules. They often disagree in front of the children, who then lose respect for the authoritarian parent. This undermining of authority aggravates the disciplinarian, who retaliates by attacking the more passive parent, which further undermines each parent's authority. This produces a vicious circle with the kids caught in the middle.

Money: Who makes it, controls it, spends it, saves it, invests it, and allocates it are all issues surrounding money and finances that can cause problems for couples. Money is the most common subject over which couples argue.

Work: Should both spouses work? Whose job is more important? Who pays for each of the various household expenses? What are each spouse's expectations of his or her own roles and the role of the other spouse for kid and household duties? When does "working hard for the family" become "hard work for the family"?

If you're having trouble solving these types of conflicts, get professional help. A neutral third party can help you sort out these issues and reach some common ground for working together. But do it now, before too much water passes under the bridge.

Sex is Love—Not!

Men feel that sex is a necessary expression of love and perhaps the most important one in a marriage—remember, men are "action-oriented"; they relate to others through action or activities. Women however, want to be shown affection first and then sex will follow; relating emotionally is more important to most women than physical contact. A man might think, *If she loves me she will want to have sex with me.* For a man, sex equals love. However, a woman might think, *Show me that you love me (help with the kids, provide my family's security [home, financial support, etc.], do the chores, romance me) and I will want to have sex with you.* For a woman, sex doesn't equal love. Sex is the byproduct of love, not love in itself. Therefore, most women don't need to make love to feel loved, whereas most men equate the two. This explains why having sex is often a much higher priority for men than women.

Let's imagine that a woman and her husband each start the day out with a list of the ten things they want to accomplish that day—their "Ten Things to Do Today" list. It is almost a given that he will have sex somewhere in the top three and she will have it in the bottom three (if it's on her list at all!) Obviously, that's not true of every day, but it would be true of most days. Most married women just don't see sex as that important, particularly if they have children. But, right or wrong, men do. You can also see why being chronically fatigued or trying to maintain too rigorous a schedule can knock sex off a woman's "Ten Things to Do Today" list a lot quicker than it would a man's. Men often don't understand that a busy schedule makes sex difficult for a woman, because it doesn't have the same effect on him. Unless he's in a body cast, a man is always ready to make love: "We had seven minutes last night. . . . Where were you?" He doesn't understand that a woman doesn't just need enough time to have sex; she needs enough time for sex *to happen.* Which is a whole lot longer than seven minutes! If my wife has had her usual sixteen-hour day and I give her twenty to thirty minutes alone to "get in the mood," she'll fall asleep! Of course, once that happens and I wake her up from her nap, she'll do what I do when someone wakes me up from a nap—become grumpy—and the moment can be lost. This is why it is critical for the woman complaining about decreased libido to schedule time to allow sex to happen without feeling that it is being forced on her. The Hurried Woman needs to clear unimportant things off her schedule, take time to relax, get some of the stress and pressure out of her life, and save some time each day (or at least a few times each week) to reflect on "physical matters." Otherwise, unpressured sex simply won't happen. More on this subject in part 4.

Substitutions

Most couples get married because they really love each other—*they really do!* When a man and woman fall in love and get married, they establish a primary love relationship; a lifelong bond between two people—"to love, honor, and cherish each other until death do you part" (at least, *I think* that's what I said). But as the years go by, two unhealthy substitutions frequently occur in this primary love relationship: a man will substitute work for the relationship with his wife, and a woman will substitute their children for the relationship with her husband.

It is a natural consequence of reproduction that the husband will have to stand back somewhat and allow his wife to raise and nurture their children—a mother's bond with her children is a secondary love relationship. This nurturing requires virtually all of her time and energy at first, but then the center of her affection should turn back toward her husband, as he is the focus of her primary love relationship. Obviously, she now must share her affection among all the members of her family and the primary relationship between husband and wife will never be quite the same again once children arrive on the scene. (*Amen!*) But, a strong and unique relationship must be carefully maintained between Mom and Dad to prevent too complete a substitution from occurring, which could injure the primary love relationship. Many couples wake up when the kids are gone to discover that they are both married to a stranger. They've both changed through the years but have not tended to their primary love relationship and have grown distant, somehow unfamiliar.

In the old days, this led to lives of "quiet desperation." Nowadays, it leads to depression, alcoholism, extra-marital affairs, and divorce. Let me make it clear that this phenomenon is not the woman's fault. In nature, it is very common for a female to guard her offspring and even shun the father to protect them. (After having my own children, I know now why some species eat their young!) However, it is equally as "natural" for the shunned male to go off and impregnate other females once his reproductive work is done at one location. I find neither of these scenarios very "adaptive" for humans—both lead to marriage failures. So, let me encourage you to rise above your instincts and not push your husband away once you have children, just as I would encourage your husband not to be offended by your temporary loss of interest in his reproductive power. He needs to be patient and supportive of you and your role as mother to his children. Equally important to preserving your primary love relationship is for the husband to not allow work to dominate his life. This used to be more difficult to accomplish in the past. Corporate America is beginning to see the value of including spouses—remember, women also have careers outside the home now, too—in the careers of its workers, including family at corporate events, encouraging paternity as well as maternity leave, and providing more financial security for the family through insurance and retirement plans. Yet substituting career for home is a classic "man thing" to do and must be constantly guarded against. If he's like most men, this substitution is not necessarily a conscious effort to withdraw from the family but a natural consequence of his male need for gratification through competition and "prize winning." Work is where most men choose to compete.

Work provides constant "prizes," such as a paycheck, social interaction, and potential promotions, and perhaps "perks" like a car, meals, entertainment opportunities, and vacations. Crossing the finish line and winning the prizes at work builds a man's self-esteem. Of course *work* is a four-letter word and, as such, has its unpleasant side, too. Long hours, deadlines, tough travel schedules, and ultimately fear of failure may make your husband feel he has to turn away from you and your family at times to "get the job done." It's critical that you and your husband communicate to know when these tough times arrive so that you can be supportive and not critical of his efforts. However, it's important at these times to gently remind him that the home "prizes" he's already won (your love and the love of your children) are always going to be there for him and that they are the most important ones to keep. Did you catch the paradox in that statement? On the one hand, he needs to know that you and the kids love him and support him in his efforts away from home and that he can be confident that your love will always be there. But, on the other hand, he has to acknowledge that if he takes you for granted or if he turns away too far and ignores you and his family, he could lose your affection. There's a fine line between "working hard for the family" and "working too hard for the family to take." There's an equally fine line between reminding him that his family needs him and criticizing him for working too hard, which will tear down his self-esteem. I've found this to be a sensitive area for most couples and one in which they both feel inadequate at times. My best advice to wives is to always make the prizes at home appear as attractive and important as the prizes at work and sprinkle them with just a pinch of guilt—too much guilt will spoil the recipe.

If you both work outside the home, this becomes a much more difficult issue. You must sit down together and discuss the goals each of you hope to achieve in your respective careers and find the areas where these goals merge (common ground) and where they clash (trouble spots). Enjoy the common ground areas first; then tackle the trouble spots one by one. Prayer often helps in these tough situations. Thankfully, there's somebody smarter than me to help answer the really tough questions that confront us. Ask Him on a regular basis to help you sort out the problem areas, reassess your goals and priorities, and show you the best way to get there safely.

A Final Note

Sometimes your relationship is simply too far gone for you to retrieve it without professional help. If you read through this chapter and you haven't got a clue as to what I'm talking about, get counseling. It's not that you're stupid or not trying. You are obviously pretty bright—you bought this book, right? It's just that you need more help than a "self-help" book can provide.

If your husband reads this book and doesn't have a clue, remember, he's genetically deficient and will have to be spoon-fed the information. No real surprise, huh? But, seriously, if he just doesn't seem to "get it" after a few times through, I recommend counseling. It often takes a neutral third party to sift through your troubles and help you come up with a solution that works for the both of you.

17

Low Sex Drive—Suggestions for Women

OK, now it's time to get down to the "nitty-gritty." You understand that men and women are different in many ways and particularly in how they approach sex. But rather than trying to make women out of men (that would be a lot like the "silk purse out of a sow's ear" trick) or vice versa (that would be a lobotomy, right?), both men and women need to agree to be different and learn how to make these differences work to the couple's advantage.

1. Analyze Your Health

If you suffer from a medical condition that is out of control and needs treatment, get to your doctor for help. If you have painful intercourse, have never been able to achieve a climax, or question whether there is some other physical problem keeping you from being satisfied sexually, consult your gynecologist. If you scored poorly on the mood test in Appendix A, you must seek help from your family doctor or gynecologist for possible treatment or referral.

A lot of primary care doctors don't like to give their patients antidepressants or hormones. They may feel that another doctor who has a special interest or extra training in this area will do a better job of monitoring and adjusting the medications. They may be just lazy, but I hope that's not the reason. Either way, don't be shocked or offended if your doctor refers you to a psychiatrist. You have to be crazy to see a purple cow, but you don't have to be crazy to see a psychiatrist. They are the doctors with the most expertise in prescribing antidepressants and other medications in this area. Also, and often just as important, they are usually better able to hook you up with a counselor or other stress management programs than your lowly generalist or gynecologist.

126

2. Analyze Your Marriage Relationship

Are there other problems that must be solved first? If you are married to an alcoholic or an abusive husband, nothing will work for you until you get these problems out of the way. Go for counseling immediately.

Are you angry with him over something, perhaps not too obvious at first glance? Does he side with his mother when you argue with him? Did he have an affair three years ago and you haven't really forgiven him yet, even though you thought you had? Do you feel neglected because he spends too much time at work and/or "with the boys" hunting and fishing? These conflicts aren't always apparent on the surface. Counseling may help here also.

If you aren't happy with your partner, you will not want to have sex with him. Find and fix the problems in your marriage first; otherwise, a happy love life is difficult at best.

3. Unhurry Your Life

"Well, thank you very much, Doc, for that simple answer to all my prayers!" Actually, it *is* a simple solution because it is easily understood, yet it will not be a simple task to accomplish. However, no matter how hard the task may seem, it is critical for you to realize that this is probably the most important aspect of solving the problem of a low sex drive and a subsequently unhappy sex life. You must unclutter your schedule with the things that in the long run don't really matter, so that healthy sex will have time to happen. The last part of this book focuses on how to analyze, prioritize, simplify, and organize your life so you can get the happiness back into your love life, and the rest of your life, too. Many women don't believe me at first when I tell them how important this is. The good news is they usually get it right with their *next* marriage. Don't wait until then. Change things now.

4. Schedule Quality Time Together, Away from the Kids

Many couples routinely schedule a "date night," perhaps twice a month. This is a night that the two of you can go out to a movie or dancing or dinner and just talk (relate). Most couples having problems in their love life have trouble communicating in other areas, too. Spending time together, as a couple, is very healthy and builds communication. Relive some of your experiences from dating. Gossip about your crazy relatives. Talk about the kids, your future together, and the good times you've had in the past. It may be a little awkward at first, but anything worth having is worth working for. Most couples tell me that this technique really helps strengthen their relationship.

Try to schedule a weekend or overnight trip away from home, just the two of you. Couples' retreats at church are sometimes good because the speakers at these events can give you ideas about improving your relationship. However, when it's time for activities, many times the men go one way and the women go the other. This is not "quality time" with your spouse. A little of these meetings goes a long way. The other reason I encourage time away with each other is that it helps reverse the common substitutions that occur in our marriage relationships. Finally, this is not a "once-a-decade" event. Make these times away a priority and schedule them as frequently as you can blackmail Grandma into keeping the kids. In fact, many couples support one another in this effort by keeping each other's kids for the weekend—not the *same* weekend, of course. Swapping kids for a weekend isn't going to help your marriage that much unless your kids are a lot worse than theirs. But you get the idea.

5. Try to Spice Up Your Love Life

Sometimes a woman becomes so bored with the way her husband approaches making love that she just really isn't that interested anymore. I've heard patients complain about this frequently, and I believe that it comes after years of frustration and lack of communication. Even couples with a healthy sex life complain about this a little bit—I mean how many pairs of boxer shorts covered with hearts or skimpy silk panties does it take to reach the saturation point? This must be a common concern among couples, because every time I'm in the check-out line at the grocery store I see at least five different women's magazines with banner headlines on the cover graphically describing how to improve one's sex life. I'm embarrassed to take my kids to the grocery store anymore.

What I really want you to do here is try to add a little romance back into your love life. Leave little notes for him in his underwear drawer. Surprise him one night when he comes home from work by greeting him at the front door wearing only one of his dress shirts, with the kids away at Mom's house for the evening. Call him at work and tell him you are thinking about him. Remember those little things you did when you were dating to make him want to be with you? Even though they may *seem* silly now, most men will appreciate your thoughtfulness in doing them again. Besides, it will give you something to talk about if you're having trouble getting things started. The whole point of these suggestions is to refocus both of you on having fun together and helping you to remember the things about each other that made you fall in love in the first place.

6. Let Him Know That You Love Him

"Oh, come on, Doc! He knows that I love him—I wash his clothes, keep a clean house, cook for him, and do most of the child-raising around here." You're right, those are important things that show your love, but if you think about it, none of those are really personal *to him.* In fact most of these things are more important to *you* than they are to him. He probably wouldn't care if the house were a little less neat or if you ate out another meal or two each week if you would be more responsive physically. The point is, the things you feel show your love don't necessarily mean the same thing to him. Each of us sends and receives love differently.

If you want to make him feel loved in ways other than sex, you have to appeal to the little boy that's inside all men. Remember, "the only difference between men and boys is the price of the toys." How do you show your children you love them? I know, I know . . . you cook, and clean, etc. But, until your kids move away from home and have to do these things for themselves, they will never fully appreciate your sacrifices. No, if you want to show love to a child you encourage him, you cuddle him, you make a special effort to tell him/her, "I love you—not mumbled in passing as he or she walks by in the hallway, but you stop what you're doing and tell him or her eyeball to eyeball. Try it on your husband. Oh, he may not know how to react at first, so give him time to digest what's happened. I almost guarantee (of course, I don't ever guarantee anything to anyone these days) you will find him more likely to begin responding in a similar way, not in anticipation of sex, but because you love each other independent of your physical relationship.

129

7. Encourage Him

If you want him to help around the house more or take a more active role in the kids' lives or if you want him to just talk to you more (relate), then you must encourage him. Tell him what you want and reward him for doing it. "I shouldn't have to do that, he's a grown man!" Is he? Is he *really?* At the heart of every man is an insecure little boy who needs to be encouraged, to know that he is still your hero—your "knight in shining armor"—and that you think of him as a "big man" (even though you and I both know he's still a little boy inside). Besides, men are genetically deficient and need extra care and watering. You may still say, "It shouldn't be that way"—*but it is that way.* And the sooner you realize it and stop trying to change him to be like you, the happier you *both* will be.

Some women, when I explain all of this, think I am suggesting that women are somehow superior to men. (Well, you are, but don't tell anyone I said so! I'd have to deny it.)

18

Low Sex Drive—Solutions for Men (Yes, You!)

OK, guys. You've heard about it, and now you're going to read about it. It's time for you to learn why there's been less "heat between the sheets." These are the facts as we know them: "It's all your fault!" No, I'm just kidding. It's not necessarily your fault, but there are some things that you can do right now to improve the situation.

First, go back and read chapter 14 on how men and women view sex differently. This will give you some background information that will help you apply the "nuts and bolts" approach to improving your love life that is discussed here. I would also advise you to read chapter 11 to understand why her work and home schedules are probably a major factor in making sex a low-priority item for her. Finally, you really ought to read chapter 13 to know the real reason that you're in this predicament. It explains why it's really *not* your fault, but the facts revealed there aren't too pretty. You've been warned!

After you've read the background chapters suggested, look carefully at the five major suggestions outlined in this chapter. Let me encourage you to spend some time by yourself thinking and praying about them to see which ones pertain to you and how you might adapt the suggestions I've made to your particular situation. For you to be successful in this planning phase you'll have to take a candid look at yourself and rethink your goals and priorities for yourself, your marriage, and your family. This is no easy task, particularly since none of us is very good at predicting the future. Ask God to show you what's really important in your life. He created you and the world around you, so He knows what's best for your ultimate happiness. Ask Him to help you as you make your plans. It's possible that you might need to let go of something you think is important, so you can hang onto the things that really are important. A wise man once said, "The most important things in this life aren't things." This is an important concept to remember as you try to focus on reordering your priorities.

Before you think this another of one of those "blame it on the guys" books and you've got to do a lot of changing to fix things, you must know that I asked your wife to do the same things I've asked you to do here and much more! Low sex drive is a "couples" problem that requires a "couples" solution. You've both got to meet in the middle somewhere for things to work out right.

Enough said! Please take the time to read the background chapters I have mentioned and the following sections. Once you've done your "homework," take some time to think and pray about what you've read. Then draw up your battle plan, get your gear together, and *charge!* Good luck, Pilgrim. It may be tough at times, but the rewards of victory should be well worth the struggle. Besides, it really can't hurt to give this a try, right?

1. Stop Feeling Sorry for Yourself

Doing this one thing will probably help you more than anything else. Your wife is in a difficult predicament and needs your help—OK, all you "knights in shining armor," it's time to saddle up your trusty steeds and go slay the dragons. No, don't kill your children—you'll never get away with it! One of the grandparents would probably fink on you anyway. Instead, you need to analyze your wife's situation through her eyes and then help her by gently offering a different perspective. She's not undersexed; she's overworked! But you have to help her fix it by offering to *help her* fix it.

2. Pitch In and Help

Support her efforts to prioritize, simplify, and reorganize her schedule. Offer your time and energy to help her get her work (at least her work at home) done. Help with the chores, offer to barbecue or take her out to eat more often, make an extra effort to help with the kids, and encourage her that she's still an A-1 mom if she doesn't volunteer to be homeroom mother or Cub Scout den leader this year. This support is particularly helpful if she works outside the home, too. In that case, you need to pitch in even more. You surely don't have the excuse "I have a job." So does she. Approaching the family chores as a team encourages

132

esprit de corps, a sense of belonging and togetherness. I have never been closer to my wife than in the times we have had to struggle together to get a job done.

3. Learn to Relate to Her

I really hate this phrase, but it is so commonly used that I find myself saying it, too. It sounds so "sixty-ish" to *relate*, man. Wow! Cool! But that's what you need to do. Learn to give her a hug and say, "I love you," without any hint that sex is on your mind. Just as Garth Brooks sang, "Tell her you love her somewhere other than the night." This lets her know that you love her even though sex is out of the picture.

Call her at work (whether that's in or out of your home; remember, keeping a house and kids going is a full-time job with no readily identifiable rewards—no paycheck, no bonuses, no vacation, and no five-and ten-year service recognition awards) and tell her that you're thinking about her. Try to remember how you used to sit on the phone and talk to each other when you were dating. It's not easy to do at first and probably not a good idea to "force it," but a quick call can mean a lot to her. A word of warning—there is a right and a wrong time to call. Don't get angry when she tells you it's a bad time; just make a mental note of it and try again another day.

4. Tell Her You Appreciate Her

A little of this goes a long way, and a lot of this may help her go "all the way." Seriously, women need encouragement, particularly women who work at home. The workplace has its encouragements—a paycheck, a job title, a pension plan, employee evaluations, service awards, etc. What encouragement does she get at home? If she's like my wife, the kids thumb their noses at half the food she spends hours preparing, we leave the house a wreck four out of seven days each week, there truly is an *endless* amount of dirty laundry available at any given time, and the only recognition she gets is when the blouse my daughter wanted to wear to school today didn't get ironed. If I worked at a job like that, I would have quit a long time ago. I thank God my wife is committed to us, and I hope she won't get committed somewhere else (like the asylum) until the kids grow up. Realize what she does for you and your family and recognize her for her efforts. If you don't understand how difficult her job is, try it for a while. No, one Saturday is not enough. You have to take it on for a good week before you realize that it's a job *you do not want.*

You can also help her by organizing the older children into a work force to help get the chores done. You have to reward them with an allowance if you want them to perform effectively. This also helps teach them responsibility and the reward of working for a goal, even if it is money.

5. Romance Her

Your love life is in the toilet not only because she's overworked, but she's underromanced, too. You have to help her reorganize her schedule to allow sex to become a priority again. You can accomplish this in two ways: (1) you can help her un-hurry her schedule by pitching in and helping out to keep sex from being pushed off her "List of Things to Do Today," and (2) you can make her feel so special, important, and sexy that *she* wants to push sex *up* on the priority list. We've already talked about the first option, but the second is important, too.

Learning to talk to her, letting her know you are thinking about her, and showing her you appreciate her are all good ways of encouraging a change in her priorities regarding making love. But it is also important that you let her know that she is special to you and that you still find her attractive. Compliment her looks, the way she does her hair, a dress you find particularly attractive. Noticing these little things tells her you look at her and that you still find her comely. "You don't sweat much for a fat woman," won't cut it, fellas. Your wife is still the girl you fell in love with on the inside, no matter what's happened on the outside—don't forget; you've changed some, too, since then. She wants to know that you still find her attractive, not in a lewd sense but in the way you first looked at her—when she caught your eye the first time. If you can make her feel that special again, she will respond to you.

One final word of warning: Most women are very sensitive in this area and they can smell a fake a mile away. Faint praise may do more harm than good. Don't be patronizing or make the mistake of coming off as insincere in your complements or your strategy may well backfire.

Then you'll probably wind up in the doghouse and blame me somehow for your misfortune. Remember, be sincere and honest as you approach your wife, and everything else for that matter. It will pay off in the end.

Set time aside for just the two of you. Many couples find a "date night" very effective. Perhaps two nights a month, go out to eat or catch a movie together. You may find conversation awkward at first, but after a few dates you'll probably find more and more to talk about. Talk about your past dates, the kids, and your dreams of the future. It sounds hokey, but it really helps couples reestablish meaningful communication. As you get into it, you may want to sometimes give up one of these nights to interact with other couples, but don't do it without discussing it together first. Remember, it's not "your night" to give away—talk to her first. I also recommend setting these nights up on a regular schedule so you can keep them free from other commitments. Nothing will anger her more than for you to allow work or activities with your buddies to interfere with this special event. You would get mad if she scheduled a Tupperware party with the girls on your date night without consulting you first, right? Give it the importance it deserves by making an effort to preserve it for each other.

Schedule a weekend away—all by yourselves. It doesn't necessarily have to be a romantic location. In fact, be careful not to assume that sex is even part of the plans. Many women get put off if they think they are expected to perform. Remember, you have to allow time and opportunity for sex to "happen," not force the issue by putting pressure on her to "put out." Don't pout or get angry if it doesn't happen on the first night or even the first trip away. Give her room and time to come up with the idea herself. "Good things come to those who wait." Enlist your mother, mother-in-law, or friends to help keep the kids. Some couples trade weekends to help keep children. If you are really sporting, you can surprise her with a night away from home. Get one of her girlfriends to help plan the child care; you arrange for a hotel room and dinner or a movie (not the "adults only" movies in the hotel room!). Remember, don't expect sex, but by all means provide ample opportunities for it to happen.

Sadly, gentlemen, your wife has read all about your strategy to improve your love life. The good news is that you can learn to work together as a team to un-hurry her life and bring her energy levels back to near normal. The bad news is that if you follow my recipe like a cookbook, the Russian judge will take points off for originality, which might mean the difference between you taking home the gold versus the bronze medal.

I hope you've gained some insight into the underlying problems and how to fix them. Hint: Wait about two weeks after reading the book before you implement any of my suggestions. After about ten days with nothing changing, she'll think you haven't learned a thing. Then, right before she gives up and declares you hopelessly ignorant (or, as we say in East Texas, "ignant"), you can start to "shine." Maybe she'll think you came up with some of it on your own. I hope it works.

P.S. Please take the time to read the preceding chapters on the differences between men and woman and the suggestions I made to your wife in chapter 17. It will help you help her make your relationship better.

Of course, you might think that you don't need any help improving your love life. "This stuff is for other guys," not you. You might be right, but just remember one thing: Your wife gave you "this stuff" to read for a reason. Maybe she thinks you can improve things a bit. Either way, "if Mama ain't happy, ain't nobody happy," so it might be a good idea to take a look at it anyway. You can trust me on this one; I used to be a man . . . now I'm a gynecologist.

19

FAQS and Statements

"Can birth control pills lower my sex drive?"

They certainly can and do for about 10 to 15 percent of my patients. Most authorities think that birth control pills tend to lower the amount of testosterone in your bloodstream, which can in turn lower libido or sex drive. Pills that have a relatively lower dose of progesterone will be less likely to cause this side effect. Ask your doctor about changing pills if you have this problem. If you are still having problems after three months on the new pill, you should consider either checking your testosterone level and starting replacement if indicated, since there is no reason why you can't receive testosterone replacement while on birth control pills if you need it, or getting off birth control pills for about three months to see if the symptom goes away. If your libido doesn't improve after three months off the pill, you should definitely check your testosterone level if you did not already do so. If it's normal, you need to look for another cause of your low sex drive. I suggest reviewing the information in chapters 10 through 16 and then discussing the problem with your doctor again.

Birth control pills can actually improve sex drive for some patients, particularly those with severe PMS, endometriosis pain, or excessive fear of pregnancy. One of the main consequences of these conditions is decreased libido. Helping the other symptoms, such as painful intercourse go away, will often improve sex drive, too.

"Will taking estrogen make me gain weight?"

There are different levels of estrogen therapy. Birth control pills have estrogen and progesterone, but both are in higher dosage than those used in menopausal hormone replacement therapy (HRT). Most women will gain about five to ten pounds when they start taking birth control pills. However, this weight gain can be avoided. Recent studies indicate that the increase in weight generally comes from an increase in appetite, i.e., the "munchies." Women who watched their food intake when they began taking the pill did not gain more than five pounds, and the pill's effect on appetite went away after two months. Therefore, the weight gain from birth control pills can be anticipated and controlled by diet.

Most studies on initiation of HRT don't show any significant weight effects, because much lower doses of estrogen and progesterone are used. Now I know that many of you out there are shaking your head, saying, "I didn't gain all of this weight until I had my hysterectomy and started taking estrogen." And you're right, you've gained weight since your surgery, but so have most women you age, whether they had a hysterectomy or not. In fact, I have gained weight since your hysterectomy, too! The plain truth is, most women tend to gain a pound each year after the age of thirty. Of course, they don't actually gain one pound each birthday, but when they wake up on their fiftieth birthday, they generally weigh about twenty pounds more than they did when they went to bed on their thirtieth. In fact, most women rock along at about the same weight for several years and then suddenly gain seven pounds at age thirty-five or so and wonder what happened. That's when they usually ask me to sort it out for them. We've all heard about "the middle age spread" and, trust me, it's a real phenomenon. Fairly good scientific studies have followed groups of women through these middle years, one group with hysterectomy on estrogen replacement and another group without estrogen replacement—the weight gain is the same in both groups. As we discussed in the section on weight gain, the rules on weight control change (without your permission!) sometime after thirty, making it difficult for most women to keep the weight off as long as they continue to eat at the same level, unless they can compensate by increasing their activity levels. I know it's not fair, but the fair comes in October—this is life. You've got to deal with the realities of the situation if you want to successfully take back control of your weight.

"Does it actually hurt my husband not to have sex regularly?"
Every man in America wants me to answer "yes" to this question! For years the condition called DSBU or Dreaded Sperm Build-Up, was reported to exist and even claim the life of a poor unfortunate young man every now and then. But the answer to the question of physical harm from lack of sex is really "no." This rumor should probably be classed with the one concerning "teeth in the vagina." Every junior high

138

school boy *hopes* it isn't true but would simply like to confirm it for himself (or maybe have someone else do it for him first). Most experts agree that men have a more basic physical need for sex than women, but proof that physical harm occurs from avoiding intercourse is lacking.

Men often do become a little moody, start kicking the cat, yell at the kids, and generally pout when they haven't had enough "attention" in this area. But physical pain? I doubt it. A man who has been aroused for a prolonged period of time may experience some pelvic and even scrotal discomfort if he does not ejaculate afterward, but this is not quite the same thing.

"Is there a medication or an herb I can take to make me want to have sex?"

Another way to ask this question would be, "Are there any true aphrodisiacs?" The answer to this one is also "no." Although many chemicals, herbs, and foods have been touted off and on again as sex stimulants, nothing has yet passed double-blinded tests against a placebo. These studies require that both the researcher and the patients themselves do not know who gets the medication and who gets the placebo ("sugar pill"). This is the only way to factor out the power of suggestion from a study of this nature. Besides, if a true aphrodisiac existed, you can bet that those dirty old men in Washington, D.C., would pass legislation to have it added to the food we eat. The words *fortified* and *enriched* might take on a whole new meaning.

"Will I grow a beard if I take testosterone?"

No, not if you have your blood levels tested to be sure they are within the normal range. Of course, you may suddenly be unable to ask for directions, start scratching yourself in public, and start letting out embarrassing gaseous eruptions, but otherwise there are very few side effects.

Let me add here that I have not been overly impressed with the long-term results of testosterone supplementation in my patients complaining of low sex drive. About 30 to 40 percent of my patients with this complaint actually have a low testosterone level. I only give testosterone to patients with a documented deficiency and replace them with doses that bring them into the normal range. Most patients see some improvement initially, but after about six months a large portion of patients take themselves off the medication because they don't think it's working anymore or they are afraid that they will develop side effects.

Our current knowledge of testosterone and its role in promoting sex drive in women is still in its infancy. Hopefully, more information and better options will be forthcoming.

"What about "natural estrogen" that come from soybeans or yams? Are they safer than the synthetic estrogen pills or patches that most doctors prescribe?"

This has been a hot topic for the past several years. I approach it with patients by asking a couple of key questions:

1. Do you think estrogens are safe?

It is clear that the large amount of available scientific evidence strongly supports the use of estrogen to prevent osteoporosis and heart disease in women. Using estrogen increases the risk of developing only one cancer—cancer of the uterus—and this risk can be eliminated if progesterone is given at the same time. Based on the overwhelming majority of currently available scientific data, estrogen does not cause breast cancer. There are a few zealots who claim that estrogen does cause breast cancer, but there are also a handful of people who think that the *Apollo* moon walks were faked. So, you must answer the question for yourself. If your answer is "no," you should refuse to take any estrogen, including the estrogenlike substances found in plants (phytoestrogens). It makes sense that if you really think estrogen is bad, you shouldn't take any estrogen, whether it comes from plants or not. Right? If, however, you think the benefits of estrogen outweigh the possible risks and your answer to the question is "yes," then why not take an estrogen that has been scientifically tested and shown to be effective at preventing osteoporosis, lowering heart disease risks, and manufactured with adequate quality controls to ensure that the right amount of medicine is in each pill or patch, no more and no less?

2. Which estrogen is better?

If you agree with me that the benefits or estrogen outweigh the risks, you must now decide which estrogen is best for you. First of all, as mentioned earlier, use one that has been proven effective and safe. Second, if you think "natural is better," then which estrogen is more "natural," the one produced by your body the day before your ovaries stopped working (estradiol, branded as Estrace, Estraderm patches, and generic) or one produced by a sweet potato? You decide.

"Are there any FDA-approved estrogens that don't affect the breast tissue yet still provide protection against heart disease and osteoporosis?"

Yes, there are. Scientists are always looking for a better mouse trap as well as better estrogens. The newest type of estrogen replacements called SERMs (selective estrogen-receptor modulators) are those that selectively stimulate the different types of estrogen receptors found throughout the body. The estrogen receptors found in the bone and heart are different from those found in the breast, the lining of the uterus (endometrium), and the vagina. These "designer estrogens" seek to selectively stimulate one set of estrogen receptors while leaving the others alone. Originally, they were developed to cope with vaginal bleeding, the most common complaint of women on hormone therapy in menopause. Remember that progesterone must be given along with traditional estrogen replacements to avoid overstimulating the lining of the uterus. However, when progesterone is added, many women begin to experience vaginal bleeding. This bleeding will eventually go away in 80 to 90 percent of women, but if it stays beyond the first six months of therapy, it is a common reason why many patients want to stop taking hormones altogether. You can't really blame them—after cycling regularly for *40 years,* most women are glad to see their periods go away and don't really want to welcome them back! Evista *(raloxifene,* Eli Lilly) is a SERM that has been proven to help prevent heart disease and osteoporosis risks, but does not stimulate the lining of the uterus and therefore doesn't cause vaginal bleeding. Additionally, Evista doesn't stimulate the estrogen receptors found in breast tissue and some women feel "safer" using Evista than traditional estrogen replacements. However, Evista doesn't stop hot flushes and night sweats or help with vaginal lubrication—two very important symptom areas for women in menopause. (You knew there would be a catch, didn't you?) Women who choose Evista can use vaginal estrogen cream, usually one-half of an applicator two or three nights a week, to help with vaginal moisture and preserve vaginal elasticity for intercourse. Hot flushes and night sweats can often be controlled with

Bellergal-S tablets (*phenobarbitol*, ergotamine, and hellodomma, Sandoz) at bedtime—although many women find this medicine leaves them "hung over" in the morning—or one of the newer antidepressants which have been shown to decrease these vasomotor symptoms in post-menstrual women. I still feel that that traditional hormone replacement therapy with estrogen (and progesterone, if needed) provides the best overall benefit with the fewest complaints. However, for the woman who won't take estrogen because she thinks she's at too great a risk for breast cancer or has problems with persistent vaginal bleeding on traditional hormone therapy, a SERM may be the best answer.

"If a man says something in the forest and there's no woman there to hear him, is he still wrong?"

Probably so, but at least he won't be *told* he's wrong more than once, if at all.

"Our eighteen-month old baby still sleeps in our bed at night. It's really affecting our love life. What can we do?"

A child sleeping in your bed is a great contraceptive but a lousy aphrodisiac. The best way to prevent this situation from happening is to never start it in the first place. It's a common mistake couples make, particularly with their first baby. Having the baby with you in bed is convenient for breastfeeding, it makes Mom feel more secure that she can monitor her baby more closely during the night, and it seems to strengthen the bonding between parents and child. However, once the newness wears off (which doesn't take long by the way—about one night after the six-week post-partum visit when the doctor says that sex is OK again), having little "Missy" or "Bubba" in bed with you is a real romance killer. I've had several couples tell me that they must wait until their toddler falls fast asleep (right!) and then slip into another room to make love, always watchful that the baby might wake up. Now, how much fun can sex be under these conditions?

If you're already in this predicament, ask your pediatrician how to wrestle your life back from a two-year-old, but be ready for some restless nights until you can overthrow this dictatorship. On one level it sounds "homey" to have the baby in your bed, but it causes a lot of trouble for a marriage and it's a hard habit to break.

"Does having infertility affect your sex drive?"

It certainly can. Many couples get tired of the emotional roller coaster they experience in trying to get pregnant each month. Instead of just letting sex happen, you must time it to match ovulation. This is usually accomplished with basal body temperature charts or an ovulation predictor kit, which both require daily monitoring around the time of suspected ovulation and "forced sex" to hit the right day for pregnancy to occur. This turns making love into a home science experiment, which takes a lot of the fun and spontaneity out of conjugal relations.

In addition, each month has its own emotional cycle as well as an ovulation cycle. Ovulation occurs with a lot of artificially timed sex, which sounds good at first but loses its luster and becomes more desperate as several months go by without success. Ovulation is then followed by two weeks of hopeful anticipation (and sometimes flat out worry!), which go by slowly, along with imagined symptoms of early pregnancy or impending menstruation until either success is achieved or, more commonly, failure is announced, i.e., a period. After a few days to a week of despair, the final days before the next attempted impregnation drag by until the excitement of ovulation is predicted again and more forced sex occurs, starting the cycle all over again. The emotional ups and downs that accompany this cyclic ritual as well as the loss of sexual spontaneity that goes with it make the infertile couple a prime set up for trouble with loss of sex drive for both the woman and her man.

"Do you ever recommend divorce for your patients?"

Since I'm not a marriage counselor, I don't make recommendations like that. If a patient tells me that her husband is physically abusive or that she and her children are in immediate danger at home, I recommend that she leave and go to a safe shelter or to stay with family or friends immediately. She can then contact a lawyer and perhaps the police to sort out the details once she's safe. But thankfully, most marriages don't have this kind of trouble.

I think that divorce is all too common in America today. In fact, more than half of the marriages in this country end in divorce. To me that is a startling statistic. I think that one of the major reasons divorce has become so popular is that it has become very easy and socially acceptable to get one. When a couple hits a rough spot in their marriage (and even the most happily married couple will hit rough spots along the way) they often try counseling for a while, then perhaps a trial separation.

143

If things don't work out pretty quickly, they get divorced. One, two, three! It's that simple. Of course, it's not that simple for the kids and the rest of the family or the new families formed by remarriage, but when things are at their worst in the marriage divorce may appear to be the easiest way out.

I have often pondered why people who were so in love with each other at the beginning of a marriage are so "out of love" at the end of it. What happened? Did they "grow apart?" Did they change so dramatically through the years that they have nothing left in common? I can't solve this mystery in the short course of two paragraphs, but most of what I hear from the women (of course, I usually hear only her side of the story!) relates to a lack of agreement on priorities between husband and wife. Finally, either the man or the woman (or both) will decide that the other one is "wrong" and acting selfishly. This is when feelings get hurt, resentment and anger build, and relationships are torn down. In most instances, no matter who started it, both spouses have contributed to the problem. Major areas for mismatched priorities include raising kids, money, sex, work, friends, other family, and leisure activities.

My wife and I have four children, and we agreed a long time ago on a way to prevent divorce in our marriage—the one who files gets all the kids! You've got to really want a divorce to take on that responsibility by yourself!

"My husband says that he needs to have sex to feel 'loved,' but I don't feel that way at all. How do we handle this?"

Earlier in this part of the book, I told you that most men feel that "sex is love" or at least a necessary expression of love. However, I must admit that I have oversimplified the facts a bit. In his book *The Five Love Languages* (Northfield, 1995), Dr. Gary Chapman explains that there are five basic ways that we express love and receive love. He calls these "love languages." Each of us has a primary love language—the language that speaks love to us most effectively. Many of us also have a secondary love language, but the primary love language is our "mother tongue" and is always the way we receive love most effectively. The five love languages are:

1. Words of affirmation—verbal compliments, words of encouragement or congratulations, requests rather than ultimatums.

144

2. Quality time—a sense of togetherness, genuine conversation (relating!) listening as well as talking, sharing feelings and emotions, playing together.
3. Gifts—both giving and receiving gifts: physical gifts and money, gifts of time, attention, and yourself ("being there").
4. Acts of service—doing chores, helping each other, acts of chivalry (opening doors), keeping the kids for a night out with friends.
5. Physical touch—this includes sexual intercourse but, more important, holding hands, kissing, giving back rubs, brushing against each other in the hallway, sitting close to each other in the car or on a couch.

Dr. Chapman feels you must learn to speak your spouse's primary love language in order to make him or her feel loved. Your mate's primary love language is often different from yours and may be difficult for you to "speak" naturally, but if you don't learn how to express your love in a way that you can each understand, your attempts to communicate love to each other will be much like an American and Chinese businessman attempting to negotiate a contract without an interpreter—utter chaos and frustration.

Dr. Chapman explains in great detail how to determine your primary love language as well as that of your spouse and how to use this information to improve your marriage. I simplified his approach in my explanation about how men and women view sex differently, as well as in the chapters on ways to improve your marriage—I included recommendations that "speak" in *all* of the five love languages! That way, no matter what your spouse's primary love language, you will be able to communicate that you love him effectively. When a couple know how to communicate love in a way that provides fulfillment for both partners, the end result is a happy marriage. I highly recommend Dr. Chapman's book to couples who find themselves feeling un-loved and struggling to communicate.

"Doctor, have your recommendations for improving one's sex life worked for you at home?"
You may not know this, but male gynecologists don't have sex. Well, they do allow us to have sex twice a year, but only to have children. We certainly aren't allowed to *enjoy* it, that's for sure!

Seriously, LaNell and I struggle with many of the same problems you do. Fortunately, God gave us some insight into what was causing the trouble and how to improve things. Throughout the book, I've shared with you some of our experiences in the hope that you may benefit from our successes as well as failures. We haven't achieved perfection yet and probably never will, but we've come a long way together and look forward to steadily improving our relationship with God, each other, and those we love. Our sincere hope is that you can, too.

Part IV
Becoming an Un-Hurried Woman

20

The Beginning of the End

We've spent a lot of time together, you and I, looking at how stress and, more specifically, hurry impact the three primary symptom areas of the Hurried Woman Syndrome: fatigue, weight gain, and low sex drive. The interrelationships among these problem areas may not be apparent at first, but as you look beneath the surface you will begin to see, as I did, that they build upon one another. Let me summarize what you've read thus far and then try to show you ways to take the hurry out of your life so you can become an Un-Hurried Woman.

Hurry, particularly the chronic persistent variety—the type of stress that comes from work, kids, husband, friends, etc., and the constant strain of trying to juggle their needs and schedules—can wear you down physically, as well as lead to a chemical imbalance in your brain that looks a lot like depression but not quite as severe, called pre-depression. This chemical imbalance compounds your physical fatigue, leaves your mood much lower than expected, and cheats you and those around you out of much of the joy you've previously experienced. Lower energy levels lead to a lack of desire to participate in activities, causing you to withdraw from exercise, and consequently you gain weight. This weight gain is further compounded by your busy schedule, which leads to more meals on the run, which are anything but low-calorie, and a further withdrawal from exercise because you no longer have the time or energy to do it. Your overall lack of energy, lack of time, and gain in weight all make sex less attractive to you. Perhaps you feel less sexy because you've gained weight or you are beginning to feel unappreciated and resentful about all of the work you do that often goes unnoticed, or maybe you feel at the end of most days that you've taken what my momma used to call an old-fashioned butt whippin'; i.e., you're "just too tired to tango." Whatever the reasons, making love becomes a lower-priority item for you (it wasn't that high a priority to begin with). However, your husband's priorities have *not* changed and he sees your withdrawal from sex as a sign that you are rejecting him—that perhaps you don't love him anymore. This mismatch of desire for sex can lead to hurt feelings, guilt, and a lot of resentment for both of you.

At this point, many women begin to feel that they are failing everyone around them. They feel that they are not supporting their kids, their husband, or their friends enough, certainly not like they used to. They may begin to struggle at work, too. All of this leads to feelings of guilt and often anger, which can flare up unexpectedly and sometimes undeservedly, leading to more guilt and hurt feelings. Many women who are already down on themselves begin to suffer from an even lower self-esteem, which leads to further withdrawal, and so on and so on. This is a vicious cycle—a "death spiral"—and it is very hard to break out of without help and virtually impossible to escape without insight into its cause.

The main thrust of the first three parts of this book was to point out the symptoms of the Hurried Woman Syndrome, how these symptoms are related to one another, and how they impact your life and the lives of those around you. Now that we've described the syndrome, we should look beneath the symptoms to its cause. Stress is the common thread that links all three components of the syndrome—fatigue or pre-depression, weight gain, and loss of libido. It is important that you go through the medical work-up for any of the three components that are troubling you (each of these work-ups is described in detail in the preceding chapters) and get treatment as your doctor suggests. But even though you may feel better with your newfound insights and appropriate medication or diet, you still have not gotten help for the underlying problem—hurry. Until you relieve some of the stress in your life, you are really only treating the symptoms and not the disease itself. It's like having bacterial pneumonia and only taking cough syrup and Tylenol. These medicines will help make you feel better by easing your symptoms, but they absolutely won't cure your lung infection—only when you treat the underlying infection with antibiotics will you finally get well. In fact these "symptom relievers" will only help lessen your symptoms in the early phase of the illness. Once the bacteria get firmly entrenched in your lungs, you could very well die without the appropriate antibiotics for the underlying pneumonia. Similarly, dieting successfully, taking hormones or antidepressants to help reverse the chemical disturbances that cause pre-depression, and exercising regularly will make the woman suffering from Hurried Woman

Syndrome feel better, but they won't fix the problem in the long run. Only lessening your hurry or stress levels will result in long-term success.

I wish I could give you a cookbook approach to remove stress from your life. Believe me, if I had one I would do it. But everyone's situation is different, every woman's priorities are different, and every person has different abilities and resources available to solve the problems she faces. Because each woman's situation is unique, no one solution is right for everybody. However, there are four basic principles that will guide you as you begin to sort through your circumstances and work out a solution that fits your individual needs. I will cover each of them in the next three chapters.

21

Prioritize—Put the Big Rocks in First

Know Your Limitations

It's time for what psychiatrists call a "reality check." There is only one of you (and, at times, only a piece of you) to do all the things that you currently do. And for the moment, trying to make one person do all the things you do is killing that person, namely—you! If you are a single parent, the problem is compounded exponentially, because even if a husband is a "dud" (instead of a dad), he probably at least helps out by doing the yard, watching the kids sometimes, or carting them to a few activities each week. Single moms don't even get that kind of help. Whatever your situation, you must realize that there is simply not enough of you to get it all done at present, and the way you feel now is proof that what I am telling you is true. You are mortal flesh and blood, and even though you have worn the "Supermom" uniform proudly, it's time to admit that you—yes, you—have limitations just like the rest of us. There is a limit to the amount of attention you can give to any one project, only so much time you can devote to any one problem, and a limit to the amount of emotion you can pour into any given relationship or situation before it becomes unhealthy.

Since you are finally willing to admit that you do have limits, it's time to prioritize what's in your life so that you can get the most important things done first, because it's quite possible that—dare I say it—you may not be able to continue squeezing sixty-five minutes out of each hour, twenty-seven hours a day, 8.75 days a week, 33.33 days each month, 392 days a year! Something's gotta give, right? My advice along these lines will be best explained with a story.

A noted inspirational speaker—one of those guys that either snows you or tells you a bunch of stuff you already know but can't quite seem to accomplish in your life very effectively (in fact, your mother probably

152

already told you most of it)—once gave his audience the following demonstration. He produced a large jar and put several big rocks in the jar, stacking them to the top as tightly as he could. He asked the group if the jar was full, and they obediently said, "Yes." He then brought out some gravel and began to pour it into the jar, filling up the spaces in between the rocks. He again asked the group if the jar was full, and they again said, "Yes." He then whipped out some fine sand and poured it into the jar, apparently filling in the smaller nooks and crannies around the rocks in the jar. This time, when he asked whether or not the jar was full, the group sensed where he was going and said, "No!" He agreed and then poured about a quart of water into the jar and then asked the group if anyone could tell him the purpose of the demonstration. The gist of what the audience offered was that you can always work a little harder and do more, even when you think your time, energy, and resources are used up. His response was, "No, put the big rocks in first." Most of the stuff a motivational speaker gives you could easily have come out the south end of a bull facing north, but this one stuck with me. You have to put the big rocks in first—if you don't, once you let the gravel, sand, and water into your jar there will be no room left to add them in later. You have to make the decision about the big rocks now, before the rest of it gets dumped in.

What are your "big rocks"? What and who are the most important priorities in your life and how do you determine what they are if you don't already know? More important, how do you reorder your priorities as things change? One thing is absolutely certain about the human condition—nothing ever stays the same, at least not for very long. Our lives, our wants and needs, our interests, and the people around us are constantly changing. They sometimes change very subtly, but they change nevertheless.

It is impossible for me to tell you what your limits are and what your priorities should be—only you can make those decisions. But I would like to discuss some of the biggest problem areas that confront most women and how many of them have resolved these issues. I hope by sharing these examples I will help you find solutions you can live with.

N.b.: To my friends and patients, if you recognize yourself in one of these examples and aren't happy about it, *don't tell anyone* and they will never know it's you. If you go around telling everyone, "That's me!" it's your fault. Don't blame it on me.

Kids

I believe that children are truly a blessing from God, but they are also a challenge. The issue of how to raise children is the second most common reason couples in America fight. Although "the little dears" don't mean to do it, they add an incredible amount of hurry to your life. And in my opinion, children are the most important source of unnecessary hurry for most women. Kids wear us down to some extent, because they are "anti-adults." Sort of like matter and anti-matter—they can't exist together without an explosion. Adults and "anti-adults" (kids) just create trouble when we force them together. How are kids "anti-adults'?? Look at all of the things that we as adults would love to do and our kids hate to do: "Clean your plate," "take a nap," "stay in your room (and read a book or just hang out), and "go to bed, *early.*" Oh, the agony! You'd think that they'd been shot when you give them one of these wicked commands. They hate all these things. Adults, of course, would love to do them all, probably as often as we could get away with it! Just more proof that children are "anti-adults." (Perhaps they're actually aliens sent here to destroy the Earth!)

Let me give you some background about my family—I think it well help make the examples I give more meaningful. We have four children between the ages of seventeen and nine. My daughter is the oldest, and the three boys are ages fourteen, ten, and nine. Yes, the two youngest are close in age, actually ten months apart. That's an interesting tale in itself.

My wife and I decided to adopt our third child after about a year and a half of trying for pregnancy unsuccessfully. (Of course, since male gynecologists are only allowed to have sex twice a year, it usually does take them a lot longer to get their wives pregnant, but we were getting impatient and decided to adopt.) Well, about a month after bringing our new baby home, we found out that LaNell was pregnant! Yes, even people who know better get caught by statistics. It's really my fault; I should have known that my wife could never resist a bargain: "buy one, get one free." As you can well imagine, it was very busy around our house for a couple of years, but we survived. My wife says that the best thing about our adopted child was that I had the episiotomy—right under my wallet. Ouch!

With four children, things can get hectic around our house pretty quick. In fact, traveling in the car on vacation can be a party, let me tell

154

you. One of the worst things is trying to synchronize everyone's "pit stops." (Of course, I have to stop the car every two hours for a potty break, too. After four kids, my bladder control is not what it used to be!) But LaNell and I have noticed something very interesting through the years about the anxiety levels in our home when it comes to our children. When one of them is gone, the level of commotion drops by 50 percent. At first glance, it doesn't make sense that decreasing the number of kids by only 25 percent (one out of four munchkins) would decrease the household angst by 50 percent, but it does. And not to pick on any one of my children, it really doesn't seem to matter which one is absent; when one kid's away, the mice will play—and with a lot of less anxiety. Why? I'm not absolutely sure, but the best reason I can come up with is that the number of possible combinations for conflicts between children and their schedules drops exponentially when one of them is out of the picture. Look at the following table and see if it makes sense.

With all four kids at home (A, B, C, and D), you get the following possible combinations for conflict:

2 kids = A+B,A+C,A+D,B+C,B+D,C+D   (6 possible combinations)
3 kids = A+B+C,B+C+D   (2 possible combinations)
4 kids = A+B+C+D   (1 combination)
                    Total possible conflicts = 9

Whereas, with only three children at home (A,B, and C), you only have four possible conflict situations:

2 kids = A+B,A+C,B+C   (3 possible combinations)
3 kids = A+B+C   (1 combination)
                    Total possible conflicts = 4

If you think about it mathematically, it actually *does* make sense that having one less child around will significantly decrease the amount of conflict in your home and the accompanying noise, emotion, and anxiety that follow. But I didn't make this point to encourage you to get rid of one of your children! (Besides, someone would catch you if you "offed" one of the rugrats—although there have been times when the thought has crossed my mind. In fact, this is the main reason one of my good friends says he doesn't carrying a handgun!) Nor did I mention it to discourage you from having more children. That kind of talk could put me out of business! I give this example to show you how much

155

children complicate your life—exponentially. Don't make the mistake of underestimating the amount of hurry children add to your life and, more important, how adding only small amounts of hurry results in much higher stress levels than expected.

Children's Activities

Children choose their activities like they pick food off the cafeteria line. If left to their own devices, kids would pick out more food to eat at the cafeteria than a truck driver with a tapeworm. The blue Jell-O looks good and so does the pudding with whipped cream and a maraschino cherry on top. Oh, yes, and the salad (right!) and the chicken or chopped steak—whatever protein they decided to have *with their ketchup* that day has got to be part of a balanced meal, right? (My kids smother every meat on the planet in ketchup. In fact, there is no way that they can possibly taste the flavor of the meat with all of the ketchup they put on it. My poor daughter lost ten points on her nutrition test in the fourth grade because she thought that chicken and beef were both vegetables—members of the ketchup family, I presume. And once they get past the entrées, there are of course, the dreaded vegetables! Aaarrgg!!!! They only eat a few of these awful (healthy) things even on a good day, so they may not select too many of these. Then they scurry on to the bread and—oh, yeah—the desserts! At the end of the line, where the checkout lady with the hairnet sits, is your child with a mountain of food. You and I both know that there is no way that your child could possibly eat all of the food he or she has picked out—it would take three Jethroes from *The Beverly Hillbillies* to eat all of that grub. We also know that after a few bites, when your child's hunger begins to fade, that the food won't look nearly as enticing as it did when he or she was in line picking it out, and he or she will lose his or her appetite very quickly. It's a sure bet that the child won't want to "clean his or her plate" and absolutely won't want to *pay* for all of that food. The fact of the matter is, he or she really only wanted a taste of each of the things picked out, but the cafeteria requires that you buy a bowl or a big scoop of whatever food you want. You can't get "just a bite" of anything on the menu—it's a whole serving or none at all. Aren't your kid's activities pretty much the same as the food at the cafeteria? The food (activities) look good when you're in line (signing up to participate), but when it comes time to "clean your plate" (make all of the practices and play to the end of the season), you lose your appetite (desire to keep playing).

Like most children, mine had a big appetite for *starting* activities. They wanted to play soccer in the fall (which never really worked out for us; the games took up every Saturday for fifteen weeks and I just couldn't make sense of it with my schedule; whether it was instinct or providence, I never agreed to let my kids play soccer), basketball in the winter, and baseball in the spring. In addition to sports, my daughter wanted to take gymnastics and dancing lessons, and one or two of the boys were in Cub Scouts or Indian Guides. Then we added music lessons and church activities like Mission Awareness (Baptists have RAs [Royal Ambassadors] for the boys and GAs [Girls in Action] for—you guessed it—the girls) and choir. And when homework was added in on top of everything else, our family schedule got dreadfully busy very quickly. When you tally it all up, each child had a minimum of two practices and one or two games each week plus two nights a week of church activities plus one afternoon or evening of Scouts or dancing (depending on whether the kid had "indoor" or "outdoor" plumbing) plus a music lesson each week for the older kids, and because some thoughtful (osteocephalic!) parent thought the season might be too short for the kids to really "sink their teeth into it," the different sport seasons often overlapped for a couple of weeks. Of course, this wrinkle allowed us to have *two* sets of practices and games to juggle for a couple of weeks each year. (The "it" that they were sinking their teeth into was, of course, our schedule!) With four kids and this level of activity, it was a rare night when we were all at home together as a family. On most days, there were at least two kids away from home, usually heading in opposite directions and at conflicting times. Unfortunately, my work schedule often kept me from helping out with shuttling the children about, so this difficult task fell almost completely on my poor wife, LaNell. Now, I do realize that having four children is a self-inflicted wound to some extent and you shouldn't expect a lot of sympathy for those, but even couples with only two kids experience the same almost insane scheduling problems at times. This hurried schedule almost killed my poor wife—and our marriage. After one particularly difficult baseball season, I finally noticed how tired and grumpy my wife and I were both becoming and how our crazy schedule was affecting our marriage. At that point, I resolved to change things and LaNell agreed that something needed to be done.

After a lot of prayerful thought, we realized that, as parents, we had to set limits on the activities our children could be involved in and not leave it for them to decide. Children don't come into the world knowing what's best for them; they have to be taught. Children, particularly young children, have no concept of time or the future—they see things only in terms of "now" and particularly "right now." They don't understand the long-term consequences of their decisions. Have you ever made the mistake of telling a four-year-old that you were going to take him or her to the fair *next week?* What happened next? You most likely spent the next seven days in pure torment, counting down the days one-by-one and telling your poor child over and over again, "No, not *tomorrow.* We are going to the fair *next Tuesday.* That's six days from now."

Not only are children locked into the present; they also see themselves at the center of their universe; i.e., they are incredibly selfish. Of course, we are all selfish at times, but in their defense, they are often unaware of their selfishness, whereas most adults should be. Kids simply don't think that what they do could possibly have an impact on anyone else—they never stop to consider it. When we sit down at the dinner table and my wife and I are serving up plates of food to our four Tasmanian devils, the fourteen-year-old still asks us to "make my plate first." He really doesn't mean to be selfish; it's just that he doesn't stop to think that if he gets his plate first the other three will be hungry a little longer—the thought that he might be acting selfishly never even crosses his mind. Of note, my daughter, who is seventeen going on twenty-five, will usually defer to having her younger brothers served first, and often pitches in to help Mom get the boys served, particularly if Dad's not home yet. She is much more in-tune about the effect her actions have on others. It comes with age and experience. Once you've gotten sand in your eyes, you become a lot more careful about where you kick dirt. Put simply, children lack the maturity to understand concepts like "you reap what you sow," "pay now or pay later," and "put the big rocks in first." Because they don't have a full understanding of time and its management and since they lack a global perspective on the family, they will continue to choose what pleases them individually at the expense of everyone else. Remember, it's not that they are particularly selfish—they just haven't learned to think about others first and to look beyond today for tomorrow (much less next week, next month, or next year!) You have to be the one to teach them these concepts. They aren't born with this knowledge; it has to be learned and, once learned, it must be reenforced.

Before you allow your child to participate in any activity, you should ask three very important questions:

1. What goal or goals does the activity serve?

The conflict will usually be between (a) family versus individual goals and (b) long-term versus short-term goals. (A) Family versus individual goals: Does the activity benefit other family members or just the individual who participates? Another way of looking at this question is to assess who really "pays" for the activity, in terms of time and effort—the child involved or the other kids and parent(s) who sit on the sidelines and watch or perhaps miss other opportunities for growth or fun themselves. For most families, a day at the park or the beach is better than a day at the ballpark watching Janie play soccer. The first examples build relationships among family members and also create common memories, which are really all we have left when the kids grow up and leave home and each other. Common memories are a substantial part of the "glue" that binds family members together. (B) long-term versus short-term goals: is the activity something that will benefit your child later in life or does it simply entertain him or her today without any clear future benefit? Learning teamwork and cooperation are important goals for any child and are probably the most commonly cited reasons that children should participate in team sports and group activities. But are there other less "expensive" ways (in terms of time spent and anxiety produced) to get the same benefits now and later? It's OK to participate in an activity that is purely for entertainment, but don't be quick to pay too high a price for entertainment alone. If letting your child participate costs the family too much relative to the joy received by the individual, then I wouldn't recommend sacrificing the rest of the family's happiness to do it. Besides, doesn't participating as a family in chores and helping neighbors and extended family with their needs teach your child teamwork, responsibility, and cooperation? I think it can, if properly structured. It may sound trite, but the family is actually a "team" or an "organization," with specific roles and duties for its members. And its members must interact and cooperate with one another to achieve a goal. Children need to have chores and be expected to participate in the work of the family because it gives them a sense of belonging and self-worth. Allowances are certainly reasonable and can be used to motivate proper behavior, but a child should be expected to give back something to the family just because it's his or her family. I am not saying that individual goals should be squelched. Some of these goals can be quite important to your child's development. After all, we are not all alike and we have different talents, needs, interests, and abilities that often change as we mature or our circumstances change. But other family members should not be asked to sacrifice unreasonably for any one person to achieve their individual goals. It has to be "give-and-take." Of course, some people want you to do all the giving while they do all the taking!—but you must not let that happen, particularly with your children. Life doesn't allow any of us to always be a "taker," so teach your children how to cope with this fact by denying them occasionally. They will be happier in the long run and you might live longer, too! Learning to play a musical instrument such as the piano, guitar, or flute would clearly be a personal goal and may be very beneficial to the individual. It may provide a lifetime of entertainment for the individual as well as his or her family; it may help promote a sense of self-worth and confidence and help inspire creativity in other areas of the participant's life. As such, it represents a long-term goal. Another example of an activity with long-term goals might be a summer reading program. Improving a child's ability to read may make doing homework easier, improve writing skills and vocabulary, as well as encourage a love of reading and knowledge in general that inspires the child to reach for higher goals. This type of activity is much more likely to be useful in the future than learning how to dribble a basketball better, do a cartwheel, or pitch a tent in less than two minutes. It is important that you establish what the family's long-term goals are and the individual goals you feel are important for each of your children to achieve. Although I think your child should have more and more input into these decisions as he or she gets old enough to make logical choices, you shouldn't necessarily expect him or her to be able to see the differences in these different types of goals at first or be willing to hold out for long-term goals when short-term goals look good at first glance. You must teach your child how to do this. In fact, we all need help in this area.

2. What are the benefits versus the cost of the activity?

How much does participating in the activity cost in terms of time, money, energy, and emotion? What other opportunities did the participant and the family give up to allow participation? Economists call these opportunity costs. Who ultimately benefits from participation and how much? For example, when you compare costs and benefits, will brother Johnny's (age eleven) benefit from playing Little League baseball through June and July because he made the All-Star team compare favorably with the week-long vacation at the beach the family (Mom, Dad, and Tiny Tex, age eight) will lose because there isn't enough time left in the summer to go since sister Sue (age sixteen) starts drill team practice in late July? These are tough questions to decide sometimes, particularly if both kids think that their activity is "like so like important that like I would like *die* if I didn't like get to like do it!" Of course, nobody said being a parent wound be *like* easy; "motherhood ain't for sissies," right? Let me analyze the preceding scenario further, because it may help you sort through similar (although always somewhat different) situations confronting us as parents. Brother Johnny is a pretty good ballplayer. He's probably the fourth or fifth best hitter, and he can play shortstop and first base as well as any kid on the team. In fact, the coach says that he will probably start Johnny most of the games because he "likes him." It sure sounds like Johnny will have a good extra season if he participates, and Johnny says he wants to play. These are the benefits, and they mostly fall to Johnny. The team will benefit, too, right? (Sure, Johnny is a good ballplayer, but do you really think that he's "irreplaceable" or that the All Stars won't play their extra season if you say no to the coach? Not on your life! There's too much testosterone flowing through the coach's veins to let the season hang on some *woman's* decision. Trust me, the team will go on with or without brother Johnny's bat and glove.) Don't make your decision based on motherly pride or guilt about the hurt feelings of someone outside your family—they don't count for much in this situation. You must be the one who provides rational perspective and defends the *family's* best interests in this decision. Johnny's Little League baseball coach is most likely not going to be at your family reunion in twenty years or at your fiftieth wedding anniversary, either! What are the costs to Johnny if he chooses to play? There will be at least two practices a week and two or three games each week in June and July—that's four nights and a Saturday each week for nine weeks. There are really only about ten and one-half weeks of summer vacation these days in Texas because the legislature, in its infinite wisdom, decided several years ago that SAT scores were falling because the school year was too short. (Surely it's not because the curriculum has radically changed away from the basic "3Rs" of reading, [w]riting, and [a]rithmetic, or that a lot of the teachers who would [hush!] *fail you* for being lazy and/or stupid have long since died, quit teaching in frustration, or realized that no one really cares anyway and stopped bucking the system, or that parents and the court system don't allow good ol'-fashioned discipline [or prayer for that matter] in schools anymore. Nahhh! It couldn't be any of those things—could it?) With only ten and one half weeks available for family vacation, you've got to make a mental effort to plan long before summer comes around if you want to preserve time for a vacation. Moreover, once your children reach high school age, if they are involved with organized sports or band, drill team, cheerleading, etc., your summer will be even shorter because early practices or rehearsals usually begin a few weeks before school starts. But back to the analysis: If Johnny plays ball, he will have to stay in town nine of the ten and a half weeks of summer and commit himself to a minimum of eight to ten hours of baseball per week, which also ties up four nights per week and every Saturday. Of course, he'll have time during the day to "goof off"—called *unstructured play* by the psychology types—sleep late and play with his friends, chat on-line, torture small animals, etc., but playing on the All Stars will be a serious time commitment for brother Johnny and one that he may be seriously underestimating at the moment. (The old "your eyes are bigger than your stomach" problem rears its ugly head again). Since Johnny can't drive (except you crazy), you'll be carting him back and forth to practice and sitting in the stands for all of those games. (Have you ever wondered why you would "sit" in the "stands"? It just doesn't seem logical.) Realize that Johnny's time commitment to a great extent will also be *your* time commitment. Besides practices and games, your evening meal plans will need to be altered to accommodate baseball four nights each week. You'll have to either fix a second meal for Johnny (soups and sandwiches look good to me for brother J., but since you're "Supermom" I'm sure you'll go whole hog and fix him something like a real second meal most nights, thereby doubling your evening workload) or do what most busy moms do—eat out at the ball park or grab something fast on the way. There go your diet plans, by the way (well, maybe not, if you follow my suggestions in part 2). Certainly some or all of the rest of the family will be forced to come to most of the games to show their support and will have to fit them into their schedules, which will add a little stress here and there. These are all opportunity costs that should be factored into the decision about whether

Johnny "plays or stays," but the most important opportunity cost in this scenario is the loss of the family vacation. This one will hurt everyone involved, including Johnny. To paraphrase a popular thought, "the family that plays together stays together." God created family vacations for a reason. They let working parents get away from work, which is always helpful, but they also allow (force?) parents to interact directly with their children away from the distractions of work, friends, telephones, computer games, etc. Vacations are a great opportunity for one-on-one interactions among family members and for group interactions as a family. Many people say that they find these situations stressful, probably because they are not used to communicating with one another so directly or for so long—like being forced to sit beside someone on a waiting room couch or talk to somebody in an elevator. It's uncomfortable in the beginning, but once things get rolling, these interactions can often be quite pleasant and, more important, build better relationships. My wife and I went to Vermont one October a few years ago to see the fall foliage. (We both agreed that we had obviously "gotten older" because we thought it would be exciting to see leaves change colors!). My week at work prior to leaving town had been particularly grueling with several evenings away from home and LaNell's had also been very busy with school projects and activities. (It was the middle of football season and our daughter was on the drill team—we never knew what "busy" was until we had a sixteen-year-old daughter on the drill team. Wow! Those girls can think of more stuff to do for and to one another than I could have ever imagined. They give one another cards and presents and pictures, have surprise breakfasts and sleepovers, wrap yards with toilet paper, go to special practices, have swim parties, etc. On and on and on it goes, each girl and each mom trying to outdo the last one's kindness or clever trick. It's simply amazing.) I really think that LaNell was angry at me for being gone most of the week before we left and I was upset with her for being upset with me—a classic "no-win situation" if I ever saw one. As we drove to the airport, the conversation was a little awkward. I was afraid, as I'm sure she was, that we would have a bad time, not only because we were a little crossways with each other but also because we were going a little early in the season and the leaves might not even be turning yet. As it turned out, we drove all over the state of Vermont that weekend looking for trees turning colors and the quaint little wooden bridges that are the *sine qua non* of the "Green Mountain State." I guess we spent about six hours in the car together each day, searching for the bright red, yellow, and orange leaves that would be there in full glory about three weeks later—yes, true to form, I had scheduled us there about three weeks too early! But instead of being miserable, we had one of the best weekends together that I can remember, and by the end of the trip she was even laughing at my silly puns, instead of rolling her eyes, and sighing a lot, which is how she usually receives them when we're home "at the Russian front." That weekend together in Vermont reminds me of three important facts: (1) vacations with family encourage time together, which helps build relationships through better communication and common experiences, (b) married couples need time away from work and children to simply have fun together, which keeps the fire burning that brought them together in the first place, and (c) that I love my wife very much and even though my work and our busy family schedule tend to pull us apart, there is something between us that is very special and worth holding onto—worth fighting for. Make the effort to plan meaningful family vacations and arrange regular opportunities for "quality time" alone with your spouse. These are important to developing and sustaining a healthy primary love relationship. Returning to the example of brother Johnny's extra baseball season, the loss or serious curtailment of a family vacation in my opinion would be a critical mistake for most families. I seriously doubt that Johnny's loss from not playing on the All-Star team would be as big as the total losses incurred by the rest of the family in forgoing their vacation together. Also, this is a good time for Mom and Dad and even Johnny to take a reality check: the odds that Johnny will be a major-league baseball player are almost a million to one, so why should the entire family trash their vacation for one person to meet a short-term, individual goal? You might argue, "Team sports provide for physical conditioning, stress discipline and teach the importance of working together as a team. These are long-term goals, right?" Sure they are. Remember, I said that none of the activities most of our kids want to participate in are bad in themselves. In fact, many of them are very good things for our children to do, *but* . . . you must look at the overall situation and evaluate the cost versus the benefits to everyone involved before deciding whether or not to allow your child to participate. If baseball is the only activity Johnny will participate in all year or if you think Johnny really is good enough to play at the college or professional level someday, it might be worth sacrificing the family vacation to allow him to play ball. Under these circumstances, playing ball this summer looks more like it meets some long-term goals. But, for most kids, this All-Star season would be the dessert at the end of the cafeteria line. Their tray is already full of more food than they can eat or even want to eat, so why let them put it on their tray, and more important, why should you and the rest of the family have to pay for it? It's not an easy task to fully assess a situation for all of the costs and benefits, assign a realistic value to each one, and then total up the positives and negatives to decide whether an activity is really worth doing or not. Besides, unless you are clairvoyant and can see the future, you can't always know what's really important now and what's wasted effort, but you need to grasp hold of the idea that every benefit has a cost. Some costs are direct and easily seen, such as money for uniforms and equipment or the hours spent each week in meetings, rehearsals, practices and games—you can count these things. Other costs are indirect and much more discreet but perhaps more important to the overall health of your family, like the mental stress of juggling "just one more thing" into an already busy schedule and the extra wear and tear one more activity will have on your family and particularly your marriage.

3. Can I realistically take on this extra commitment?

Most of us don't set out to make ourselves miserable by becoming over-burdened with hurry; it creeps up on us slowly. We usually make the mistake of adding things to our schedule like we add charges to a credit card. If I'm at the mall and I see an item I want, sometimes premeditated and sometimes on impulse, I charge it. It's not very painful at this point because I can't really keep track of what I've charged (at least not for very long), and if it *seems to me* that I can afford it, I'll get it now. (I have been amazed many times when I received my credit card statement at the end of the month to see how much stuff I had charged in one month. It's obvious to me now that I can't "eyeball it" and keep track of my spending on a credit card.) I think most of us, to a varying extent, feel that as long as there's room on the card, we can buy more stuff. What we forget when we think this way is, of course, that eventually we are going to have to *pay for all the stuff we've charged.* That is the harsh reality of the situation. And to add insult to injury, we are going to have to pay a lot of interest charges if we don't pay it off quickly. Moreover, the credit card companies know our tendency to put things off, particularly painful things like paying our bills, so they set the minimum monthly payment due on the card very low. In fact, so low that it would take you around ten years or more to pay off a balance of $5,000 if you made only the minimum monthly payment and didn't charge anything else! The Hurried Woman often adds activities to her schedule in the same fashion. If there's room in her schedule and the activity appears to have merit ("Johnny wants to play and baseball is good") she'll let her child participate. And, to make matters worse, moms are perfectly willing to sacrifice themselves for their kid's benefit. So, even if she realizes its going to be a squeeze to fit it into her already busy schedule, she'll do it anyway by rationalizing with one or more of the following reasons: "he *really* wants to play"; "the season *only* lasts for ten weeks" (unless he makes the All-Stars!); "it won't be *that* bad"; or "all of her *friends* are doing it" (peer pressure, hers and yours!) But remember, just like the credit card, *you* eventually have to pay for all the activities you've let yourself get involved in, *and with interest.* Interest charges in this case are things like having extra energy at the end of the day to do something you want to do, losing your time to exercise and gaining weight, the extra stress that comes from juggling another thing into your schedule, and maybe some resentment that gets directed inappropriately, causing you to be short-tempered and lose your desire for intimacy with your husband. Unfortunately, unlike the credit card, you can't pay just the minimum monthly payment; you've got to pay all of the current charges now. This situation reminds me of the *Ed Sullivan Show.* "Why?" you ask? When I was a kid, we would always try to watch the *Ed Sullivan Show* on Sunday night. It was live TV back then, so you got to see the "bloopers"; they weren't edited out. I remember one night seeing a juggler. This guy juggled everything; juggling pins, plates, baseballs, knives—everything! At one point in his act, he started juggling two pins and had his lovely assistant (they always had a lovely assistant back then) toss him another one every few seconds. He juggled three pins, then four, and then five pins. He had a little trouble with five pins, but he kept 'em going. I mean this guy was a "jugglin' fool"! But when she (you know, "Lovely") threw him the sixth pin, he dropped them all. How embarrassing for him. She had finally found his limit, and when he went past it, he fell apart. I think this example teaches a very valuable lesson—never let a woman throw you *anything*! No, that's not it; how about, "A woman can always find a man's limitations"? Well, although that certainly is painfully true, it's not the message I wanted to put here. No, the take-away message from this story is that we all have limits, and the Hurried Woman tends to let her kids, husband, and even herself "toss her juggling pins" (take on activities) until she is struggling but making it (five pins) or falls apart (six pins). Of course, most women don't "fall apart" under the strain of their busy schedules, but they begin to struggle. Life loses its flavor. Easy things become hard. They give up their personal time for enjoyment and self-development to meet everyone's else's needs. This is not a healthy situation, and if it continues over time, it will eventually lead to symptoms—the Hurried Woman Syndrome. Therefore, it is important to take a step back and take a realistic look at your schedule as a whole and your child's schedule for that matter, before taking on any new commitments.

Putting it all together, before you let your child take on any new activity, and also when you are trying to decide whether or not to let him or her continue in an activity, you should first determine what goals are being met by participating. Second, decide whether the benefit of the activity outweighs the costs to the child and to the rest of the family. Third, take a look at your schedule as a whole and decide if you and your child can realistically fit the activity in or if something of greater value going to suffer because of the addition. If the activity passes on all three parts, you should be able to add it with little worry.

It is valuable to periodically rethink each activity you and your family are involved in to see if your goal priorities, the costs and benefits of participating, or schedule commitments have changed. If so, you will want to consider dropping activities that don't fit anymore. You (and your husband, if you're married) must establish the priorities for your family, and a very important part of that process is setting reasonable limits on your children's activities.

This is a very tough area for a lot of parents today. For any number of reasons, children's activities have left the neighborhood and become very organized, very competitive, and available in many venues virtually year-round. Children are presented with a number of opportunities for extra-curricular participation in athletics, music, gymnastics, and added educational experiences. It's probably good that kids have more opportunities for participation available to them today, but it's bad when these activities lose their primary focus—fun or mastering important skills—and become a burden to parents and children alike. It almost seems as if mass hysteria or mass hypnosis has produced a drive in our culture to participate and compete at everything we can, as long as we can, and as often as we can—often to the detriment of many families. Identifying priorities and setting goals is important for the Hurried Woman, but it's also important for parents to teach these skills to their children.

Your Activities

You should ask the same three important questions when attempting to assess the value of your own activities: (1) What goal(s) does it serve?; (2) Is the benefit greater than the cost?; and (3) Can I realistically fit it into my schedule? If the activity measures up, then you should feel free to do it, and reassess the situation periodically, maybe twice a year. However, there are a couple of key points I want to stress when assessing your activities versus those of your children.

First, let me say that you deserve to have a life also. *Really!* Don't be willing to sacrifice all of yourself for the sake of your family. It is a noble gesture, one that we should applaud—*but don't.* Think twice before you accept new responsibilities. Moms who stay home are particularly subject to abuse because they are the first people others think of when they need a room mother at school, Cub Scout leader, or volunteer for the book fair. Of course, none of these are bad things to do, but they can be bad for you, and your family, if you don't have room for the extra hurry they produce. You may feel that you need to "take your turn" at these chores, and rightfully so, but don't feel prodded into doing it by the other mothers, teacher, or children. There were several years when my wife was the room mother for at least three of our four children. Those were some very hectic times. Not only was it hard to get all the stuff needed for the parties and activities throughout the year, but she often had to run back and forth between parties because she needed to be in two places at one time. (I've never been able to swing that one, either.) I'm sure that she felt rewarded to have provided the kids with a good party, but she had several evenings of hard work getting ready. She "had to " get party favors and balloons, bake cookies and cupcakes, get party bags together, etc. Many of those evenings were not particularly "joyful" for her or for the rest of us at the Bost house, I assure you. I wonder if any of those children will remember the great cupcakes they had at their third-grade end-of-school party when they are fifty years old or if the taste of those wonderful chocolate chip cookies will resonate in the mouths and hearts of those kids when they grow up and have their first job interview or buy their first home. Perhaps on some unconscious spiritual level chocolate can transcend time and space and "bring forth life where there was none before" . . . but I doubt it. I suspect my wife, God bless her, busted her tail (and ours) for not a whole lot of gain in the long run. Now, I know what all you moms out there are thinking: *"How can he be so callous about bringing joy to a child? It's the little things that are important!"* My only challenge to you is to think back on your memories of those early school years and try to remember what you ate at your second-grade end-of-school party? I'll bet you can't. If you can remember anything about it at all, it would probably be some of the decorations or activities or an isolated event like spilling red punch on your white dress, not how good the homemade cookies were. Of course, this is only a minor example of the hurry moms heap on themselves. But the reason I bring it up is to stress that you must try to balance the amount of effort (cost) you put into an activity with the benefit to be received, and always be aware of the long-term effects of your choices. Volunteer work, whether through school, church, or Junior League or other charitable organizations, is important and certainly not "bad" in and of itself. But you have to place it in its proper perspective with the rest of your obligations—to yourself, your spouse, and your family. Remember, you have to put the big rocks in first; then you can add the gravel, sand, and water later, if you want. Don't let other people, however well intentioned, pressure you into doing things that divert you from what you need to do. Nancy Reagan said it best: "Just say 'no!' "

Earlier in this section, I explained the importance of family time to play together and, specifically, vacation. Begin to think about your family vacation for next summer—a year in advance. Think about what you want to do, how long to take off, and what it will cost. After making a few inquiries, come up with a tentative decision, but leave it on the back burner until around Christmastime. Rethink it through then; maybe even investigate your second choice with a few phone calls; perhaps discuss your plans with a friend for feedback. Then make a final decision and start to schedule it. If you don't, it may get pushed around by unexpected things that may not be so important but seem so when they get here. Decide early when you can be more objective about your choices, rather than having to look brother Johnny in the eye and say, "No baseball, *just because.*" It's easier to say, "We've had this vacation scheduled for months. I'm sorry you can't play. Maybe next year." Of course, some vacation spots require reservations long in advance, even a year ahead of time, so if you're thinking about one of those places, you'll have to move your timetable up some.

I also recommend scheduling family events, like reunions, graduation parties, etc., as soon as you can set a date and posting them on the calendar where all family members can see it. This avoids confusion later. Also, I would make a rule that no one can calendar an event except Mom and Dad. This keeps the calendar neat and allows you to decide what is important for the family and what is "fluff."

Save Time for You

You must save time for yourself. If you don't think to do it, no one else will. People are inherently selfish, and they will continue to ask you to do more and more for them, if you let them. They don't necessarily mean to harm you by their selfishness, but it harms you just the same. Men usually have a hobby—some activity that they can do apart from work or the family to help them relax. Men play golf, tennis, or softball. They go hunting or fishing, read, or write goofy books about women's problems. Whatever they choose, most men find a hobby of some kind that gives them time to themselves (or perhaps with other guys) to get away from the stresses of work and home. However, I have found through the years that most women, particularly women who work, don't have a hobby. (When I first wrote this sentence, I mistyped it "through the tears"—I might have been right the first time!) Most women won't take time away from the family for their own enjoyment. I guess they feel guilty about being so selfish as to ask for time away from the kids to do something by themselves—for entertainment! Can you imagine that? Women need time away from work and family to be by themselves and relax just as much as men do. Until you do keep time for yourself, I predict you will never be truly happy.

I recommend that you begin saving time for yourself with time for exercise. Now, I'm sure that you are thinking, *What a stupid (MAN) idea! Exercise is not relaxing!* But it can be. When I run, I have time to think, pray, and sometimes just clear my head of the things that are troubling me. I don't have to answer the phone, wear a beeper, or answer any questions. Time for exercise is my time, plus it gives me energy later and helps keep my weight down. Schedule your exercise time just like you would schedule a doctor's appointment, and be faithful. Exercise is important treatment for the Hurried Woman Syndrome.

In addition to exercise, I recommend setting aside time by yourself to think and pray. Everyone needs time to think through problems. Complicated issues are difficult to resolve with kids screaming in your ear or being constantly asked important questions like "what are we having for supper?" and "where are we going this afternoon?" (and tomorrow and the next day and the next?). It wouldn't be so bad if they would only ask a question once or if they could just remember the answer you gave them the last time they asked the same question.

On a recent road trip with our three boys, the youngest asked where were we going to eat lunch that day and LaNell answered him. Not five minutes later, the oldest boy asked about lunch and she dutifully answered him, reminding him that his brother had already asked that question. He even acknowledged that he had heard the exchange but "just forgot." Then, you guessed it, about three minutes later the middle son asked, "Where are we going for lunch?" Fortunately, this exchange struck both of his parents as funny or we might have asked him to step out of the vehicle (which was going about seventy miles per hour at the time) and check the back tire.

Kids add so much commotion and confusion to our lives that I am convinced that I have lost about ten IQ points for every child I have. That's forty IQ points I've lost thus far. When you consider where I started from, that puts me about even with the ficus tree in our entryway! I need time away from work and family to refocus, think through complicated issues, and pray for wisdom and help. And I am sure that you do also. You may have learned to juggle your schedule enough to squeeze it in here and there, or you may be trying to struggle along without it. Wherever you are now, make a commitment to reserve some quiet time each day for yourself and for prayer. Even though it may be just ten minutes, it'll help you stay focused on your priorities and goals. If you continue to try to struggle along without time for reflection and prayer, you'll be like guys stuck digging in a deep hole. All they can see is dirt. They keep digging and digging, sometimes harder and sometimes slower, they might even pick up a different tool and dig for a while, but when they stop, all they can see is more work ahead of them—more dirt. That can be very discouraging. After they've been digging for a while, they may begin to lose their bearings and veer off course, digging in the wrong direction. Remember, all they can see around them is dirt. The only way they can keep digging in the right direction—to reach their goal—is to occasionally get up out of the hole to be sure they are staying on course. Quiet time allows you to "get up out of the hole" for a few minutes and check your bearings, to stay focused on your goals. Otherwise, you might get discouraged that you haven't accomplished much from your efforts or lose your bearings and waste time digging in the wrong direction. That might cause you to miss your goal altogether. I find my prayer time to be the most meaningful time "alone." Who better to bring your problems and concerns than the one Who moved mountains, put the stars in the sky, and created us in the first place? If He can do all of these things, He can certainly help you solve your problems, whatever they are. I find that my relationship with God helps me most with keeping my priorities straight and staying focused on the "Big Picture." Once you have a handle on your priorities, you won't let the "little things" that sometimes look like "big things" throw you off target. You can keep your goals in focus.

Is There "Life after Children"?

Yes, I've heard about it! Not for me yet, of course, but others have told me about it. But I am convinced that it exists! Actually, this is a serious area of concern, because many women make raising their children their life. Virtually everything they do focuses on the kids and their happiness, activities, etc. Of course, if raising her kids has been the primary focus of a woman's life for over eighteen years, what happens when the last child leaves home? Her world collapses. Often called the Empty Nest Syndrome, it's really a form of depression. Much of what gave the woman who suffers with this problem her a sense of worth or self-esteem has been removed from her day-to-day existence. Phone calls and even frequent visits help, but these are no substitute for the constant interaction of having a child living in her home. If she has failed to maintain a close relationship with her husband (because of death or divorce, she may not even have a husband), has not established firm social contacts with other adults, or has no significant activities to occupy her emotional energy and time—like a hobby or work—when "her baby" leaves home, she has lost everything in her world that gave her a sense of purpose. This is a devastating loss. Now, I am not suggesting that you should distance yourself from your children to avoid this problem (other than a "healthy distance"—the umbilical cord won't reach more than about three feet, certainly not from Houston to Sacramento!), but I am saying that you need to spend some of your energy today investing in your relationship with your spouse and other adults, as well as developing interests other than child ranching, as my wife calls it. You may think that I'm crazy and that this couldn't possibly happen to you and I hope you're right. But I have seen it happen over and over again to women who I thought really "had it all together." And when it hits, it can bust up a marriage, cause suicide, and wreak havoc on the lives of everyone involved.

To help avoid the Empty Nest Syndrome, and because I think it is healthy for you in general, make time for your spouse. Certainly you should spend quality time together with the kids, but without them also. Have a "date night" each week if you can or at least once a month. This will help keep the fire burning in your relationship. Schedule a weekend away once in a while—I suggest at least every two or three months. Grandparents usually want to see your kids (as soon as they get the cast off from the last visit) and are a good source of baby-sitting for this kind of trip. If grandparents aren't able to keep the kids, get a friend or friends to keep your children for a weekend and you can pay them back later. It'll be a small price to pay to keep your marriage relationship healthy.

You also need to keep and nurture relationships with other adults. They may also have children, which is the main reason most of us have the circle of friends that we do—our kids are involved in the same activities, church, or school together. Nurture those adult relationships also, and not just the women but also the men if they are compatible. When the kids are gone, these friends will become very important to your emotional health. Have friends over to eat or play games (not strip poker—behave!) sometimes with the kids and sometimes without. Our Sunday school class schedules a party every other month. Sometimes we have our children with us, but most of the time we organize stuff for them to do at church, which gives the adults time to interact without all of the extra commotion kids cause. Baptists call these events "socials" instead of parties. They're afraid to let anyone know that they might be having *fun*. Heaven forbid! Actually, Baptists aren't that bad; I just like to pick on them because I am one. Fortunately, they don't have excommunication as an option for irreverent members like me.

Setting your priorities and being able to value them one against the other is probably the most difficult task any of us has to master. Most of us, even old guys like me, still have trouble keeping our priorities ordered correctly and staying focused on our goals. This is an area of my life that requires almost constant attention. Don't forget to use the most powerful tool available to you to help keep it all in line—prayer.

22

"Simplify, Simplify, Simplify"

Henry David Thoreau's words are as important now as they were when he penned them over a hundred years ago. Our lives are often unnecessarily complicated by a lot of clutter, which confounds us and adds worry and extra hurry to our lives. Most of the clutter I am referring to comes from our activities and our possessions. I'm afraid most of us make some bad choices in this area based on two faulty assumptions: (1) more [stuff] is better, and (2) always get the best. I would propose that you rethink these two assumptions, as I am trying to do, and realize that (1) more stuff is more trouble, and (2) to paraphrase Voltaire, the enemy of "good" is "better."

The First and Second General Rule of Things

I can't remember whether it was a preacher or a psychologist who said that "worry comes from fear of loss." If you've got nothing to lose in a given situation, then you don't worry about what happens. If you think about it, when there are two possible solutions to a problem and neither one costs you anything, you won't care which way it turns out. You don't lose either way. If, however, a situation has two possible outcomes and one costs you something and the other costs significantly less (or perhaps nothing at all), you'll obviously prefer the solution that costs less. And, here's the important part, if the difference in costs between the two alternatives becomes large enough to reach your own personal level of significance (it matters to you), then you will *worry* that the more costly outcome will occur. I know this is too philosophical an argument for a "potty book" (a book you frequently pick up and read while you're in the bathroom), but it's an important concept to grasp. Simply stated, the more stuff you have, the more worry comes with it. This is the First General Rule of Things.

Certainly, if there is a *First* General Rule of Things then there must also be a *Second* General Rule of Things. Otherwise, the First General Rule of Things would instead be called the General Rule of Things. There would be no need for a "second" rule if there were only one rule, right? Anyway, the Second General Rule of Things states that the more you have invested in an object, in terms of either money or emotion, the more you will worry about losing it. Once the lightbulb goes on in your head on this point, the proof to support it becomes almost ludicrous, but let me give you a couple of examples anyway.

If you had to leave your car on the side of the highway overnight because you couldn't get help to fix it until the next morning, you would be a lot more worried about your brand-new BMW than a 1989 Toyota Corolla—duh! And when it comes to people, you would be a lot more worried if your husband told you that he was leaving you and never coming back than if your yard man told you the same thing. Unless you are romantically involved with your yard man (and don't tell me if you are, because I don't want to know), the thought of your husband leaving and all that goes with it (him) would prompt a great deal more worry and stress than the notion of replacing Tiny, the yard guy. It makes sense, doesn't it? The more you value something, the more you worry about losing it.

In the earlier example, if a car is simply a means of transportation to you, then the Toyota is a "good" car. It gets you where you want to go, keeps the rain off of your head while you drive, and does an adequate job of carting the kids and your stuff around town. It would be hard to argue with the notion that the BMW is the "better" car if for no other reason than it costs more and therefore has a higher economic value. However, in terms of its function, what does the BMW do for you that the Toyota wouldn't? It might ride a little smoother, and it might make you feel more "worthy" somehow, but it is a lot more expensive and costs a lot more money and trouble to maintain (you don't take a BMW to Bubba's Garage for repairs), and the insurance and taxes are much higher, too. With the price of the vehicle (value of the item) comes more trouble (things to worry about and cost to maintain). That's what I meant when I said that the enemy of "good" is "better." A good car is simple to own because it is functional and much less bother to take care of than the "better" BMW. Furthermore, the more "better" things you have, the more total worry you have to endure. In summary, the First and

176

Second General Rule of Things can be restated as "more stuff equals more worry" and "better stuff equals more worry, too."

So, after decreasing the hurry in your life by realizing your limitations and reordering your priorities, another secret to decreasing stress is simplifying and organizing what you own. By "simplifying" I mean decreasing the quantity of things you have to deal with in your life and also reducing the amount of money and emotions you have invested, or will continue to invest, in them—particularly the things that aren't that important to you (after you have reassessed your priorities, of course). Remember, the most important things in life aren't "things." Also, organizing will free up resources that you can use elsewhere to greater advantage. This is particularly true when it comes to time.

I often find it difficult to separate simplifying from organizing in the examples I give, so I won't always attempt to make a distinction between them. What I will now attempt to do is provide suggestions to help you in several of the major problem areas that have caused unnecessary stress for my patients, friends, and family through the years. I have borrowed some of these suggestions from *Simplify Your Life* (Hyperion, 1994) by Elaine St. James, modified somewhat by my own experiences and those of other authors. Although I find some of her suggestions impractical, her book is entertaining as well as thought-provoking, and I highly recommend it for your "potty book" collection.

Problem Areas—General Stuff

Most of us hesitate to throw anything away that we perceive has some value. If it's got any life left in it, we tend to keep it. Men leave these things lying around the house until someone trips over them. Women tend to put them away somewhere—usually where their husbands can't find them! In any event, we just don't like to throw anything out that might have a use someday. The problem with this strategy, of course, is that through the course of time we accumulate a whole bunch of *stuff* that we can't possibly use and that clutters up the house, filling up all of our available storage space. Have you ever seen a house with an *empty* closet?

Some people are worse than others about keeping everything. I call them pack rats; my wife calls her Mother. (I'm sure I'll pay for that one!) They keep old magazines, broken stuff they intend to fix, someday, calendars from 1968 (it was a very good year!), any present that they've *ever* received no matter how much they hate it, etc. Elaine St. James suggests that if you haven't used something in a year, get rid of it. You can sell it, give it away, have a garage sale, donate it to the Salvation Army—whatever! Just get rid of it. You obviously don't really *need* it or you would have used it within the last twelve months. This strategy makes a lot of sense to me, and I hope you will try it out. I'm not suggesting that you sell everything and live in a tent. Surely no one expects you to part with your fluorescent picture of Elvis painted on black velvet, sometimes referred to as a "Black Velvet Elvis," or "Velvis," by connoisseurs of such fine art. If something brings you pleasure, by all means don't get rid of it. But if you can't find a good reason to use it in a whole year, I doubt owning it for the sake of simply possessing it is that important to you—let it go.

Shopping

Sit down before you go grocery shopping and plan out meals for the next week. Look at the calendar to be sure you accommodate nights when you'll be eating out or you know some of the children or Dad will not be eating with the family.

Ms. St. James recommends that after deciding on a meal plan you mark your grocery "punch list" for the items you need. She suggests that you create a master punch list of any item you might buy when you go shopping, arranged in the order in which they are laid out in the grocery store. (This little exercise obviously takes some serious effort! Can you say, "Obsessive-compulsive"? I knew you could!) Run off several copies of this list for later use. Then, when you sit down to make your shopping list each week, you can just check off the items you need on the punch list. This will help you to not forget things when you go shopping and not waste time constantly going back and forth to the store during the week.

I would also recommend that you never shop without a list and never go to the grocery store when you are hungry. When I do either of these, I come home with a lot more stuff than I'd planned on picking up—and it's usually the fattening stuff, too! I also recommend buying items in bulk if you have enough storage space and you can use up the items before they spoil. You can take advantage of volume discounts, and once you get it home, you've got a lot less to pick up each week when you go shopping. Plus, there's just something about buying a twenty-pound box of detergent or perhaps two huge boxes of Frosted Flakes slapped together with duct tape that makes you feel *grrrreat!!!*

Laundry

Wash big loads when possible to save water and detergent, and try to buy clothes that don't need ironing. Ironing clothes is a huge pain! Unfortunately, more and more designer clothes require ironing or dry cleaning, which St. James also encourages her readers to avoid.

At my house, kids seem to make a disproportionate amount of dirty clothes. When my middle son was younger, he would change clothes two or three times a day for no apparent reason. In fact, we had to make a mental note of what he was wearing at breakfast to catch him changing clothes in mid-morning and sometimes again in the afternoon. You'll have to keep reminding younger children to hang up or refold clothes that they've worn but aren't really dirty yet. This way the kids can wear them again later, until they *really do need* washing. Make bringing the dirty laundry to the laundry room one of the kids' chores, and let them all share in it by rotating the "lucky tot" on a regular basis. This will give them an appreciation of just how much dirty laundry there is each week and perhaps encourage each of them to do their part to keep it under control.

I also recommend having a policy that everyone use one towel each week. My mother used to wash bath towels every Saturday and would then issue my brother and me a new towel for the week. (Not one towel for everyone, but everyone got their own towel!) Have everyone in the house change towels on the same day so you can keep track. And if you have a swimming pool, find an out-of-the-way place to let towels air-dry for reuse. Assign each child his or her own towel for swimming so he or she can use it all week, too. Perhaps a towel hook with each child's name on it would help them cooperate.

Clean out your closet and give away clothes that don't fit, are worn out, or you just haven't worn in a year. They are cluttering up your closet, plus they might do someone else some good. Don't buy a lot of extra clothes that you will only wear rarely, and try to simplify your wardrobe. I think most women like to have some variety in what they wear, much more so than men—have you ever seen a man with a "summer" and a "winter" wallet? (And shoes! Men have five or six pairs, max. Women have as many shoes as there are stars in a summer sky. It's awesome to look at all of the shoes in my wife's closet. I counted each shoe once, and she had forty-seven shoes in there! Hmmm, that's odd. . . .) Try to get by with as little wardrobe as you need to be happy and get rid of the things you don't wear anymore.

Housework

This is another duty in which children should actively participate. Obviously, small children aren't going to be of much help at first, but as they grow up, kids can help by taking out garbage cans from bedrooms and baths, straightening up their rooms and picking up their toys, making their beds (if you're into that sort of thing), keeping pets clean, etc. I think as soon as they can hold a vacuum cleaner or power a bottle of window cleaner, kids should participate in keeping the house clean. They won't be able to do it as efficiently or as effectively as you could—after all, you are Supermom, right?—but if they can get it 80 percent clean, the other 20 percent won't take you nearly as long or stress you out as much as doing 100 percent of it by yourself.

If you can afford it and don't already have one, you might consider getting a maid to do the stuff you absolutely positively hate to deal with but can't trust the kids to accomplish. Even just a half a day each week would free you up to spend time on more important activities for the family and help make you a happier camper at the end of the work week. However, out of the other side of my mouth let me say if you can be happy with a smaller home—simplify!—perhaps you won't need a maid and can save some money in the process. You'll have to decide for yourself what's best for your situation and budget.

Television

I recommend turning your TV off. I know it sounds scary at first, but hear me out on this! At least limit the time your kids spend in front of the television. I think it saps smaller children of their creativity and makes them want a lot of things that they normally wouldn't even care about. Madison Avenue has gotten very smart about how they advertise to their target markets, and kids are a huge market. My children ask for a lot less when they watch television less—I'm convinced it's the effects of advertising.

During the school year, we generally turn the TV off when the kids get home from school. When we didn't do this, we had a lot more struggles with the kids about getting their homework done. Before we enacted this dictum, they would get home from school and go immediately to the television (by way of the kitchen of course). Then, after letting them "unwind" a little bit, we would attempt to start on homework—and with four kids, you have to start on homework *early* to get it all done. The fussing, the squawking, and even temper outbursts were really unbearable some days. That's when LaNell and I decided to change things and turn the TV off each day *before* it became an issue. It was amazing how much quieter and calmer our house became without it. Oh, sure, there were still protests. Not too many children relish doing their homework—except boys in fifth-grade health class when they're reading about *reproduction!* Once in a while LaNell and I loosen up and let them watch a show here and there, but sticking to this rule has really lowered the anxiety levels at our house where homework is concerned.

Now, before you think I'm totally against television, I'm not. Television is one of the greatest inventions of the twentieth century. It has made the world a smaller place, brought different peoples and cultures closer together, and informed us as well as entertained us. But like mineral oil, it is best taken in moderation. I definitely recommend that parents carefully screen what their children are watching and set reasonable limits on the amount of viewing time each day. Encourage your kids to read, play outside when the weather's good, and play games as a family rather than subjecting yourself and your loved ones to prolonged mass hypnosis in front of the "one-eyed monster."

Entertainment

Going to the movies used to be a big event at my house when I was a kid. We probably went four or five times each summer and maybe two or three times during the school year. I remember going to see *Mary Poppins* as a child (of course, I was still nursing) and the tickets cost $.90 each, which my mother complained was inordinately high at the time. I wonder what she thinks now when she takes her grandchildren to the movies at $6.50 apiece! If you buy popcorn and drinks, you can spend a small fortune taking your family out for a show.

We have gone more and more to trying to wait until a movie comes out on video before seeing it. Taking my family of six to the theater costs about thirty-five to forty dollars, if you don't include snacks. However, even one of the high-demand movies only costs about three dollars to rent, and you can watch it twice if you want to. (Kids really like to do this, for some unknown reason.) That's a big difference in cost. We still like to go to the movies just for the sake of getting out and some movies are just better viewed on "the big screen," but we now think twice before heading out to the show, and we usually eat dinner at home or on the way to the theater to cut down on excessive snack costs.

Meals

Most moms complain about mealtime. In fact, even the Hurried Woman who is in deep denial (and I'm not talking about a river in Egypt!) will usually admit mealtime is stressful—particularly with small children. It's difficult to find a time when the whole family can gather together consistently to break bread. Either the kids complain about eating out too much or they don't like food you cook for them. Of course, they often love something one week only to hate it the next, but to sum it up, coordinating meals for a busy family is a real hassle for most women. Here are a couple of hints I hope will make some of these common mealtime worries less stressful.

If you find that there's just not enough time to get a meal ready between getting home from work and the evening's activities, consider preparing some meals in advance. There are two good ways to do this. One, is to "cook ahead" when you see a busy week ahead of you. Perhaps on Saturday morning or Sunday afternoon cook lasagna or a casserole or bake chicken and freeze it in the appropriate freezer-proof storage bag or plastic container. Then when the tight part of the week's schedule hits, you can put the frozen main dish out to thaw when you leave for work and be able to pop it in the microwave or oven when you get back home with minimal prep time. You can then heat up a few veggies and/or bread to go with it and be ready to feed the masses with less hassle. Alternatively, you may want to occasionally prepare twice as much of a main dish as your family usually eats and freeze half of it for a meal later.

This will work just as well as the first scenario and may suit your schedule better.

I also think that you should teach your children to cook when they are old enough to learn effectively, even the boys. My mother had two boys, and she taught both of us how to cook a variety of dishes. I'm certainly no chef, but I can make most casseroles, fry chicken and beef, and prepare most breads and vegetables. (But if you know my wife personally, my children have requested that you don't tell her I said this because she'll expect me to start helping in the kitchen and they're afraid that the quality of the food at our house will drop dramatically.) Let your children help you get meals ready, particularly if they get home in the afternoon before you do. They can start things for you, which can save a lot of time and lower your stress levels, too. Admittedly, sometimes it seems that training them will be the death of one or all of you, but the time spent teaching your kids to help you in the kitchen and around the house is time well spent.

Also, don't forget to ask your husband to cook on the grill more often. At least you won't be responsible for the main dish, which will help you cope better with a busy schedule. Remember that we are trying to limit eating out, which is how many Hurried Women attempt to adjust to a hectic schedule, but it causes trouble for them because it's hard to eat out frequently and not gain weight.

Meals Out

We've already discussed the vagaries of fast food when it comes to your diet. The general rule is that any place with a drive-through window is not "diet-friendly." However, if you're going to eat there anyway, just be sure to leave room in your daily calorie count to accommodate the additional calories.

A money-saving trick one of our friends with a big family uses when they go out to eat is to order water for everyone with their meal. This saves my family about seven to nine dollars each time we eat out—remember, there are six of us. It's also healthier to drink water instead of soft drinks. Simplifying your lifestyle doesn't have to be less expensive, but it often does save money to "go simple," and lessening your money worries helps lower your stress levels overall. Also, as part of your meal planning each week plan the meals you will eat out and account for this in your budget. This will help you stay within your budget each month and also plan in advance your calories in for the day rather than being surprised, in which case you either blow your diet by overeating or have to go hungry to stay on track.

A final note about eating out at restaurants: There is no such thing as diet Mexican food. I am not making any kind of ethnic slur, but I cannot go into a Mexican restaurant without consuming my weight in chips and hot sauce and then struggle trying to find something on the menu that isn't wrapped in starch and smothered in cheese. The sad fact is that it's impossible for me to keep my weight down and eat Mexican food on a regular basis. You can keep trying if you want to, but I predict failure for your diet plans if you don't put limits on the burritos and tortillas. *Comprende?*

Stop Junk Mail

At my house, junk mail is a royal pain. We must get close to a thousand catalogs each year, and virtually all of them are unsolicited. Direct marketers share our names and addresses among each other just like hobos share a cheap bottle of wine. Actually, mail-order companies buy lists of names from credit card companies and other catalog retailers. I have to agree with Elaine St. James's recommendations to stop junk mail by getting your name off the numerous mailing lists that you are undoubtedly on. She says that you can write to: Stop the Junk Mail, PO Box 9008, Farmingdale, NY 11735-9008 and request that your name (all variations of your name that appear on mailing labels) not be sold to mailing list companies. She then recommends that if you request a catalog, ask the company to not sell your name. Last, she recommends that you sort your mail over the waste can. Unless you really feel that there's something in a particular catalog that you've been looking for, throw it away. Otherwise, old catalogs will stack up and clutter your house. I can testify personally to the importance of throwing this type of correspondence away immediately unless you have a specific need. Leaving catalogs—particularly toy catalogs—lying around encourages needless consumption and makes keeping the house clean and orderly more difficult.

I would also recommend stopping your junk e-mail, too. I recently returned to my PC after a five-day vacation to find 129 e-mail messages waiting for me! It took me well over an hour to sort through them all. More than three-fourths of the e-mail messages I receive are jokes, most of them forwarded to me by friends, who are actually friends with one another, which oftentimes causes me to receive the same joke from two or three different people. I have started telling my friends to please be a little more selective about the e-mail messages they forward to me to avoid cluttering up an hour each day sifting through a bunch of lame jokes just to get my messages.

Telephone

It used to make me angry when I called someone and got an answering machine. I hated to leave a message, often hanging up a few times until I got the hang of what to say. Now that I've learned how to leave a good message as well as use my own answering machine to screen calls, I don't mind them anymore. We use our answering machine to screen our calls, particularly during mealtime. Unfortunately, when I am on-call for my group I can't do this very well, but most nights the answering machine allows us to better use our family time together and avoid annoying interruptions.

Beepers and Cellular Phones

I remember when I first started medical school and saw the faculty members and chief residents carrying beepers on their belts, no one else had them. Back then, a beeper was a status symbol. You were important if you carried a beeper—you were "somebody." Nowadays, everyone has a beeper. Even the janitor has one! And after fifteen years of carrying one, I wish I could get rid of mine.

However, beepers can be very convenient and many moms are getting them to be more mobile but still accessible. Cellular phones allow for much of the same mobility and quick access to a "safe" phone, particularly on the highway. My only caution is to not give your cell phone or beeper number out to just anyone. Once someone has your number, he or she has quick and unfettered access to you at all times. This can become quite annoying, particularly if you occasionally want to get away from the person who has your number, usually memorized of course.

I am amazed at the number of children who now carry cell phones and beepers. My daughter carries a cell phone in her vehicle for emergencies, which I think is a good idea. However, she can only use it for emergencies and I monitor the bill each month to make sure it's not being used for chitchat. But I cannot for the life of me understand why parents would allow a teenager to use a beeper. You might think that "a beeper allows my children to go anywhere they want to go and still stay in touch." And that's precisely my argument against them. Where exactly is your kid when you page him or her and what is he or she doing? Do you know? I like the old-fashioned but effective method of "call me from Jane's [or Joe's] house when you get there," because your kids are not stupid. They know that you can verify if they are there by simply calling them back after they hang up, so they are much more likely to toe the line and be where they are supposed to be if they are required to check in once in a while. I know it's more convenient to issue them a beeper and "just page 'em when you need 'em," but who said that being an effective parent would ever be "convenient"? In fact, it's probably an oxymoron. Of course, most kids think that their parents are morons at some point in their lives. Why not an oxymoron? Mark Twain made the most revealing comment on the parent–child relationship when he wrote: "When I was 18, my father was a fool. When I was 21, I was amazed at how much the old man had learned in three years." Your kids may think you're boorish and old-fashioned, but just smile and agree with them and keep providing them with firm yet loving guidance, because they are not born knowing the right choices to make in life. You have to teach them.

Finances

This is the number-one problem area for married couples in America, and surveys show that it is the primary issue over which husband and wives argue. In fact, Jesus speaks more about money in the New Testament than any other subject, including sin, heaven, hell, teaching people about salvation, or auto repair. Money is important to people in almost every facet of their lives—often it's too important. Learning how to effectively handle your money, rather than letting your money handle you, is a very important key to being happy in life. I wish I had more space to devote to this topic, but I don't wish to digress too far. Perhaps it will be the subject of my next book, but here are a few key steps to achieving peace about your finances and harmony ("har*money*?" with your spouse when it comes to the green stuff.

1. Get out of debt

I listed this first because it is the most important single step you can take to reduce stress in your life when it comes to money. *Debt* ought to be a four-letter word for you—well, I guess it actually *is* a four-letter word already, but you know what I mean! You ought to hate going into debt and try hard to avoid it when you buy anything other than your house or perhaps a car. Paying interest to a bank or credit card vendor is basically money you have given up for the privilege of purchasing something now. Depending on the interest rate on your card, this "own it now" privilege can cost you anywhere from $15 to $25 for every $100 you charge. Instead of the familiar "20% OFF" sale, it's like having a "20% ON" sale! Sounds pretty rotten when you think about it in these terms, and the interest charges add up to a lot of money over the course of time. For example, if you carry an average balance of $500 over five years at 20 percent interest, you will have given the bank over $500 in interest payments. Was what you bought worth an extra $500 just so you could have it now instead of waiting? Besides interest charges, the monthly payment obligations can start to stack up if you have more than one credit card, and most of us have several. In fact, we often decide whether we can afford a new purchase based on whether we can meet the monthly payment rather than what the item actually costs or, more important, what the total cost of the item will be when we pay all of the interest charges, too. Most credit card companies know that we view our capacity to buy things in this fashion; that's why they schedule our monthly payments as low as they can. On average, a credit card with a big balance may take several *years* to pay off if you just send in the minimum required payment each month. You might be thinking, *If I make my monthly payments on time, then I'm okay.* That's true to a point, but look at all of the extra interest expense you've paid to do it your way. What will happen if you have an unexpected big repair bill, like replacing the air conditioner, or get sick and are not able to work, or suddenly get laid off?

Your bank account will very quickly look like the *Hindenburg* in flames. Furthermore, what about saving for retirement, your kid's college expenses, a safety net for your parents, or even early retirement for you? You cannot adequately prepare for any of these possibilities if you are floundering in debt. Jerrold Mundis in his book *How to Get out of Debt, Stay out of Debt & Live Prosperously* (Bantam Books, 1990) provides a proven system for getting out of debt. It is not a quick fix, but there is no easy way to get out of debt except through discipline and determination. However, his book offers you your best shot at fixing the problem by yourself. If you think you're in over your head, seek the help of a professional credit counselor. Many offer their services to you at no cost because they either are subsidized by the credit industry or make a margin off of the discounts they get from your creditors. Most of these services are listed in the yellow pages of your phone book under "Credit-[or Debt]-Counseling Services." They will advise you to go to a bankruptcy lawyer if you need one, but this alternative should be used as a last resort. Bankruptcies tend to hang around you like bad tuna—it takes a long time for the smell to go away.

2. Cut up all but one credit card

Some people do better with no credit cards at all, but most of us need one credit card for catalog or phone purchases and to avoid carrying around a lot of cash. Pick a card with a low interest rate, no interest penalties if you pay off this month's purchases on time, and perhaps some lagniappe for your purchases such as air miles or points toward a purchase of a new car and always pay the whole balance off each month. This is a good time to realize that nothing in this life—other than your mother-in-law's opinion—is free. To some extent, you *are* paying for the card's bonus program. However, most of the bonus you get from the credit card is predicated on the fact that the majority of people *don't* pay off their balances in a timely fashion. So if you do pay your card off each month, you are probably gaining something from the bonus schedule. However, if you let balances stay on your card for more than a month or two, then you will be paying for the bonus you ultimately receive. They're pretty smart, aren't they! Just be honest with yourself—a novel concept for many of us—and go for the lowest rate card rather than the one that pays a bonus, if you don't think you can keep it paid off each month. If you decide to use a credit card, then budget the amount you are going to charge *and pay it off* each month. Be disciplined and don't charge over the self-imposed spending limit. Put a sticky note in the front of your checkbook to keep track of your current charges. Alternatively, you can use a portion of your checkbook ledger to do this if you wish. Jot down the date, the vendor, and the amount of the charge on your sticky note, and keep a running total if you charge a lot of little things. When you hit your budgeted amount *stop using your credit card* until the statement comes and you pay it off. This system will keep you in budget and out of trouble with your credit card. I have some "high roller" friends who use their bonus-style credit card like a checking account. They run everything through their credit card, including groceries and the like, and rack up big bonus points each year. In fact, one of our good friends flew his whole family first class to Hawaii this summer on the air miles he got from his credit card bonus program. But—and it's a big but—he makes a lot of money and can afford to overcharge sometimes and even make mistakes keeping track of his charges without getting busted. Most "real people" can't afford to do that. As in most things, the KISS philosophy works best—keep it simple, sister!

3. Change your buying habits

Don't be an impulsive buyer. Only buy what you set out to get in the first place and learn to be patient before you purchase. Going to the mall looking for "nothing in particular" with no budget and room on your credit card(s) is a recipe for financial disaster. It's like going to the grocery store when you're hungry—there's no way you're going to get out of their economically. If you stumble upon something you think you need, ask yourself, *Self, do I really need this or do I just want it now? Is it worth what I'm going to have to pay to get it?* If you're not really convinced that you need it at this point, you probably don't need it. Go home and think about it. Sometimes the excitement of buying something clouds our rational thinking. If you really need it, you can pick it up the next time you go to the mall. If you do this, you'll be surprised by how many things that you would have previously thrown into the shopping card (and, ultimately, the back closet) stay at the store and off your credit card statement. Delay any major purchases for one month. This will give you time to think them through and to shop around for the best deal, should you decide to buy. You might also look into borrowing or renting the item rather than buying it, or purchasing it secondhand. This is especially true of equipment used for leisure or hobby activities. I have personally owned more exercise equipment than World Gym but rarely used any of it for more than a few weeks. Once I discovered that whatever it did was still *exercise* (you know—hot, sweaty, and no fun), I immediately stopped using it, marked it "50% Off," and declared it ready for the next garage sale. Now I know not to purchase new exercise or sports equipment without first trying out a friend's gear or consulting my psychiatrist. Osteocephaly strikes again!

4. Rethink your big ticket items

Elaine St. James recommends that you "get a smaller house, . . . drive a simple car, . . . and get rid of the damn boat." Of course, what she says makes a lot of sense if you can detach your emotions from the decision. Remember the Second General Rule of Things: the more it costs you, the more you worry about it. A simple car is less expensive to operate and maintain than a "fancy-schmancy" foreign car. A smaller house usually costs less, has lower property taxes, and has fewer things that need repair than a bigger house. Also, a smaller house has less room for stuff than a bigger house, therefore lowering your stress through the First General Rule of Things—less stuff equals less worry. Of course, that is not always the case, but it is usually. After I had been in private practice for about four years, we decided to build a house. We had two kids at the time and wanted more room. My practice was growing quickly, we had finally paid off my practice loan, and the money was really starting to come in. So, we made the mistake a lot of people make who are new to money: we spent too much of it on a huge home. I mean, it was H-U-G-E! Something like 7,200 square feet huge. It was a positively splendid, well-built home, and we really liked it, because it had been built for us from house plans that we drew up and our neighbors were very good friends. However, as you can well imagine, the monthly note that went with this big house was huge, too. We lived there very happily for about two years when we began to realize that this big, wonderful house was really a lot more house than we needed and that perhaps it sent the "wrong signal" to others about our values and what we thought was important. Yes, we were making good money and we could have afforded to stay there and wrestle it away from the bank, but at what cost? My children (we had four of them by this time) were beginning to think that Dad was flat and five-by-seven, just like my picture in the hallway. I was at work all of the time trying to pay for "the Big House" (isn't that what they call prison?) and all of the headaches that came with it—$600 monthly electric bills, property taxes of $12,000 per year (can you imagine?), eight big rooms of even bigger furniture, fancy light fixtures, and several hundred dollars each month of repairs and "improvements." Our big, lovely home was adhering to both the First and Second General Rule of Things—more stuff is more stress and better stuff is more stress, too—causing us a lot of extra worry. Eventually, God showed us that what we needed a house to be was a shelter from the weather, a secure place to keep our belongings, and enough room to live in and raise our children in reasonable comfort. We also realized that the big house that we thought would be perfect for us was really only a house and, as such, was an incredibly expensive one. So, after much prayer and a lot of soul- and goal-searching, we sold it—at a huge loss, I might add. But except for missing our old neighborhood, we have never really regretted doing it. It was the right move for us. Of course, I spent a lot of time telling you this tale to encourage you to rethink what you need in a house, and if you can downsize, a smaller home will probably provide the same shelter, security, and reasonable comfort you have now, but with a lot fewer worries. Perhaps you've been thinking about getting a bigger house or buying your first home. Just be sure to rethink it and order your priorities carefully before making the move up. Where and how you choose to live are some of the most important decisions you will have to make in this life. Recreational items like boats (I'm talking about big boats), travel trailers, and beach or lake homes are wonderful things to have if you use them enough to warrant the time and expense involved with maintaining them. Most people I know who have owned boats, fall in love with them at first. They can't wait to get through the work week and "get on the boat." They may spend three out of four weekends each month joyously "on the boat"—swabbin' the decks, blowing out the bilge pumps, and "keeping her in tiptop shape." However, after a few months to years of this activity—particularly if the first mate (Mom) and the crew (kids) don't share the captain's lust for a life at sea—the weekends spent on the boat become fewer and further between. Also, "keeping her in tiptop shape" becomes "fixing the darned boat, again." That's when, if they're smart, they finally sell it. I would propose selling the boat *now* if you're not really using it. It's costing you a lot of money, concern, and time away from home. I would also propose, for those of you who don't have a boat, don't get one unless you're absolutely sure that you and your "crew" are really going to use it. You can always charter a boat if you like to occasionally go deep-sea fishing, or perhaps you can find a fishing buddy who has a boat. You can offer to bring the food and pay for the gas each time you go fishing together. It's a whole lot cheaper than buying and maintaining a boat. The same is true for recreational vehicles (RVs). We went on a tear a few years ago and decided that we needed to take the kids camping. They were younger then and a lot less involved in their own activities, and we thought nothing could be better for them than to gain an appreciation for "the great outdoors" through spending a couple of weekends each month at the lake. Of course, we didn't want to OD (overdose) on the "outdoors" part, so we decided to buy a trailer. And being the yuppies that we are and buying wholly into the concept of "bigger is better," we bought a *big* trailer. In east Texas, we call it a "Big-Dog" trailer. It was thirty-two feet long, which is about the length of an average adult killer whale, and had a room that slid out after you were parked. This "home away from home" weighed about 9,000 pounds fully loaded (and you *know* that we fully loaded it!) and was, to say the least, a little tricky to pull with a regular Suburban—it would have been a little tricky to pull with a Humvee, too. Of course, like most of the best-laid plans of mice and men, ours also went awry and we wound up going camping in it about twice a year. About two summers ago, we took it (we lovingly called the trailer *It* or sometimes *The Thing*) camping on the Frio River, near Uvalde, Texas, with a group of friends from church. The trip out there was uneventful, although every time we took it on the road, my palms got sweaty, my respirations doubled, and my neck and shoulder muscle tone got cranked up about 80 percent higher than normal—and we were still sitting in the driveway. On the road, The Thing had a bad habit of swaying back and forth, to and fro, hither and yon. . . . Yes, Dad, I had the anti-sway bars on, the weight balanced correctly on the trailer hitch, the electric brakes hooked up, etc. The plain fact was that it was just too big for my Suburban to pull (and it was also possessed by demons, but that's another story). On the way back home from the Frio, the trip was progressing as usual (I was scared to death, but I hadn't wet my pants—yet) when an 18-wheeler decided to pass me. I was going about sixty mph and he must have been doing eighty when he went past me on my right side; it was a four-lane highway. As luck would have it, I had just run into a patch of sand on the road—where it came from is still unclear to me—when the air blast of his backwash hit us from the side. The combination of the side wind, the slippery road, and the trailer's demonic desire to kill all of us caused me, my wife, our four children, the Suburban, and It to slide back and forth across the two lanes heading east. I didn't panic and oversteer, which might have caused me to lose control of the vehicle and flipped us over (which I am sure would have pleased the Trailer Demons immensely), but I was clearly not in control of where we were going. As we were floating back and forth across the road, I thought of two things: if we made it home alive, I was going to (a) sell the trailer, and (b) throw away the pants I was wearing! We put an ad in the paper on Monday and sold it by Friday. We got back about two-thirds of the purchase price we had paid for the trailer four years earlier. Now, when we go camping once a year, we rent a much smaller trailer for about $300 a week. We use a trailer so seldom that renting, rather than buying, makes much better sense for us. Besides, when we owned a trailer, we had $15,000 tied up in an asset that was depreciating more each year than the cost of renting a similar asset, based on our level of use. OK, do the math yourself: the trailer lost about $5,000 in value over four years, or $1,250 of value was lost each year. Our cost to rent a trailer for one trip a year was only $300, so until we rented a trailer more than four times a year ($4 \times $300 = $1,200$), we would come out ahead renting a trailer rather than buying one. In addition, if we owned the trailer we would have to pay for maintenance and repairs, licenses, road use fees, insurance, and interest charges if we had bought it on credit. Also, since we didn't have a garage big enough, we had to pay about $25 each month for a place to store it. The hidden costs of owner-ship were pretty substantial. Remember this when you are trying to make a decision on buying a boat, RV, or vacation home.

5. Get in the habit of saving

A wise cowboy once said that the best way to double your money is to fold it over and put it back in your pocket. Believe me, after having invested in a few too many "dumb doctor deals" (doctors are notoriously astute businesspeople!), this is good, albeit a little too simple, advice. However, we have all been told to "learn to live within your means," but what does this statement really mean? I think it means you must learn to save some of what you make now for later and not buy things with money you don't have, which we call credit. You can't look at your paycheck and think, *This is how much money I can spend this month.* You have to condition yourself to take the total on your paycheck and first, subtract your tithe (10 percent for Baptists), then take out the amount you will set aside for savings and debt reduction—I recommend 20 to 30 percent—and then learn to live off the rest (which is 60 to 70 percent). You may think at this point that I'm crazy: "Look Doc, there's no way I can live off of sixty to seventy percent of my current paycheck." If that's true, then I propose you are currently living beyond your means and you need to cut back on spending. You must begin to look at your savings as another "bill" that must be paid each month. The good news is that this bill is paid to yourself! This is the money you will need later to pay for retirement, cover education costs for your kids, care for your parents if needed, and provide "rainy day" protection against unexpected expenses. It's easier to start this new approach to savings when you are young and haven't yet committed yourself to a lot of financial obligations. But, even if you think you're "up to your eyeballs" in debt, you can change over now. You may have to use most of the 20 to 30 percent savings for debt reduction at first, but decide right now not to take on any new debt obligations and you will, slowly but surely, pay your way out of debt. As your debt load decreases, you can then begin to shift more of the 20 to 30 percent portion of your money into savings. A credit counselor, as discussed earlier, or a financial planner, as mentioned in the next section, can help you set up a schedule to pay off your debts and begin saving now. As parents, we owe it to our children to teach them how to manage their money effectively and learn how to save for their future. Encourage your children to establish the savings habit now, so it can become a habit before they get into trouble with overspending and debt as adults. Besides, we need to be sure that they become good savers now so they can help us with our retirement if we didn't save enough!

Investments

An in-depth discussion of investment strategies to minimize stress and maximize wealth is beyond the scope of this book, but I would make a few suggestions.

1. Have a plan

Even if you think you're a "low-roller" and don't have much to plan in regards to your retirement, kid's education costs, etc., you can still benefit from the advice that an independent financial planner can give you. Many life insurance agents are also trained as certified financial planners (CFPs), but you have to remember that they were life insurance agents first, then became financial planners. They often look to life insurance first when trying to implement a financial plan because it is familiar to them and they know it will get the job done. However, it also pays them to use insurance for a financial plan because they often receive commissions from the insurance you buy. Most of these financial planners are reputable people who honestly want to help you achieve your financial goals, but I would recommend that you use a certified financial planner who is paid a fee rather than by commissions or one who is independent of an insurance company. When you call to make an appointment you can ask the planner how he or she is reimbursed for his or her services. If the planner won't tell you this information up-front, try someone else. You can find a listing of CFPs in your area on the Internet from the Certified Financial Planner Board of Standards at *www.cfp-board.org* or the Institute of Certified Financial Planners at *www.icfp.org/plannerse-arch/*. A financial planner will help you think through your short- and long-term financial goals—handling debt, planning for retirement, college expenses for your children, and other needs—then show you different options for achieving those goals and help you line out an action plan for getting there. He or she will also offer periodic reviews, usually yearly, to monitor your progress and offer advice on how you are doing and update the plan as needed. A good financial planner will earn the fees he or she charges, if you let him or her help you.

2. Use "low-maintenance" investments

Once you have defined your overall financial goals, have your financial planner help you meet those goals with investments that don't require you to do a lot of direct maintenance. For example, the investment portion of most variable life insurance policies is basically a group of mutual funds, just like a 401k retirement plan. Mutual funds are professionally managed stock portfolios, classified by the type of return expected and the amount of risk the investor wishes to bear. They are low-maintenance because a financial service professional manages the money in the fund for you. Your financial planner can give you the details of the various types of mutual funds and the mix of fund types that will best suit your investment needs. Trying to pick individual stocks to adequately diversify your portfolio and effectively manage risk and return is difficult even for seasoned market veterans. Unless you enjoy constantly monitoring the stock market and the economy in general, it will be difficult for you to manage your investments more effectively than a professional money manager. Of course, if you really enjoy watching the market and "running your own show," then go for it. Otherwise, lower your stress level about three notches by investing your money in mutual funds and letting the "pros" handle it. Similarly, don't get involved in unconventional investments that can't be easily monitored or are difficult to sell when you get nervous or tired of worrying about them. Don't invest in Cousin Lenny's reindeer farm, any unsolicited investment (you didn't call them, they contacted you), or anything sold over the phone. You might occasionally miss out on "the deal of a lifetime," but most likely you will keep your money and keep it growing steadily and safely. Most "get rich quick schemes" only work for the guy selling them to you. You are the one who usually gets left holding the proverbial "bag." Stick to investments that are tried-and true.

3. Reevaluate your plan at least annually, and stick with it!

At least once a year, you need to take some time to sit down with your trusted adviser and review the progress you've made toward reaching your financial goals. Don't be upset that in the first few years it looks as if you'll never make it. The power of savings and investing comes through the compounding of interest, which builds slowly at first and then finishes strong. If you invest or save money at 10 percent compounded interest, it will double every seven years. So if you have $5,000 invested at age thirty that is earning 10% interest, when you are sixty-five you will have over $160,000! Isn't that amazing. If you don't believe it, let me show you how it works. Remember, money doubles every seven years at 10 percent interest, so if you had $5,000 at age thirty, here's how it will grow:

Age	Amount Saved
30	$ 5,000
37	10,000
42	20,000
49	40,000
56	80,000
63	160,000

This is the amount of money you would have at age 63 from the initial $5,000 you invested without having to add any more money to it. Think how much more savings you would have if you added a little money to the initial $5,000 on a monthly or even yearly basis. Start saving now!

Work

Few topics stir a woman's emotions as much as work. Women who work outside the home are defensive about their time away from the family. Women who stay at home with their children are sensitive about not having "a career"—did some idiot say that raising kids is a hobby? When the subject of work comes up, both camps draw their swords, ready to defend their positions. Let me start out by making a couple of affirming statements—to gird my loins against attack from both sides—and then discuss work and how it affects the Hurried Woman.

First, I think women who want to stay at home and raise their children should feel free to do so. The presence of a caring parent in the home during a child's formative years is very beneficial. Often children raised this way are much more verbal (an early sign of intelligence), perform better in school, and tend to stay out of trouble better than children raised by others outside the family.

Second, I feel that women who seek a career outside the home should feel equally free to do so. Work is honorable, and women who have the skills and abilities to work should enjoy the same opportunities as men in the workplace.

Each couple, husband and wife, must decide for themselves the place work holds in each of their lives and how to balance their work goals with their family's goals. This is not an easy task. I have found through the years that most women suffer from the "grass is always greener on the other side of the fence" perception of how "the other half lives." Women who work full-time often wish they could stay home more, and women who stay at home, particularly those with small children, frequently long to get out and work with adults.

I think the best way to sort out the question of work is to answer for yourself the three questions discussed earlier in evaluating other activities: (1) what are your goals for family and career, and how will working outside the home serve these often competing goals, (2) what are the benefits and costs associated with working, and (3) how will (or does) work affect your schedule?

Women who stay at home and have symptoms of the Hurried Woman Syndrome often complain of the monotony of life at home with children and feel that they are "trapped" by their circumstances. They feel that they are "missing something" by not working. If these women can arrange for economical child care, they often feel rewarded by working part-time. Part-time work allows them to earn money, get out of the house, interact with other adults, continue in a career, and still have quality time at home with the family. I have two accountant friends who "job-share," splitting a position between the two of them. They both work about twenty to thirty hours each week and can come in to work more frequently in a pinch.

Hurried Women who work need to be honest with themselves about why they work, the importance for the family of the money they bring home, and how much they need to work, if at all. Could you be happier working less hours, perhaps part-time or in a job-sharing arrangement? Would a less stressful job make you easier to live with at home? Would you be happier working in a job that paid less but gave you more time off or more flexible working hours? If you are a single parent, you probably don't have many viable alternatives, but if work is adding a lot of extra hurry to your life and you don't need the money or feel the need to work full-time, you might have more energy and feel better about yourself if you cut back your hours. Ask yourself these questions: *Self [how else would you address yourself?], am I working so I can have a bigger home, a better car, and better "things"? Are these benefits worth the extra hurry and anxiety my current workload is causing?* My former pastor, Bob Bateman, told me that in his many years of service he never once heard anyone on his deathbed say that he wished he had spent more time at the office! What are you getting from work and what is it costing you?

These are deep, soul-searching questions that require concentrated mental effort to sort through. The right answer is not always obvious at first glance. Because of the importance to you and your family of answering these questions correctly, I strongly recommend getting away for a few days or for a few hours every day to think about these questions and pray for help in answering them.

23

Get Organized Now

Now that you've reset your priorities and simplified what you can, it's time to get organized. Because of time constraints, I will only mention the major areas that most women want help with. Once you get started organizing, you may see other areas where you can improve. Feel free to experiment.

Schedules

Get a family calendar and post it where everyone can look at it, but only Mom and Dad can write on it. Everything the family needs to concern itself with should be on the calendar. As soon as the date for a major event such as vacation, trip, school event, recital, rehearsal, etc. is announced, it should be placed on the calendar. This will allow scheduling conflicts to be discovered as early as possible and avoid confusion about commitments.

My wife told me this last summer there were several day trips and activities that she wanted to do with the kids, but before she knew it, summer was gone. She had made a priority list in her head for summer activities but didn't write it down and schedule them. If she had put them on the calendar, she would have probably done most, if not all, of them, because once something is on the calendar, she schedules other activities around it. As it was, on any given day one or two of the kids would have found something else they wanted to do or be away from home spending the night at a friend's house, etc., which made it hard to place any substantial activity—overnight trip, afternoon drive out of town to look at wildflowers, shopping trip to Houston—into the schedule at the last minute. When it comes to scheduling family activities, you have to put the big rocks in first or the sand and gravel will fill up your jar instead. Keep an accurate calendar of events for the family, and schedule things as soon as possible.

Assign Chores and Responsibilities

Make out a written list or schedule of each child's duties and responsibilities and post it on the refrigerator, where it will be seen frequently. Sit down with each child and review what his or her duties are and what you expect from him or her each day. Discuss what you consider to be good and bad performance and how you are going to reward each. I recommend a set allowance each week for good performance and withholding some or all of the allowance for poor performance. People need incentives to modify behavior, and your children are no exception. Give each child an allowance that is appropriate for his/her age and spending needs and pay them on time. That's what you expect from your employer, right?

Anticipate that you will have to frequently remind your children to do their chores. This is one feature of parenting that drives both me and my wife crazy. Why should we have to continually stay on the kids to do their work? My poor wife often gets frustrated because she has to constantly stay on the kids to do their chores. Of course, she's with them most of the time, so this duty falls on her—and so does the chore if she fails to get the kids to do it. But, after constantly reminding one of our little cherubs to do something I have heard her often say in frustration, "It's easier to just do it myself!" I understand how she feels. We get tired of reminding kids over and over again to do what we've asked them to do. But if you don't force kids to follow through and do their work, they will never learn to do it. In our shortsightedness, we sometimes take what appears to be the easy way out and do the chore for them. But, if we take the long view instead and call them back one more time and make them do the job right, this process will help them: (1) establish a work standard for them to follow ("the job isn't done until it's done right,") (2) learn how to manage their time ("don't do tomorrow what you can do today,") and (3) realize that there are consequences for their actions or lack of action ("you reap what you sow"). The problem most of us have as parents is that we get tired of their childishness at times and we give up or rather give in to it. This is where persistence pays off. Motherhood ain't for sissies, right? You've got to be consistent, even when you're tired—"I want it done right and done right now!" There also needs to be a penalty for not doing chores in a timely fashion. Otherwise, your children will think doing things right and being on-time aren't that important.

Before you give up and diagnose them as having terminal Osteocephaly, remember that they are immature; that's why they're called children. They are going to be forgetful, preoccupied with their own concerns, and have a short- rather than long-term focus in their decision making. Hopefully, after a few weeks of constant beating . . . I mean gentle reinforcement . . . they will begin to perform with less prompting. *Hopefully!*

Children's Activities

Set reasonable limits on children's activities, because they won't—they don't know how to do this by themselves. You must help them learn how to do this effectively. Of course, if they see you running around from place to place with your hair on fire all the time, they'll think that being frazzled is normal and seek to be just like you when they grow up. Chances are they'll be successful at it, too—and just as tired and miserable as you are.

At the start of every school year and every new sport season, my children wanted to sign up for almost every activity available to them. They started out each new activity with great enthusiasm, particularly when it came to picking out a new uniform or updating their equipment, e.g., spending money. But by about the third week of the new endeavor, their initial enthusiasm had waned and they soon began searching for any excuse not to go.

"My stomach hurts."
"My hat gives me a headache."
"Some ugly kid is always drinking from my water bottle."
"My uniform makes me look fat."
"I don't like [you can insert anything you can think of here; they did!]"

It didn't matter what the sport or activity; my kids usually wanted out within a few weeks. But, of course, in the finest traditions of parenting, we never quit anything. We didn't want our children to become "quitters", right? What a terrible lesson to teach them! So, we plodded along dutifully, week by week, season to (overlapping) season, with our kids "bellerin'" (a southern expression for complaining; I know it's a colloquialism, but no other word quite expresses the persistent, gut-wrenching, bitter whining that I wish to describe here) all the way.

In the middle of one particularly bad baseball season, I finally recognized this pattern of behavior and vowed to change it. After considerable prayer and many long discussions with my wife during that summer—although she had "come close to the edge" a few times that baseball season, she was not a believer at first (denial is one of the classic defense mechanisms of the Hurried Woman)—she agreed to give my plan a try *only one* extra-curricular activity per child, per year. I know it sounds harsh, but our family was quite seriously falling apart and we knew we had to do something to slow everyone down, particularly Mom.

Just before school started that August, I assembled the troops for a family briefing. I announced that their mother and I had discussed things and we thought that the best thing for our family would be to limit each kid to one sport or other activity outside school each year. They were initially in shock; then they began to bellyache. Thankfully, there was a lot less wailing and gnashing of teeth than I expected—it actually only lasted for about twenty-four hours! After that, whenever it was time to sign up for a previously chosen but now forbidden sport, the kids would ask again if they could play, just to be sure Dad hadn't changed his mind, and that would be the end of it. I obviously didn't want to damage their little lives by taking something away from them that gave them pleasure, but the reality was, and still is, that the main reason they wanted to play most sports was simply for "a taste"—what we used to get as kids by playing in the neighborhood with our friends after school and on weekends—certainly not a whole bowlful! They had little desire to make a serious commitment to regular practices and games that would cut into their time off away from school. They really didn't want to play the sport; they just didn't want to let *the opportunity to play* get past them. Let's face it; no one likes to burn bridges or close doors by saying no to something. It's against our human nature. It makes us uncomfortable. We always seek to keep opportunities available, not turn them away. But one of the most important skills we all have to learn in life is to let *unimportant* opportunities go by and to not look back. To do this effectively, we have to use a decision-making process like the one described in chapter 21 on setting priorities. We have to learn to ask ourselves those three little questions before we say yes to anything: (1) what are the goals?, (2) what are the benefits versus the costs?, and (3) do I really have time to do this right? If any of your answers don't make sense to you, then say no instead.

Why have children's sports become so organized and competitive anyway? When I was a kid, we used to ride our dinosaurs to the school ballfield or to a neighborhood vacant lot and play baseball, football, tag, kickball, and, believe it or not, croquet! The only organized sport back then was Little League baseball, and only the kids who were any good got to play. I tried it, of course. I managed to maintain the warmest seat on the bench for two seasons, until it was painfully obvious to everyone that I was not going to play major-league ball either. So I retired to the neighborhood league. However, sandlot baseball was a lot more fun for me, because there weren't enough guys on our street for them to play without me, so I always got to start. I played every inning, and sometimes I even got to pitch!

Today's Little League baseball and other sports, for that matter, have become even more organized than they were when I was a kid. Current estimates put the number of American youth participating in various organized sports at 40 million. That's about 15 percent of the entire U.S. population, men women, and children! With the average sport requiring eight to ten hours of total practice and playing time each week, that equals about 400 million hours our kids cumulatively spend playing organized sports each week. (I wonder if this might be part of the reason why SAT scores keep going down?) I know that there are benefits to be gained by participating in organized sports, but when do kids have time to be kids? I personally feel that unstructured play can be good. It forces a child to use his or her imagination. My kids had more fun playing in a load of sand we had dumped in our backyard the other day than they ever had on a ballfield. Before we enacted the "one-sport rule" at our house, we would routinely spend four nights a week and part of Saturday away from home at somebody's game or practice. On the rare nights when we didn't have a game or practice, we were lethargic—exhausted from the week's activities. Now, when my kids are in the much longer "off-season" they actually have fun at home, playing games with one another, having friends over, or even reading a book. Imagine that! And, needless to say, Mom and Dad are a lot less tired than they used to be and a lot more fun to be around. It shocked my wife all right, but Dad finally did have a good idea! The one-sport rule really worked for my family. Perhaps your kids really are the best ones on their many teams and maybe they really do enjoy playing the sports they've chosen. And, who knows, maybe they can land a college scholarship or even play professionally if they (and you) work hard enough. This is a subliminal dream shared by many parents who push their kids into organized sports, often at the child's insistence. However, the sobering fact is that according to the National Center for Educational Statistics, fewer than 1 percent of the kids participating in organized sports today will qualify for any sort of college athletic scholarship—less than 1 percent. That's not fewer than 1 percent of children your kid's age; that's fewer than 1 percent of *all* the kids in your Little League program, age six through high school. Time for a reality check, Mom and Dad. The odds are overwhelmingly stacked against little Johnny starting for the Astros someday or even playing for your local college. So what are the *real* benefits of Johnny's baseball and what are the costs to you and your family? Think about it.

Now, don't throw this book down in disgust and tell all you friends "that jerk Brent Bost says that organized sports are a waste of time and we shouldn't allow our kids to play!" That's not what I said. I think that participation in organized sports is exactly what some kids need to feel a sense of belonging, learn teamwork, and find discipline. I simply want you to take a long hard look at what sports and the other activities that your kids want to participate in cost you in terms of scheduling hassles, time away from home, and lost opportunities for other activities that might be important to you and your family as a whole. What does all of the hurry do to your energy levels, weight loss efforts, exercise program, and sex drive? Be sure the benefits of the activity outweigh the costs when you evaluate it in the long run—"the Big Picture."

If you think that your children's activities are having a major negative influence on you or your family, you may want to enact the "one-sport rule" at your house, too. At least try it one year and see if it helps. If you keep your kids out of basketball or baseball or soccer *for just one season,* what real harm will it do to their chances for Olympic Gold? The answer is, "None!" But it just might save your marriage. The other thing to remember is that about three-in-four "kiddie athletes" drop out of organized sports by the age of thirteen. Is it "burn-out" or do they find that the pressure to compete at the higher levels of play takes the fun out of the game? I'm not really sure which it is, but in any case, all of your current struggles to get sister Sue to soccer practices, games, and a week-long camp in the summer are 75 percent likely to wind up not for much. Remember, fewer than 1 percent of all participants in today's organized sports will receive any type of financial aid for college and far less will achieve professional status in a sport. Don't try to "live the dream" and wake up in a nightmare instead. Think it through.

Discipline

There's nothing harder than being a parent to your parents. The role reversal that many adult children experience when their parents get older is frustrating for both the adult child and the parents. It's probably felt hardest emotionally by the parent who must now look to his or her son or daughter as care-giver, counselor, and even provider in some cases. But it's also very difficult for the child, because, in addition to raising her own children, must now "raise" parent as well. This situation can be very stressful for the child caught in between two generations and responsible for both of them. Since this role reversal is so difficult for everyone involved, I would suggest not starting it now while your child is still in grade school or perhaps even in diapers!

If your child decides where he or she will sleep (like *your* bed), the child is in control of your life. If your seven-year-old decides when and what she will eat, then she is "large and in charge" and you are "small and not at all in charge." If your four-year-old son can throw a temper tantrum in the grocery store in order to get a toy and you crater and give in, then you should also give him a cigar and offer him your congratulations—he just became a new father and you're his "first-born child." Pretty harsh words, huh? But in a way, they're true. If you let your strong-willed child run the show at your house, he or she has in essence become your parent and you have become his or her child. Admittedly, this role reversal is quite common later in life, but your child's decision-making abilities will improve with time, particularly if you provide a good example to follow now. In addition, a strong-willed child, if left "in charge," becomes a strong-willed teenager with a whole new set of troubles, many of which are a lot more serious. Noted child psychologist Dr. James Dobson has written several wonderful books on how to discipline children lovingly and effectively. I highly recommend starting with the first book in the series, *The Strong-Willed Child: Birth Through Adolescence* (Tyndale House, 1983) and reading more from there as you need. He

206

takes a very practical approach to childhood discipline and give lots of useful recommendations and anecdotes to guide you through the process.

Sit down, first with your husband and then with the kids, to set rules in trouble areas such as television, shared toys (like video games), homework, bedtime, cars and curfews for older kids, chores, and allowances. Enforce the rules persistently and as a unified parental team. *Never argue with each other on this issue in front of the kids.* Retire to a quiet place, just the two of you, then squash him like a bug! No, no . . . I mean listen to his opinions, thank him for his time, and then agree to do it *your* way. Seriously though, dads can often be stricter than moms in a lot of areas. Use this fact to your collective advantage. Never undermine your husband's parental authority by openly showing disrespect for his decisions in front of the children. Just as important, he must show you the same respect. One thing that'll make your job easier is that the younger kids will fink on the older ones if they break the rules. Thank God for little brothers and sisters! I think He must have created them for this purpose.

Remember that raising the kids is the second most common area for husbands and wives to argue over. Consistency is the most important part of any successful approach to discipline. Get together with your husband (if you have one), set some common goals, and approach the problem *as a team.* It works!

Monitor the Process

Nothing in life stays the same. Things are changing constantly. Sometimes for the better and sometimes for the worse, but always different. In fact, the only thing that's consistent in this life is inconsistency! Unfortunately, no matter how well you've mapped out your strategy to solve the problems that bring hurry into your life, you are aiming at a moving target. What worked well for you last year or even last month may no longer do the trick. You must constantly reevaluate your limitations, rethink your goals, reorder your priorities, and attempt to simplify and organize your life based on those evaluations. It will be an ongoing process and one that you should continue to seek perfection in but will probably never attain, at least not for long. Since you are limited in your ability to see the future, you can't fully assess the true cost-to-benefit ratio in any given circumstance to decide what's best for you and your family. It's impossible for you to know everything needed to always come up with the right decision. That's one of the big reasons I recommend getting help from a higher source.

Prayer but, more important, a real one-to-one relationship with God is the key to answering the tough questions that plague each of us daily. Not only in the areas we've discussed in this book, but in every facet of your life. God knows you because He created you. That's why He understands you, the *real* you—the part you don't necessarily want other people to see—and also what troubles you. God has the vision you need to help you see your goals and priorities more clearly. He can give you the willpower to help you "gut up" and get the job done no matter how big the task may seem. Let's face it; He created heaven and earth, moved mountains, and parted the sea. . . . Now what were you concerned about again? Don't worry. God can fix your problems, too.

The Bible tells us that if we search for God we will find Him (Jeremiah 29:13). You can start by reading the Bible—I recommend buying or borrowing a newer translation and starting with the Book of Romans in the New Testament—or question a Christian friend about his or her relationship with God. Ask your friend to have his or her pastor or priest set up a brief visit or even just a phone call if you're shy. Don't put this off. Make it a priority and call tomorrow.

If you were to do only one thing that I've recommended in this book—which would be a terrible waste of time, effort, and money by the way, but if you choose to follow only one suggestion that I've made thus far—follow this one. *Make the call!* If you find God, all the rest of your worries will fall into place. Trust me on this one. But, more important, learn to trust Him.

Appendixes

Appendix A
Attitude & Mood Self-Assessment Quiz

Instructions

Here are twenty statements regarding your mood and attitudes

1. On a separate sheet of paper, number 1 through 20 down the left margin.
2. Please read each statement carefully and answer each question on your answer sheet in the way that best describes how frequently you have felt this way *during the past month.*

Answers A: Much or most of the time
           B: Often, but not a lot
           C: Occasionally
           D: Little or very rarely

3. Try to answer the questions honestly and don't look ahead to the scoring until after you've answered all of the questions. If you are currently on a diet, answer questions 6 and 16 as you would have *before* the diet.

1. I feel sad or "blue."
2. I still find joy in the things I do.
3. I cry (or feel like crying) more than I used to.
4. I get a good night's sleep.
5. I feel useful.
6. I eat as much as I always have.
7. I can make decisions easily.
8. I feel that some people would be better off if I were gone.
9. I feel good about the future.

10. I feel restless and need to keep moving.
11. I feel lonely or like to be alone.
12. I get tired for no reason.
13. I can think clearly.
14. Mornings are my best time of day.
15. I don't feel good.
16. I've been losing (gaining) weight.
17. I am happy with my sex life.
18. I find it easy to do things.
19. I look forward to a challenge.
20. I just don't want to get out of bed.

Attitude & Mood Self-Assessment Quiz — Scoring

Points for Answers

Question	A	B	C	D
1.	5	4	2	1
2.	1	2	3	5
3.	4	3	2	1
4.	1	2	3	5
5.	1	2	3	4
6.	1	2	3	4
7.	1	2	3	4
8.	7	5	3	1
9.	1	2	3	4
10.	4	3	2	1
11.	4	3	2	1
12.	5	4	2	1
13.	1	2	3	4
14.	1	2	3	4
15.	5	4	2	1
16.	5	4	2	1
17.	1	2	4	5
18.	1	2	3	4
19.	1	2	3	4
20.	6	5	2	1

Total score = _____

213

Take your total score from the self-assessment quiz and compare it with the following scale:

Score	Attitude/Mood Assessment
Below 45	Within normal range or early pre-depression
45–55	Suspect pre-depression or mild depression
56–65	Suspect moderate to remarkable depression
Above 65*	Significant depression likely

If your score fell between 45 and 65, you should consult your doctor, as medications will most likely be helpful in getting you back to "feeling yourself" again. At least discuss your symptoms with a physician to find out what treatments, if any, are best for you. If you scored anywhere between 20 and 65, you will still most likely benefit from reading this book, because the recommendations given here will help lower the stresses in your life that are making you feel less than 100 percent. And remember, although antidepressants are very helpful in reversing the ill-effects that stress has on your brain chemistry they still won't get rid of the stress that threw your chemicals out-of-balance in the first place. Only removing the stress can do that.

---

*If you scored above 65, you need to seek help from your physician right away!

214

Appendix B
Body Mass Index (BMI) and "Ideal" Body Weight Ranges

Body Mass Index—a standard index number that takes into account both height and weight in determining the amount of body fat. The federal government, in addition to putting its fingers into everything from your wallet to your rear end, has decided to issue guidelines on weight. If your BMI is:

less than 25—you're at a normal weight for your height
25 to 29—you're considered "overweight"
30 to 39—you're classified as "obese"
more than 39—you are considered "extremely obese"

Much information will be coming out in the next few years relating BMI to risks for certain diseases, particularly heart disease, diabetes, high blood pressure, stroke, and perhaps certain cancers. Of course, insurance companies will also start to rate insurance premiums based on a person's BMI, but they already do this to some extent with "ideal" weight tables (which, as we all know, are anything but "ideal"!).

You will find the BMI for your height in the "normal," "overweight," and "obese" ranges in the following table. First, find your height on the left side of the table. Then move along the row for your height until you find your weight, or the number closest to it. Now go up the column in which your weight number appears and read your BMI at the top of the column.

If your weight is beyond the numbers at the far right of the table, you're in the "extremely obese" area of the table and we need to get you back on the table quickly to reduce your risks of heart disease and diabetes, as well as other health problems. For those of you who prefer the old-fashioned "ideal" weight ranges, they're on the page after the BMI chart.

BODY MASS INDEX

BMI	NORMAL						OVERWEIGHT					OBESE									
	19	20	21	22	23	24	25	26	27	28	29	30	31	32	33	34	35	36	37	38	39
Height											Weight (in pounds)										
4'10"	91	96	100	105	110	115	119	124	129	134	138	143	148	153	158	162	167	172	177	181	186
4'11"	94	99	104	109	114	119	124	128	133	138	143	148	153	158	163	168	173	178	183	188	193
5'	97	102	107	112	118	123	128	133	138	143	148	153	158	163	169	173	179	184	189	194	199
5'1"	100	106	111	116	122	127	132	137	143	148	153	158	164	169	174	180	185	190	195	201	206
5'2"	104	109	115	120	126	131	136	142	147	153	158	164	169	175	180	186	191	196	202	207	213
5'3"	107	113	118	124	130	135	141	146	152	158	163	169	175	180	186	191	197	203	208	214	220
5'4"	110	116	122	128	134	140	145	151	157	163	169	174	180	186	192	197	204	209	215	221	227
5'5"	114	120	126	132	138	144	150	156	162	168	174	180	186	192	198	204	210	216	222	228	234
5'6"	118	124	130	136	142	148	155	161	167	173	179	186	192	198	204	210	216	223	229	235	241
5'7"	121	127	134	140	146	153	159	166	172	178	185	191	198	204	210	216	223	230	236	242	249
5'8"	125	131	138	144	151	158	164	171	177	184	190	197	203	210	217	223	230	236	243	249	256
5'9"	128	135	142	149	155	162	169	176	182	189	196	203	209	216	223	230	236	243	250	257	263
5'10"	132	139	146	153	160	167	174	181	188	195	202	209	216	222	230	236	243	250	257	264	271
5'11"	136	143	150	157	165	172	179	186	193	200	208	215	222	229	236	243	250	257	265	272	279
6'	140	147	154	162	169	177	184	191	199	206	213	221	228	235	243	250	258	265	272	279	287
6'1"	144	151	159	166	174	182	189	197	204	212	219	227	235	242	250	257	265	272	280	288	295
6'2"	148	155	163	171	179	186	194	202	210	218	225	233	241	249	257	264	272	280	287	295	303
6'3"	152	160	168	176	184	192	200	208	216	224	232	240	248	256	264	272	279	287	295	303	311
6'4"	156	164	172	180	189	197	205	213	221	230	238	246	254	263	271	279	287	295	304	312	320

Appendix B : "Ideal" Body Weight Ranges

Height (BMI)	"Normal" (19 to 24)	"Overweight" (25 to 29)	"Obese" (30 to 39)
4' 10"	91 - 115	119 - 138	143 - 186
4' 11"	94 - 119	124 - 143	148 - 193
5'	97 - 123	128 - 148	153 - 199
5' 1"	100 - 127	132 - 153	158 - 206
5' 2"	104 - 131	136 - 158	164 - 213
5' 3"	107 - 135	141 - 163	169 - 220
5' 4"	110 - 140	145 - 169	174 - 227
5' 5"	114 - 144	150 - 174	180 - 234
5' 6"	118 - 148	155 - 179	186 - 241
5' 7"	121 - 153	159 - 185	191 - 249
5' 8"	125 - 158	164 - 190	197 - 256
5' 9"	128 - 162	169 - 196	203 - 263
5' 10"	132 - 167	174 - 202	209 - 271
5' 11"	136 - 172	179 - 208	215 - 279
6'	140 - 177	184 - 213	221 - 287
6' 1"	144 - 182	189 - 219	227 - 295
6' 2"	148 - 186	194 - 225	233 - 303
6' 3"	152 - 192	200 - 232	240 - 311
6' 4"	156 - 197	205 - 238	246 - 320

Appendix C

Exercise Calorie Calculator

Calories "Burned" in One Hour of Activity for a 150-Pound Person*

Housework—100 calories

Light gardening—150 calories (this is *not* just watching the grass grow!)

Golf—250 calories (walking the course with your bag of clubs)

Tennis (recreational)—275 calories

Racquetball—300 to 350 calories

Aerobics—300 to 400 calories

Walking—100 calories per mile (assumes four miles per hour)

Exercise bike—300 to 600 calories (most bikes will calculate the calories for you)

Tennis (competitive)—425 calories

Swimming—400 to 600 calories per hour

Running—100 calories per mile (assumes seven miles per hour)

Climbing stairs—1 calorie/five steps (ex.: 50 steps = 10 calories)

Weight conversion: The more you weigh, the more calories you actually expend with weight-bearing exercise. If you weigh less than 120 or more than 180 pounds, you should convert the preceding calorie estimates to more accurately fit your weight. You can calculate your conversion factor by taking your weight and dividing it by 150. (Example: Conversion factor for 200-pound woman is 200 lbs./150 lbs. = 1.33). If the same 200-pound woman walked 4 miles in an hour, she would look up 400 calories from the preceding table and then multiply 400 by her

*These calorie amounts are estimates based on a "middle-of-the-road" pace. You may be burning more or less calories than what's listed here if you are going faster or slower than "average."

conversion factor (1.33) to calculate her actual calories expended, which would be 532 calories. (Actual calories expended = 400 cal. × 1.33 = 532 calories.)

Appendix D

The Hurried Woman Food Diary/Calorie Counter

Appendix D : The Hurried Woman Food Diary / Calorie Calculator

Week # _____	Description & Amount	*Calories In* Total	P	C	F	*Calories Out*	*Net Calories In*
MON / /						REQUIRED 1 2 3 ADDITIONAL CALORIES:	
	Sub Tot						
TUE / /						REQUIRED 1 2 3 ADDITIONAL CALORIES:	
	Sub Tot						
WED / /						REQUIRED 1 2 3 ADDITIONAL CALORIES:	
	Sub Tot						
THU / /						REQUIRED 1 2 3 ADDITIONAL CALORIES:	
	Sub Tot						
FRI / /						REQUIRED 1 2 3 ADDITIONAL CALORIES:	
	Sub Tot						
SAT / /						REQUIRED 1 2 3 ADDITIONAL CALORIES:	
	Sub Tot						
SUN / /						REQUIRED 1 2 3 ADDITIONAL CALORIES:	
	Sub Tot						
		Total	P	C	F	Calories Out	Net Calories In
	Weekly						

How to Use the Food Diary/Calorie Calculator

1. Write down everything you eat—yes, everything—as soon as you eat it. Give a brief description as well as the amount of food eaten and the total calories. Breakdown the total calories into the number of calories from protein (P), carbohydrates (C), and Fats (F). Subtotal each of these columns at the end of each day.
2. Record your exercise calories out. You have a minimum exercise requirement of three half-hours each week. When you exercise your first half hour of the week, circle the number 1 under "Required Calories Out," and circle the 2 when you finish your second half-hour. If you exercise longer than half an hour at your first session, say one hour, you can either circle numbers 1 *and* 2 when you finish or write in the extra calories in the "Additional Calories" area under the "Calories Out" column.
3. Calculate your net calories in for each day by subtracting any additional exercise calories out from your total calories in. This will show you how you are doing on a day-by-day basis. Remember though, you have the flexibility to move calories around during the week or to earn "calorie credits" from additional exercise.
4. At the end of the week, you can add up your total weekly calories in from each of the daily sub totals. This is a good time to see if you have maintained the recommended ratio of protein = 40%, carbohydrates = 30%, and fats = 30%. You can also add up the additional exercise calorie "credits" for the week and subtract these from the total weekly calories in to arrive at your net calories in for the week. This is the best place to analyze how well you are sticking to your diet plan and to make any necessary adjustments if you have reached a "plateau."
5. We haven't discussed how to calculate your target calories per week, but it's easy to do. Just take the recommended target calories in per day we calculated earlier and multiply that number by 7. To illustrate:

Target weight_____ × 11 = _____Target Net Calories
In per day

Target Net Calories In per Day_____ × 7 = _____Recom-
mended Net Calories In per Week

For more information on the Hurried Woman Syndrome, go to the web site www.hurriedwoman.com

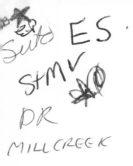

WHISPERS IN THE WILDERNESS

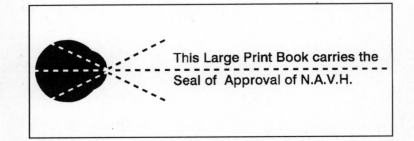

This Large Print Book carries the
Seal of Approval of N.A.V.H.

WHISPERS IN THE WILDERNESS

COLLEEN L. REECE

THORNDIKE PRESS

A part of Gale, Cengage Learning

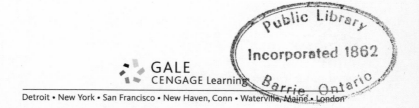

GALE
CENGAGE Learning

Detroit • New York • San Francisco • New Haven, Conn • Waterville, Maine • London

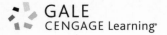

LIBRARY OF CONGRESS CATALOGING-IN-PUBLICATION DATA

Reece, Colleen L.
    Whispers in the wilderness / by Colleen L. Reece. — Large print ed.
       p. cm. — (Frontier brides; bk 2) (Thorndike Press large
    print Christian romance)
    ISBN-13: 978-1-4104-4223-9(hardcover)
    ISBN-10: 1-4104-4223-3(hardcover)
    1. Large type books. I. Title.
PS3568.E3646W55 2011
813'.54—dc23   2011033442

Published in 2012 by arrangement with Colleen L. Reece.

Printed in the United States of America
1 2 3 4 5 6 7 16 15 14 13 12

WHISPERS IN THE WILDERNESS

CHAPTER 1

Go or stay? Joel Scott slid from the saddle of his ebony mare, Querida, and let the reins drop. Trained to stand, she whinnied, rubbed her soft nose against his shoulder, then began to graze; the rise overlooking the Double J was no stranger to her.

A pang went through this golden-haired man with the face of an angel. How could he leave northern Arizona and all it offered? He gazed into the valley below — mute but appealing, it lay like a crumpled blanket carelessly tossed by a giant hand. Hills, valleys, forested slopes, and the distant rims of red canyons — they all wove invisible webs, as they had done eleven summers ago when Joel and his aunt ended their long search for Uncle Gideon. How quickly the years had flown! The seven-year-old boy, who had whooped with excitement when he first saw the Double J, lurked inside Joel's heart. Along with that was the awe that filled him

7

each time he surveyed the now-expanded ranch.

Cloudless Arizona skies smiled, no bluer than the keen eyes of the motionless man. Quaking aspens with their greenish-white trunks bent toward one another and whispered wilderness gossip. Pine, cedar, and grass rustled, alive with the sheer joy of summer.

"I can't go." Joel did not realize he had spoken aloud until Querida abandoned her grazing to nuzzle his arm. He sighed and buried his face in her black mane. Even if he could bear to leave the ranch and his family, how could he part with Querida? Ten years earlier, Gideon had called his nephew to the barn. "One of the mares is ready to foal. You need to be there."

Joel wondered at the mysterious look in his uncle's face but obediently trotted after the tall man he resembled. Even now he could remember every detail of the birth, his first to witness.

"It's a filly," Gideon told the wide-eyed boy. "Male horses are colts. She's yours, Son."

"Mine?" Joel had ridden various Double J horses, but none had been his very own. He watched the filly struggle to her feet on legs that seemed too long for her body. Within a few hours, she ran about but never strayed far from her mother.

"What shall I call her?" He thought of all the black things he could: Soot, Ink, Dark Cloud. But Aldrich, longtime foreman for Gideon, shook his head. "This filly's gonna become a real pard," he told the excited boy. "Name her something special."

"What?" Joel respected Aldrich for his range lore.

Aldrich's leathery face broke into a smile, and his eyes twinkled. "Once, a long time ago, I had a pretty little filly named Querida. That's Spanish for *beloved*." He pronounced it *Kay-reeda.*

"Querida." Joel rolled the name around on his tongue, patted his gift, and repeated, "Querida. Beloved." From that moment, the two were inseparable. By the time Querida turned five, she had reached full height and weight.

Twice, she had saved Joel from danger. Once with Joel aboard, she had outrun a visiting outlaw who had tried to buy her and had been refused. The second time was just a few months after Joel's sixteenth birthday, when Joel's foot was painfully twisted and held fast by a rock slide, trapping him. Although her eyes showed that she did not want to leave him, Querida obeyed her master's command to go home. Her arrival at the Double J, without Joel, resulted in a prompt rescue, and he loved her more than ever afterwards.

Joel's mind returned to the present. "God, I don't know what to do." He impulsively turned to his best Friend. "You know I want to serve You — it's all I've ever wanted. To take up Uncle Gideon's work and preach." His heart glowed at the prospect.

In Flagstaff, he had already earned the nickname of the boy preacher, and it was jealously defended by Lonesome, Dusty, Aldrich, and the other Double J hands. Strangers sometimes mistakenly branded Joel as soft until a demonstration of his riding or roping would convince even the strongest nonbeliever that a man could follow God and still be a top cowboy. Talk of his talents ran second only to the ripple of shock that Gideon had caused years before when he laid down his no-drinking rule for the Double J and made it stick because of who he was and the wages he offered.

Once, a new rider asked how come young Scott could talk a bird out of its bush and still be fearless and strong.

"A lot of folks think Jesus was a tenderfoot," the young preacher shot back. "But then, a lot of folks can be wrong." His frank smile took any sting out of his words. "The hills around where Jesus lived are steep and probably as rough as some of our Arizona country. How far do you think a coddled weakling would get trying to climb them?"

The rider scratched his head and allowed that it would not be far.

Ever since his eighteenth birthday, on the last day of April, Joel found himself more introspective than ever. That day, he learned the full story of his past. Joel had always known his mama died and Aunt Judy raised him. When he inquired about his real father and why he never knew him, Gideon and Judith simply said, "When you're a man, Son, we'll tell you everything." The pain in their faces stilled his boyish questions, but the feeling of some dark secret haunted him. Two years after he and Judith came to the Double J in 1877, twin cousins came along, Matt and Millie. Judith beckoned ten-year-old Joel to see the babies and told him, "They'll be more like your brother and sister than cousins, Joel, Dear." Her dark eyes shone. "I'll need you to help me a great deal now." His childish heart swelled with the trust he saw in her face, and by the time they could toddle, Joel had the twins riding in front of him.

As if conjured up by his thoughts of them, a high-pitched cry shattered the peaceful time of contemplation. "Joel!" It echoed from a nearby cliff wall but died in the steady beat of hooves when Matt and Millie burst into sight and raced toward him. How those eight-year-olds could ride! Pride rose in the waiting man and chased away the need for solitude. Since April, he had mulled over the unvarnished facts of his birth. How Cyrus Scott, unworthy of the favoritism of his father, had fallen in love with pretty Millicent Butler, married her using his brother Gideon's name, then gone away without knowing of Joel's coming.

"Are you sure he didn't know about me?" Joel had demanded when the sad story ended.

"He never knew." Judith's lips trembled. "In the message I sent to him, I only said that Millie had died."

"Then he abandoned Mama but not me," Joel said, feeling somewhat relieved.

"He also said he was sorry and asked for forgiveness," Gideon put in. Longing filled his face. "I always wanted to go back, to try again to find my brother. . . ."

Did the idea begin then? Joel wondered. The passionate longing to somehow repay the wronged uncle who rode away in bitterness when his father would not believe him innocent? Months and years had passed before God's perfect timing brought Gideon and Judith together to marry and confess the love that grew during their separation.

He would be following a cold trail, common sense advised him. *With God all things are possible* (Mark 10:27), Joel's heart retorted.

Gideon could never go. A few months before Joel and Judith had come, Gideon had been shot. The doctor who had attended him had predicted that Gideon would always walk with a limp and that riding for too long or hard would result in pain. Although he managed well, a familiar grimace of pain showed Joel the folly of his uncle's attempting the kind of riding that would be necessary in traveling the path back to the past.

The second part of Gideon's dream was to return to Tomkinsville, Colorado, where he had traveled under Cyrus's name and had fallen into gambling. "There are so many I want to tell about Jesus," he said brokenly. His strong face worked, and Joel felt his own heart bound with sympathy. Joel almost cried out that he would take Gideon's place, but caution sealed his lips. Not until he received orders from his heavenly Father could he make such a commitment.

Yes, he had considered much since April. A few more days would not matter. He hailed the twins, laughingly declared their race as ended in a tie, then mounted Querida, and rode home, a chattering child on each side. But the aspens and pines and cedars continued their tattletale whispering and filled the wilderness with soft sounds, which were increased by the early evening breeze that sprang up and set the leaves to fluttering even more.

Day after day, Joel continued helping with the endless ranch chores, his perfectly trained body busy with his tasks and his mind free to consider. To his amazement, once the unspoken idea of retracing Gideon's journey came, it settled in like butter on a hot biscuit. Suppose he could find his real father. Surely the message his father had sent to the family's Circle S ranch showed repentance! Would not Cyrus Scott's heart be softened if the son he never knew sought him out? Finally, Joel realized why the idea appealed to him so much.

"Lord, I don't want my father to die without knowing You." He paused but refused to think of all he would leave behind if he rode away from home. "Before I go, I need to know if this is just what I want or if it's Your will."

Joel settled into a time of waiting, and the knowledge that he should go firmed. Still, he hesitated, testing himself and praying for something — anything — that would justify his decision. His answer came like a clap of thunder.

One sunny afternoon, Tomkins, who had befriended Gideon so long ago, brought Judith and Joel west, then bought into the Double J and helped it grow, rode out from his home in Flagstaff. Married to a fine woman whose husband had died on their journey to Arizona, Tomkins divided his time between the ranch and various business enterprises in town. "This state will grow," he had predicted. "It's 1888, the Indian fighting's over since Geronimo surrendered a couple of years back, and the Southern Pacific Railroad's bringing more folks in all the time. Ranching, mining, farming — Arizona's got them all."

Always cheerful and forward-looking, Tomkins had lost some of his pleasant expression this afternoon. Finally, he admitted sheepishly, "I guess my foot's getting itchy. I have a hankering to see Colorado at least once more. It was mighty good to me."

15

A wistful look came into his keen eyes. "My wife's sister's been pestering her to visit her in California, and I've been thinking about heading east for a spell while she's gone." He lifted an eyebrow. "Only thing is, it'd be a lot more enjoyable if I had a traveling companion. What are the chances of Joel going with me?"

Thank You, Lord. Joel felt his last doubt slide away. "How are you going?"

"I'm game to just ride a horse and forget all the newfangled ways to travel," Tomkins drawled. "I reckon that Querida mare of yours can carry you to Colorado."

"And to Texas."

"Texas! Who said anything about Texas?" Tomkins's eyebrows arched like an angry cat's back.

"Texas?" Gideon's eyes gleamed, and he leaned forward. "What's on your mind, Joel?" His hands clenched and unclenched.

Joel's fiery blue gaze met his uncle's. "I want to go back to San Scipio and see my grandparents. Then, I'm going to find my father."

"You mean *try* to find him, don't you?" Judith looked shocked but sympathetic. The years had been kind to her; not a single gray hair marred the dark braids she still wore in a coronet.

16

"No. I'll stay until I find him."

"Impossible!" Yet, the hope in Gideon's face outweighed his words. "I tried everything. It's been fourteen years."

"Have you considered how little chance there is of your succeeding?" Judith quietly asked.

"Aunt Judy." The childish nickname came naturally. "I can't even remember the first time you taught me that God can do anything and that we must have faith." Joel straightened to his full six-foot height, young in build but with a man's steady determination in his face. "Ever since my birthday, I've known I have to find my father if he is still alive." The last words came in a whisper.

"Then you have my blessing. I only wish I were going with you," Gideon confessed. He held out a strong hand and gripped Joel's. "When you stop at the Circle S, tell Dad and Mother we already have a wing planned for them if they ever decide to sell out and come to Arizona."

"I will." As easily as that, Joel left the crossroads he had tarried beside for weeks. What lay ahead? Only God knew. He looked into Millie's and Matt's faces, quiet for once, awed by the serious grown-up talk. His gaze traveled to Gideon's face and

17

noted the mingled fear of failure and un-quenchable hope. Then to Judith, whose tranquil posture reassured him. He had known leaving would be hard, but he had not counted on its being such a wrench. All the years with Judith danced before him — the loving care, the sacrifices.

Did she sense his feelings? A small smile tilted her lips up. "God will go with you, Joel. Remember, your name means *Jehovah is the Lord.*"

This brittle moment, one to treasure, was broken by Millie's plaintive, "Aren't you *ever* coming back, Joel?"

"Of course I will." He smiled at her, and her anxious look faded. Yet, when good nights had been said and Joel restlessly sought out Querida, he wondered, *How many weeks and months, even years, might it be before I return to the Double J?* He set his lips in a narrow line and vowed, "God, You have blessed my family with the means to let me go. I am going in Your name, to set things straight for Uncle Gideon and to carry salvation to those along the way. Especially to my father. Please, ride with me. No, let me ride with You — until I find my father."

News of Joel's departure created an uproar on the Double J. "Just when I'm gettin' ya to be worth somethin', you ups and rides out," Lonesome complained. Eleven years had not changed the irrepressible cowboy who now owned stock and shares in the ranch. "Dawgone, but it don't pay to invest time in a feller."

"Aw, stop your bellyachin'," Dusty called. "Everyone knows it was me who taught Joel what he knows."

"Sez who?" Lonesome ruffled like a turkey.

"Sez me."

Joel took advantage of their good-natured warfare to escape. The last thing he needed was to let the outfit know how big a lump lay in his chest. Knowing he had to go did not make it easier. Neither did uncertainty as to when he would be back . . . if ever.

From the moment Joel declared his intention to go with Tomkins, Gideon made time to spend with his nephew. With their fair heads bent over roughly drawn maps, they endlessly discussed the route that had brought Gideon from Colorado to Arizona.

"Here's a list of folks whose names I remember," the older man said, eyes filled with a reminiscent light. "People who offered a bed or a bite to eat and never asked for a peso." He laughed gleefully, and some of the lines that the years had etched disappeared from his face. "I used to hide some money where they'd find it after I left. Always felt like a kid with a new toy, thinking about the way they'd look when they found it."

He hesitated, then said, "Joel, there are two in particular I hope you can find. The girl Lily. I helped her get out of the saloon, but I didn't tell her about God." The laughter left his face, and he looked bleak. "The other one's Eb Sears."

"The man you were accused of knifing?" Joel stared.

"Yes. If he had lied, I'd have been sent to prison for a long time. Rough and mean as he was, Eb Sears must have had something good deep down, or he wouldn't have admitted he was drunk and loud, then cleared me of blame." Gideon added, "If I hadn't been so bitter against God, I'd have stayed and tried to work on that hidden good. Tell Sears where I am and that if he ever needs a job, he has one on the Double J — that is, if he will leave the bottle alone!"

A few mornings later, just after daylight but before the sun rose, Tomkins and Joel leisurely rode away from the Double J. By common consent, they halted on top of the rise and looked back. Fog wraiths hovered in the air, waiting for the sun's kiss to dissolve them. Wisps of smoke curled from the ranch house and bunkhouse chimneys. The eternal whispering of the quaking aspens trembled in Joel's ears, calling him back, pushing him on. By the time the travelers reached the high country, the green leaves would be tinged with gold, yellower than the stuff miners sold their souls to possess.

"Whispers in the wilderness," Joel said softly.

"Yeah." Tomkins relaxed in the saddle, then reminded, "It's a long way." His gaze bored into the younger man, whose fair hair showed in front of his pushed-back Stetson and contrasted sharply with Querida's shining dark hide. "It may be an even longer way home."

"I know." Yet, when the sun burst over a hill and flooded the valley with rosy light, Joel knew he would not turn back if he could. Perhaps some of his father's restless blood stirred and came to life.

With a sense of freedom, responsibility, and urgency, he anticipated what lay ahead. His vivid imagination pictured the aspen leaves whispering *hurry, hurry,* and Joel wanted to prod Querida into a dead run. For an instant, a single dark cloud appeared and blocked the sun's rays. Joel shivered.

Again came that feeling of the need to hurry.

Should he tell Tomkins he could not go to Colorado, then strike out alone across Arizona, through New Mexico, and then to San Scipio? Were there forces surrounding the elder Scotts or Cyrus, if he lived, that demanded action and soon?

Do not be a fool, he chided himself. *You felt God confirming your decision to do exactly what you are doing when Tomkins suggested it. You cannot turn back now on the strength of a whim.* Yet, all that first day of travel, Joel found himself anxiously watching the south-eastern sky and the giant thunderheads that gathered and attacked the earth. With the ability he had possessed since childhood to sense trouble, he prayed silently but mightily that his quest, his mission, would not fail.

No one could have been a better trailmate than Tomkins. He spoke when Joel wanted to talk, rode quietly when the younger man needed time to think, and he always recognized those times. The same qualities that Gideon had discovered in Tomkins the year they wintered together on the trapline proved strong and welcome now to Joel. Yet, a difference existed. Where Gideon had been embittered and refused to mention

22

God, except to rail against him, Joel shared his early childhood faith. It strengthened them both. Around their nighttime campfires, when shadows hid expressions too private for anyone but God to observe, the men became partners. Joel would have trusted his life to Tomkins. He rejoiced that the older man had accepted Christ shortly after he came to Arizona. They spent hours talking of what the raw West would be like if only God were allowed to be in control, instead of greed and hatred.

Always, Joel carried Gideon's list. As they traveled, name after name received a heavy line through it. Some had moved. Others welcomed the young man with hearty approval and tales of how they discovered his uncle's money in the family Bible or under a plate. Joel's eyes opened wide at the stories. Time after time, those families, who had given what they could little afford to share and who secretly prayed for God's help, received their reward . . . and praised His name for using a passing stranger.

Tomkins's eyes glistened at the stories, and once he gruffly told Joel, "I reckon I had a part in helping answer their prayers, don't you think? If your uncle hadn't grubstaked me, I wouldn't have given him money." He cocked his head. "Wonder how the good Lord would have taken care of those folks in that situation?"

"I've decided I don't have to know *how* or *why* God does things," Joel said soberly. "Just that He does them."

Tomkins grunted, and Joel saw the approving look the other man sent toward him.

The feeling of urgency lessened a bit as they worked their way toward Tomkinsville. They had tarried along the way, and before they had reached the high country, fall had had the opportunity to paint the leaves with its frosty brush. Joel felt he had come home when they climbed the hills and saw his old friends, the quaking aspens. Now, their whispering leaves shone butter yellow, and with each passing breeze, some dropped to the ground to huddle in great golden piles. Miles of wilderness, broken only by a deserted cabin here and there, offered peace and a time to prepare for what lay ahead.

"It might be a ghost town," Tomkins muttered when they mounted the last hill from where they could look down into town. "I haven't kept in touch. Mining may be over."

Joel heard dread in his companion's voice and said nothing, but his heart thumped against his ribs. Tomkinsville represented the place where his real work must begin — the work of taking the gospel of Jesus Christ to those who most needed it and least realized their need.

"Aw, look at that!" A sigh of relief from Tomkins blended with a blast of loud music. "Still here and it sounds the same." He craned his neck, and Joel rode up beside him where the trail widened. Surrounded by snow-topped mountains, Joel's first parish waited.

CHAPTER 2

A tiny pulse hammered in Joel's temple. Fourteen years earlier, his uncle Gideon had ridden into Tomkinsville, sick at heart and corroded with the bitterness of false accusations. Now, Joel returned as Gideon's emissary. Another blast of raucous music desecrated the peaceful mountain air, and the young man shuddered. Flagstaff with its Saturday night cowboy sprees had been wild, but Tomkinsville roared like a wounded cougar. Would he be equal to the task that lay ahead?

He straightened in the saddle, and Querida softly whinnied. God willing, they would ride straight into the wide-open town and, if it were His plan, stir hearts for Him. Joel wondered how God felt when men invaded some of His most beautiful creations with their schemes and treachery, plotting and sin. Back home, he and Tomkins had seen mountains as high as

Humphreys Peak, north of Williams, that reached well over twelve thousand feet. Crowned with early snowcaps, they glistened and shimmered in the distance, everlastingly there as a backdrop for the layers of aspens and dark evergreens that clustered at their feet. Silver waterfalls and tumbling streams fell over rocky ledges, their water so cold Joel's teeth ached when he drank. Did the inhabitants of Tomkinsville ever look up and see the beauty? Or were they too engrossed in their quest for gold and silver, gambling and drinking to raise their gaze above material things?

"First thing we should do is find a place to stay," Tomkins advised. He laughed, but Joel could see excitement in his face. "Funny, not so long ago, folks riding in would have been asking me about lodging!" He shrugged, then shamefacedly admitted, "I guess I had to come back one more time to find out how much I have back in Arizona." He fell silent.

Joel's heart beat with sympathy. What must it be like to have a wife waiting when a man came home? A rush of color streaked his tanned face. Flagstaff had lots of nice girls, but he had never seen one yet that he would want to hitch up with for life. Double harness meant two lives blended into one,

27

each caring for the other. He had learned that from watching Gideon and Judith. They did not have to shout their love from Humphreys Peak to let people know it ran swift as a river in flood.

Tomkins shot him a keen glance. "Someday, Boy, you'll meet a special girl. When you do, make sure she's true and real, not just a pretty face."

Joel marveled again at the way Tomkins often seemed to read his thoughts. "I will." The idea warmed him. "I'll never marry until I know God approves." He felt he had just taken as solemn a vow as marriage itself, but his irrepressible sense of humor made him add, "I've never even courted anyone yet, so I'll hold off getting married for awhile. Besides, there's a long trail ahead."

Tomkins grinned appreciatively and reined in before the same log building that had housed his enterprises years before. No longer new, it hugged the ground firmly. The weathered logs brought a memory of Gideon returning to find that his old friend was now the big man in Tomkinsville. It was a thrilling story, one that Joel had begged to hear dozens of times — how only the inherent honesty of a loud, crude cowboy saved Gideon.

An hour later, the visitors surveyed the snug cabin Tomkins had rented at a price he snorted over and called robbery.

"You're lucky to get it at any price," the smooth-tongued gent in a funeral-black suit told them. "More and more people are coming into town all the time. Only reason I have this cabin available is that its owner took up a new residence."

Something in the man's voice sent a chill up Joel's backbone. "Where?"

"Boot Hill." A wave of the hand toward the window indicated a set-apart area with wildflowers blowing in the wind and a fresh gash in the earth. "The way I heard, he talked when he should have been listening and flashed a roll of bills that would choke a horse. Next morning, the sheriff stumbled over a body. The money hasn't shown up." He abruptly changed the subject. "Do you want it for the winter?"

Joel started to nod, caught Tomkins's warning glance, and stopped. He also saw a gleam in the agent's eyes he did not trust, and when the man asked a shade too casually, "Where did you say you were from?" Joel kept mum.

His trailmate looked squarely into the curious man's face. "We didn't say. By the way, they named this town after me some

29

time back. I guess that's enough. We'll look over these accommodations and let you know."

Doubt replaced the suspicious gleam. The agent backtracked. "If you want the cabin for at least a month, I can let you have it a little cheaper." He named a price, still high.

Tomkins grimaced and threw down the money. "If it's dirty, we'll come back and use you for a floor mop."

Joel's mouth dropped open. He had never seen this side of his friend, not even on the long trip west with Judith years before. The minute they got outside, he burst out with, "You sure stopped him!"

Tomkins's shrewd face gave credence to his words. "Son, this is Tomkinsville." He swung onto his horse, and Joel knew that a far deeper meaning than he had suspected lay beneath the dry comment.

Their new home sat on a rounded rise out of town and far enough away to avoid some of the clamor. A view of distant peaks from the front window, the two small bedrooms with hand-hewn bedsteads, a large living room/kitchen combination, and the semi-privacy of the cabin offered all they needed.

Tomkins's eagle gaze swept over the large room. "It will do for a meeting place until we get enough folks coming to need a bigger building." He brought in a bucket of water from a nearby creek and spluttered when the icy drops hit his face. "Your turn. We don't want to meet Tomkinsville looking like two tumbleweeds."

Joel gasped when he felt the cold water on his dirty, heated skin. His teeth chattered, but he rubbed a rough towel on his face and warmed himself up. The one set of good clothes he had brought came out of his saddlebags clean but wrinkled.

"We'll find a laundry," Tomkins promised. "First, let's go get some grub." He had changed into clean pants and shirt, then bunched his trail clothes into a bundle to take with him.

Joel thought of how they had washed out their garments as best they could on their journey. Twice, a friendly rancher's wife had insisted on doing it. He swiftly made his own bundle of laundry and followed Tomkins out to the horses. "I suppose there's a livery stable here?"

"Huh!" Tomkins's eyes glowed like twin coals. "We'll keep real close watch on our horses, especially yours. No livery stable for Querida. Some of the men around here used to have taking ways and probably still do."

They found a small eating place and

31

gorged on fresh beefsteak, mashed potatoes and gravy, corn, biscuits as light as Judith had ever made, and two pieces of apple pie apiece. Black coffee, strong enough to float a lead bar, finished off the meal.

"Well, are you ready for Tomkinsville?"

Joel took a long breath. "If it's ready for me!" he told his friend.

"Now, don't go doing anything stupid," Tomkins warned when they reached the noisy main street. They strolled along until they reached the Missing Spur Saloon. Joel's unfamiliarity with such places left him wide-eyed and wondering why Tomkins would choose a saloon as the place for making their presence known.

"There's bound to be some here who'll remember me." The answer to his unspoken question steadied Joel. "Let me do the talking." He pushed ahead of Joel and stepped inside.

The younger man's first impression mingled color and light, the reek of booze, cigarette and cigar smoke, too-loud laughter, and rough language. For a moment, he felt he had been there before. Then he realized that a replica of Gideon's descriptions, complete in every detail, lay before him. A few heads turned toward the strangers, surveyed them, then went back to their

32

gambling and drinking.

"Don't I know you?" A burly man shouldered his way from the long bar and confronted them.

"You should. I sold you your first horse," Tomkins said.

"Well, by the powers, if it ain't Tomkins himself!" The rough face broke apart into a wide smile. "I hear tell you've been down Arizony way." He clapped Tomkins on the back. "Set 'em up, boys. This is the feller who begun what made this town famous!"

A roar of approval went up. Men crowded toward the bar, but Tomkins stopped them with the wave of a hand. "Sorry, men. I don't drink."

Guffaws replaced the cheers; scowls erased smiles.

"You ain't serious!" The burly man stared. "What'd you do, git religion?"

"That's about it." Tomkins did not move a muscle. Joel had never been prouder of his friend.

"Well, I'll be . . ." The man's jaw sagged. "What about your friend?" He turned toward Joel.

"He —"

Joel cut in, unwilling to be announced as a preacher at this particular moment. "I don't drink, either. I'm looking for a man."

Stone-cold, dead silence filled the hazy room. Tomkins's acquaintance's eyes narrowed to slits. "An' who might that man be?"

Joel sensed a certain breathlessness and rushed in where the devil himself would have hesitated. "Name of Eb Sears."

"What!" The thunderstruck man shook his head as if he had not heard right. "Why in tarnation does a kid like you come marchin' in lookin' for Sears?"

"He and my uncle had a mix-up years ago, and —"

"Shut up, Joel!" Tomkins seized his arm with a steel grip.

Bewildered and unsure of what he had done but instinctively knowing it was wrong, Joel felt himself propelled back toward the door. An angry buzzing, like tormented bees from a hive, followed him. Just then the door flew inward, narrowly missing Joel. A heavyset man, carrying the smell of horse, stepped inside. He raised one eyebrow curiously at the sight of a young stranger being pushed toward the door.

"Hey, Sears, the kid's lookin' for you," someone called. "Says you and his uncle had trouble years ago. Think you c'n handle him?" A roar of mocking laughter rocked the room.

Tomkins muttered something under his breath, released Joel, and took one step to the side. "Hello, Eb."

Sears shifted his astonished gaze. "Tomkins! What're you doin' back here? And who is this kid? He looks like someone I know." He glanced back at Joel. "Who's his uncle, and hadn't you better be in bed, Sonny? It's gettin' kinda late for you to be up, ain't it?"

Eager to deliver Gideon's message, Joel ignored both the fresh round of laughter and Tomkins's muttered, "Get out of here." He asked, "Remember the name Cyrus Scott?"

"Scott? Yeah, the guy they said knifed me but didn't." Sears shook himself, and his brows met in puzzlement. "I cleared him. So how come you're lookin' for me a bunch of years later?" He dropped one hand suggestively to his gun butt. Then suspicion wiped out confusion, and he jerked his revolver out of its holster.

Before it cleared leather, Sears found himself looking straight into the steady muzzle of Joel's pistol.

Who are you, Kid?" Sears's face turned the color of old wax. "Only man I ever saw who could draw that fast was Scott."

"Put the gun on the table." Joel gestured,

his face set. What a horrible way to attract the attention of Tomkinsville! He sheathed his own gun and held out his right hand. "Sears, I'm Joel Scott, Gideon Scott's nephew."

"I don't know no Gideon Scott, just Cyrus." Some of the color seeped back into Sears's ruddy face, but he didn't take the outstretched hand.

"My uncle used that name then," Joel explained. His voice sounded loud and strange in the silent room. "He has a big ranch in northern Arizona, the Double J. He got shot up years back and can't ride the way he wants to. I've come to Tomkinsville to shake your hand, tell you he's never forgotten how you told the truth and saved him, and to let you know if you ever need a riding job, there's a place for you on the Double J."

A concerted gasp ran through the room. Sears stepped back as if shocked, then stretched out his hand and grumbled, "What a way to bring friendly greetin's." He gripped Joel's hands. "We mighta killed each other."

"Naw," a heckler called while feet shifted and onlookers sat back in their chairs. "He'da bored ya, if he wanted, Eb. Young feller, where'd ya learn to shoot like that?"

"From his uncle," Tomkins interjected. He sounded delighted at the way things had turned out, but the low note in his voice told Joel he was in for it when they got home. "Well, boys, now that you've all seen what Scott can do, I'd like to invite you to see some more of his skills."

"Can he ride? Rope?" Sears shot a significant look at Tomkins. Tomkins laughed, nodded, and said loud enough for every person present to hear, "Yeah. Preach, too." His enjoyment of the situation spilled over, and his eyes twinkled. "Come out to the old Furman cabin on Sunday morning. He preaches as good as he draws a gun."

Shock, mirth, and disbelief warred in the faces of Sears and several men who crowded around him. "This kid a *preacher?* Some of the rocks you dug looking for gold musta slipped and hit you on the head," Sears pronounced solemnly.

"If you don't believe me, come see for yourself." Tomkins nudged Joel.

Joel flashed his heartwarming smile. "Sorry I had to pull a gun on you, Mr. Sears. I had to make sure you didn't kill me before I could give you Gideon's message. See, he'd been a preacher, too, but was down on his luck when he lived here. I'm taking up the work where he had to leave off."

He moved around Sears, stepped into the crisp night air, and gleefully tasted the thrill of his encounter and the openmouthed stares of the saloon patrons at this revelation. Just maybe, out of sheer curiosity, they would come to the cabin. Joel did not care why they came, just so they did.

Responsibility downed his excitement. God had placed on him a heavy duty; he must not fail. Only through strict obedience to the Holy Spirit would the gospel's message touch and perhaps change Tomkinsville.

It did not take placards or banners to get the news out that a boy preacher had ridden into town, beat Eb Sears to the draw, invited him to ride for an Arizona cattle ranch, and would even hold a meeting the next Sunday. News ran like a spooked horse.

Tomkins said little but rounded up planks, hammer, and nails, and built some crude benches. "No telling how many folks will show up." His eyes twinkled. "Remember, I told folks you could preach as well as ride and rope and shoot." He pounded a few more nails, then eyed Joel. "I'd suggest you choose your sermon mighty careful," he added, but his eyes twinkled again.

Joel had already sensed the importance of this advice and soberly nodded his yellow head. When Tomkins refused help with his carpentering, Joel wandered off to a quiet knoll that offered as grand a view of the mountains as anything he had seen. What would appeal to the sturdy people of Tomkinsville? Certainly no watered-down message of a pallid Jesus. He closed his eyes and prayed for guidance. Warm sunlight surrounded him, and some of his feelings of inadequacy melted. Why should he fear? God had led him to this place; He would guide him.

Joel looked up at the craggy peaks above him. "I'd hate to get lost up there," he murmured, then sprang to his feet with an exultant yell. "That's it!" Thoughts raced through his brain. He pelted back to the cabin, past an astonished Tomkins. "I have my sermon," he called and bolted inside. He grabbed pencil, paper, and his worn Bible. By the time the benches stood sturdy and waiting, Joel's eyes shone and his heart thumped. "Thanks, God. This is just what's needed."

After the weeks on the trail, he felt a little strange when he donned his clean, pressed suit on Sunday morning. The night before, he and Tomkins scoured the cabin to within an inch of its life and arranged the benches. They had no songbooks, but Joel possessed a clear, true voice and would line out hymns if his congregation did not know them. By the appointed time, every bench groaned under the weight of ranchers and their families, curious cowboys, townspeople, and round-eyed children who always looked forward to a circuit-riding preacher.

"What a friend we have in Jesus," the people enthusiastically sang. No need for Joel to sing a line and let them repeat. "All our sins and griefs to bear." He looked into their faces and saw the marks that sin had left in many, grief in others. His throat felt tight, and his vision blurred. What a tremendous need existed in Tomkinsville! The song ended. He offered a fervent prayer, and with one accord, the people said, "Amen." Then, Joel opened his Bible.

"Our text today is from Matthew 18, verses 12 and 13. 'How think ye? if a man have an hundred sheep, and one of them be gone astray, doth he not leave the ninety and nine, and goeth into the mountains, and seeketh that which is gone astray? And if so be that he find it, verily I say unto you, he rejoiceth more of that sheep, than of the ninety and nine which went not astray.' "

He closed the Bible. "Friends, we all know that sheepherders aren't too popular around these parts." Cattlemen and cowboys snickered. "Now, when Jesus told this story, He could have just as well talked about a cow critter or a good horse. I know if I had a hundred horses and Querida strayed, I'd tackle the roughest country around to find her." He glanced out the door, open to the warm autumn air, and pointed to the mountains. Heads turned and nodded. Joel caught a spark of interest in tired eyes.

"Our Lord doesn't tell how tough that journey was. Most of us have tackled rivers in flood, blizzards, or heat that would fry a lizard. Jesus doesn't say He had to fight off wolves or a mean old bear to save that sheep. He leaves out how steep the canyons were and the times when He maybe had to carry that sheep that was struggling to get away. Living here, you can imagine how it was."

The spark of interest flared into the flame of concentration. Joel rejoiced. "What the Lord does tell us is that if the sheep gets found and brought back home where it belongs, the owner is happier over it than over all the other ninety-nine that didn't go wandering off where they didn't belong."

41

He took a deep breath and stepped closer to his attentive listeners. "If any of you have ever had one of your children stray, you know just what the Lord means. You'd give your life in those mountains if that's what it took to bring back your child."

A subdued chorus of agreement rippled the air.

"Friends," Joel poignantly stretched out his hands, "that's just what God did. He sent His only Son, Jesus, so every one of us could be brought back from danger and have eternal life. He loved us that much. There's not a man, woman, or child here today who isn't being trailed by Jesus right now, just like that poor, lost sheep that strayed and was tracked, found, and delivered from hungry beasts and fierce storms. Unless we accept that and invite Him into our hearts and lives, why, we're worse off than that critter all alone and bleating somewhere in a dark canyon."

Joel paused, noted the wonderment in the children's faces, a mist in some of the women's eyes, the angry brushing away of a single drop on a cowboy's face. Too moved to say more, he simply said, "We will close by singing 'Praise God, from Whom All Blessings Flow.' "

The one sad note in the song and service

was Eb Sears's absence. Although Joel had not expected him, he had hoped. All through the hearty handshakes and exclamations of gladness that Joel had come, the young minister silently prayed for Sears.

When the congregation poured out, leading the stampede were the few sheepish-looking cowboys who had bashfully perched as close to the door as possible. Joel's keen ears caught a little byplay from among the cowboys that sent him posthaste after the others.

Fifty feet from the cabin, Eb Sears sat on a stocky bay that casually browsed near Querida and Tomkins's horse.

"Hey, Sears, you're too late for the preachin'," one of the cowboys sang out.

"Preachin'? Oh, yeah, there was a meetin', wasn't there?" Either Sears was the finest actor west of St. Louis, or he had forgotten. Joel suspected the first.

"Thought I'd see young Scott's black horse everyone's talkin' about," Sears explained elaborately and scratched his head, a devil-may-care expression on his face.

A few laughed, but no one challenged him, and Sears added, "What's her handle?"

"Querida. It means *beloved.* She's the first horse I ever saw foaled," Joel told the big man, whose glistening eyes showed him to be a top judge of horseflesh.

"I reckon I rode out for nothin', huh. You're not goin' to sell her." The crowd lost interest and dispersed to buggies, wagons, and tethered horses.

Had Sears really come to see Querida? Joel did not think so. If he were a gambling man, he'd stake a lot that it had been the only way Sears would let himself get near a preacher, no matter how curious he might be. "No, I won't sell her, but I'm glad you came." For the second time, he shook hands with Sears, and the current that passed between them confirmed Joel's suspicions.

CHAPTER 3

If the gold aspens along the trails had whispered about Joel's encounter with Sears in the Missing Spur, now they sang his praises in a fluttering chorus. "Never heard a preacher preach like that" repeated itself over and over when ranchers or riders met. "That young feller talks about a God who knows Colorado and us simple folks. Never uses high-falutin' words, neither," a gnarled miner added.

Joel's second and third sermons merely added to his fame. So did the fun-loving, boyish spirit that led him into the impromptu races that Querida loved. But the test of his mettle came with the first snow.

Not everyone in Tomkinsville appreciated Joel's ministry. Business at the Missing Spur fell off when some of its patrons listened to the gospel and decided it was time to take a stand for the God who had done "a whole bunch" for them. Now, dark whispers joined the praise. Tomkins reported a growing feeling, on the part of the faithful saloon crowd, against Joel's interfering in their business.

A few days later, he stamped in out of the cold, a worried look creasing his face. "Pardner, I hate like anything to tell you, but I've got to go back to Arizona."

"Really?" Joel raised astonished blue eyes from the sermon he had been preparing and looked at Tomkins. "Is something wrong?"

"My wife's back in Flagstaff," the older man explained. "We must have got our wires crossed. I thought she'd stay longer with her sister, but she's home and lonesome." He hesitated, and Joel saw the struggle going on within him.

"It's been good to come back, but —"

"You want to get home where you belong," Joel finished. He quietly added, "I understand. When do you want to leave?"

"There's a stage going out day after tomorrow."

The words hung in the cozy cabin. Joel saw regret in the way Tomkins looked yet eagerness over seeing his wife soon. "What about your horse?"

Tomkins shrugged. "You can have him. Take him with you, or better yet, sell him. He isn't my favorite. Now, if he were Querida, it would be another story." His keen gaze bored into Joel. "Do you still have plenty of money? Tomkinsville's been buzzing because you never take up an offering."

Joel flushed. "I don't need much. I'd rather the people would use their money to get a building for a church." He stretched. "I have a feeling I'll be riding on in the spring, but if there's some kind of building and folks are coming to services regularly, it shouldn't be too hard to get another preacher."

"Folks here don't want anyone but you," Tomkins said gruffly.

"I know, and it disturbs me," Joel admitted. "It's the Lord who needs to be praised, not me. Besides, I just can't help believing there's still a long trail ahead of me, and right now this is just a tarrying place." He shook with sudden melancholy. "I'll miss you, but if I had a wife back home . . ." His voice trailed off.

Tomkins climbed aboard the stage two days later but not before warning Joel, "Watch out for rattlers — the two-legged kind who don't have the courtesy to warn a man with their buzzing."

Joel agreed, then promptly forgot it. To his amazement, Eb Sears had dropped in to see him a time or two, although he never came to the meetings. Joel still suspected Sears had heard every word of the first sermon but did not mention it, and the big man always had an excellent reason for stopping by. Once, it was to drop off a haunch of venison he said one of the ranchers had sent. The second time, he said he had heard that Joel wanted to sell Tomkins's horse. After a lot of bargaining, Sears paid a good price for it and laconically accepted Joel's offer for a cup of coffee.

"How come you're a preacher, anyhow?" he asked over the rim of his heavy mug. "Your ridin' and ropin' and the way ya handle a gun would get ya a job on any ranch."

Joel carefully blew on his coffee to gain time to know what to tell him. Then, to his own amazement, he found himself telling his whole story to Sears, who let his coffee grow cold and grunted now and then. "So your own daddy shoved off the blame on his brother," he finally exclaimed. "Still, ya want to find him?"

A longing, greater than ever before, rose in Joel. "I have to. The note I mentioned where he asked to be forgiven shows he isn't, maybe wasn't, all bad." A somber mood crept into the little cabin; he shook it off. "Maybe, because I never knew a real

48

father, my aunt Judith's teachings about my heavenly Father meant more. God also helped me not to be bitter, just sorry. Someday, if I can find my own father and tell him that, maybe he will contact his own parents before it's too late. It would mean the world to them. It would mean even more if he could find and accept God's forgiveness."

Sears abruptly stood. "You're all right, Kid. Just keep on tellin' folks about that God of yours." He strode to the door. "It's kinda comfortin' to think that He's trailin' after even worn-out cowpokes like me. Maybe someday I — some of us'll stop ridin' long enough to let Him catch up." The door banged behind Sears, but a flood of light and joy poured into Joel's soul.

It proved short lived. The next night, gunshots outside Joel's cabin sent him pell-mell into the night. The clatter of hooves sounded loud in his ears, then dwindled toward town. A light snow under a lopsided moon showed Querida tossing her head and dancing away from a huddled dark heap that stirred, moaned, then lay silent.

"God, what's happened?" Joel snatched the horse's reins, wondering how she had gotten loose and berating himself for not building a locked shelter for her sooner. He flipped the reins over a low-hanging tree branch and dropped to his knees beside the crumpled figure. Heavy breathing showed life, and Joel turned the body face up toward the moonlight. "Sears!" He ran his hand inside the unconscious man's jacket. His fingers came away warm with the sickening feel and smell of blood.

Every ounce of range-trained muscle and sinew worked together in a mighty burst of strength that got the far-heavier man onto Joel's shoulders and into the cabin. He staggered across the floor. Blood dripped down Sears's arm and left a ghastly red trail behind them. Once, Sears opened his eyes, but he did not speak. Then he lapsed into merciful oblivion.

Joel grabbed a knife and slit Sears's jacket. His stomach lurched when he pulled jacket and shirt open and exposed a smooth back that spurted blood. "Bullet must have gone in the front and come out here." He left Sears long enough to jerk a clean towel from a nail, fold it, and shove it against the wound with one hand. The other hand fumbled with Sears's neckerchief and pressed it against the man's chest where the bullet had entered. The towel soaked through. Joel wadded up the jacket and used it.

"God, I have to have help, or he will die. What shall I do?" He looked despairingly at the door. "If I leave him, he'll bleed to death. Please, send help!"

A minute or an eternity later, hoofbeats, then a call, "Preacher, you all right?" rang like heavenly music in Joel's ears. Two men, solid citizens who had openly proclaimed the need for a preacher in their town, burst through the still-open door. "We heard shots," one said as the second pushed past. "What's goin' on here?"

"Ride for the doctor," Joel sharply ordered. The first man bolted, and rapid hoofbeats sent thankfulness through the young preacher. "Hand me another towel. I can't get the blood stopped," Joel told the second man. Strong hands instantly snatched a towel, wadded it, and he said, "Let me." He held it ready until Joel slid his hands out of the way, then he pressed steadily. By the time the messenger returned with the doctor, the worst of the flow had been staunched.

"Looks like you've been butcherin' hogs in here," the doctor commented. "Get me hot water, clean rags." His dour face and matter-of-fact orders strangely comforted Joel. Obviously, gunshot wounds were a large part of the doctor's practice. He stitched and cleansed and bandaged but shook his head. "I don't recommend moving him far. Are you willing to keep him here? He's lost a lot of blood." The doctor looked dubious, and Joel's hopes fell again.

"He stays here." Joel motioned to Tomkins's room, then went in to make up the bed. "And he's going to make it." He folded his lips in a way that stopped possible argument, and thus began the long fight for Eb Sears's life.

It took all of Joel's prayers and the doctor's skills. For days, death lurked on the cabin's doorstep, grinning, waiting for its prey. Yet, Eb Sears's dogged determination coupled with the care he received, and he slowly began to mend.

Joel and the doctor had long since pieced together the story of the fateful night in the snow. Sears's delirium had loosed his tongue and revealed the heroism he would never have admitted to under normal circumstances. Sears had discovered a plot to murder "that interferin' kid preacher" and make it look like he had been shot during the rustling of Querida. Everyone knew of Joel's love for his horse. Nothing would be more natural than his rushing out to save the mare and being shot in the confusion.

Hoping to warn Joel, Sears sneaked out to

the cabin but had arrived too late and evidently had been mistaken for the victim. Not even he knew exactly who was in on the nefarious scheme, but Tomkinsville noted the significance of certain Missing Spur habitués who mysteriously disappeared in the night. A posse rode out, but enough snow had fallen to cover tracks, and they turned back.

Joel marveled at the strange paths God used to accomplish His work. Years earlier, Sears had been felled by a jealous man who had hoped to get rid of two enemies at once. Now, he had saved Joel's life by nearly giving his own. In addition, the devotion Joel showed in his care for Sears won for him even higher esteem than all of his preaching.

A greater good came from it. The people of Tomkinsville rose in their might and declared that either the Missing Spur tone down or the town would be missing a saloon. The worried proprietor, who might or might not have been part of the plot, instituted some rules and shortened the hours the saloon stayed open. An "accidental" shooting of someone was one thing, but the deliberate planning of a murder and the resultant near killing of Sears did more to clean up the wild atmosphere of the town than Joel had even dreamed of.

Not until it was safe to leave Sears in willing, protective hands did Joel hold church again, this time in the lobby of the town's hotel. It was packed, and at the end of the service, a leading citizen announced that people were contributing money and that as soon as the weather cooperated — which might not be until spring — Tomkinsville would have its own church. He added, "With all due respect, I reckon seeing you live out what you preached and watching you take care of Eb Sears has showed us what we need to do." Joel had to bite his lip to keep from letting out a cowboy yell of happiness.

A few days later, Joel returned home to a table groaning with home-canned goods, two dressed chickens, and a bushel basket of root vegetables. "What's all this?"

Eb grinned, the first real smile Joel had seen on him since the shooting. "Folks musta thought I needed more n'r'shment than I was gettin'. They brought this over." He squirmed and winced.

"When's the boys gonna bring a wagon and haul me outa here?" His face turned dull red. "I've been clutterin' up your cabin long enough."

A wild idea popped into Joel's head and out his mouth. "Why don't you stick around, spend the winter here with me? It's lonesome since Tomkins left." He saw a wistfulness in the other man's face, quickly hidden, and blandly went on. "No one's going to be out rounding up cattle until spring, anyway."

Eb opened his mouth to speak, but Joel forestalled him. "Soon as you feel like it, there's lots you could do. I'd like to go hunting but don't know the country. Then with winter about to pounce on us, we'll need a mountain of wood."

"I'll think on it. Not sure how I'd like livin' with a preacher, even one who ain't like any preacher I ever met."

Joel wisely kept silent. Sears must have thought on it, but the subject never came up again. The minute the doctor pronounced him fit to ride, however, he took Joel on a hunting trip that ended with enough venison to provide them meat for a long time.

During the weeks together, Sears became "Eb" and "Preacher" changed to "Joel." A bond forged between the two men, and Joel learned the other side of the grudge that had caused the problem between Gideon and Sears.

"Only girl I ever cottoned to," Eb said one evening when the fire roared in the fireplace and shadows hid his face. "She liked me, too, until your uncle came. I knew I wasn't good enough for her, but I never meant bad by her." He shifted uneasily and stared into the flames. "I was aimin' to ask her to marry me, so I got sore when Gideon — Cyrus then — sent her out of town. I got drunk, which I hadn't done for a long time, made some dirty comments, and got showed up in front of everyone." He sighed. "Wonder what happened to Lily? Some lucky hand prob'ly lassoed her."

"In the spring, I'm going to Colorado Springs," Joel said quietly, aware of what it had cost this private man to share his feelings. "Gideon wanted me to especially look you up — and Lily."

Eb's big frame jerked. "Whaat?"

"That's right. He feels he missed the chance to tell you about God and won't ever be really happy until he knows you've heard it. Lily, too."

Eb's breathing quickened. "Sometimes I get tired of Tomkinsville." He leaned forward and poked at the fire, keeping his face carefully averted. "Since you're goin' to Colorado Springs, maybe I'll ride along.

Not to see Lily, or anythin'," he hastily added. "When you're ridin' a horse like Querida, a feller can't be too careful."

Joel hid the twitch of his lips, but his eyes brimmed with laughter. "I'd be glad to have you. Oh, if you ever get tired enough of Tomkinsville to leave, I think you'd really like Arizona."

In the spring of 1889, over the protests of the majority of Tomkinsville, Joel and Eb Sears rode away, promising to see if a minister could be found for the little church that would be built soon. They silently halted Querida and the stocky bay that Eb rode. "Ranger's a good horse," he said, and pride shone in his eyes. "Not rustler bait like your Querida, but a good horse." He had sold the horse he bought from Joel to pay his way to Colorado Springs and to get some new clothes. "Never thought I'd wish I saved my money." He laughed, then turned the corners of his mouth down. "I guess it ain't too late. If I should take a notion to go see the Double J ranch of yours in Arizony, I don't wanta ride in lookin' like some scarecrow. Your folks'd think you took up with low comp'ny."

"They'll never think that about you, Eb," Joel said.

Admiration that had begun with the older man's willing sacrifice to save Joel and had grown during the winter months brought an unaccustomed gentleness to Eb's face, but all he said was, "Adiós, Tomkinsville. Maybe I'll see ya again and maybe I won't." He waved to the town in the valley, then rode down the trail, giving Joel a moment alone to silently bid farewell to his first parish and to offer a special prayer that the work the Lord had allowed him to begin might continue in this tiny part of the country.

The closer they got to Colorado Springs, the quieter Sears grew. Finally, Joel demanded, "Eb, something's been eating you ever since we rode out of Tomkinsville. What is it?"

A sigh came clear from the rundown heels of Sears's boots. His face filled with misery. "What if we can't find Lily? It's been a lotta years. Or worse, what if we find her and she —" He choked on the words.

Sympathy and wonder at a love that could live for such a long time without nourishment roughened Joel's voice. "We'll find her, and she'll be the same girl you knew except now she'll be a woman — nearly thirty."

"I hope so." Sears's gloomy countenance did not lighten. "Sometimes I think I oughta stayed back there." He jerked a thumb toward the west. "Fool thing. Here I am gettin' close to forty and chasin' over the countryside like a moonstruck calf."

"Who says age has anything to do with love?" Joel flared back. "Wait 'til you get to the Double J and see Judith and Gideon. They're more in love now than when they got back together in Arizona, and that's been almost as many years since you saw Lily." He pressed his point home. "Not many men are privileged to love someone the way you've done. Honestly, even though things didn't work out the way you wanted them to, would you trade your feelings and memories?"

"Not for a gold mine." Sears's eyes flashed, then he grinned shamefacedly.

Joel threw back his head, and a clear, ringing laugh brought a reluctant smile to his partner's lips. Then Eb said, "Just ya wait. One of these days some purty little filly's gonna get ya standin' on your head, then I'll be the one to haw-haw." Anticipation stamped a boyish look on his features. "Ya still ain't said how we'll find Lily."

"Don't you think that if God brought me hundreds of miles to make sure she knows about Him, He can help us find her?"

Sears cocked his head to one side. "I don't see no signposts nailed on trees and sayin', 'This way to Lily.' " A crooked grin replaced his grumbling. "But, we ain't there yet."

Joel laughed again, but a frown puckered his forehead. He gazed unseeingly down the well-traveled road they had found when they left the trail. "I wish I could be as sure of finding my father as I am of finding Lily. Eb, if Lily's married and happy, would you consider going on to Texas with me, at least for a spell? We got along over the winter." Desire for human companionship on his uncertain journey crept into his voice.

Sears grunted. "Maybe. Watch out there, Ranger!" He swerved the bay to the side of the road to make room for a wagon coming toward them. Querida followed.

"How far to town?" Joel called when the nondescript wagon pulled abreast of them.

"Less than a mile." The driver waved and drove on.

Joel felt the stiffening go out of his knees. He had blithely promised to find Lily. *God, please help us.* Such a few words to request aid. *If only everyone realized how available God is!*

It took time, in a town as big as Colorado

Springs, to find anyone who might know Lily. Joel and Eb inquired at a couple of rooming houses, some stores, and a bank. Always the answer was, "No, don't recall a Lily." Many of those they questioned were recent arrivals.

"Try the stage line," one helpful man advised. But the old-time drivers had long since moved on, replaced by young fellows.

For five days they searched in vain, then Joel came down to breakfast in the modest lodgings they had found and announced, "We've been going at it all wrong."

"Who sez?" Sears put down a forkful of flapjacks dripping syrup.

"What we need to do is find out who the old-timers are around here." Joel attacked the steaming plate of cakes their landlady slid before him. "We'll go back to the biggest dry goods store and start there." Eb eyed him but said nothing. Thirty minutes later, they marched into the emporium. "Who's the owner?" Joel asked a clerk.

"Why, Mr. Livingston." The pale-faced young man in a store-bought suit looked surprised. "His office is up there." He waved toward a set of stairs. "Go right up."

Conscious of the clerk's stares, Joel grinned and told Eb, "Soon as we find where she is, we'll get you a suit like that

61

jasper's wearing."

Eb just snorted and kept on climbing.

Five minutes later, a secretary, who could be a twin to the clerk, ushered them into Livingston's office. A sigh of relief escaped Joel. Good. The gray-haired man looked old enough to have settled Colorado Springs, but even thick glasses failed to hide his keen eyes.

"Sir, we're looking for a girl who came in on the stage from a mining town named Tomkinsville about thirteen years ago," Joel began. "Her name is Lily."

The man sprang from his chair; his glasses fell to the floor and shattered. "Lily! Who are you, and what do you want with her?" His hands shook, and he stared at the strangers.

A great leap of hope warmed Joel's words. "Years ago, my uncle helped her get here. My name is Joel Scott, and this is Eb Sears who used to know Lily."

Unashamed tears stood in Livingston's eyes. "Thank God you've come. If ever Lily needed friends, it's now."

Sears pushed past Joel and confronted the distraught man. His big hands worked. "Where is she?" he demanded hoarsely. "What are ya to her, and why is she needin' friends so bad?"

Livingston fumbled in his pocket and brought out another pair of glasses. He slipped them on, obviously fighting for control. "Lily is my daughter-in-law. I gave her work when she first came to town. My son fell in love with her, and they married. Last fall he was thrown and killed. Since then, Lily's changed from a happy woman to a little black shadow. Doctors say it's shock and if she doesn't come out of it soon, she'll die."

CHAPTER 4

"No!" Eb gave a strangled cry, then determination straightened his shoulders and snapped his head into a fighting position. Color came back to his pale face, and he wordlessly turned to Joel.

"May we see her?" Joel hesitated. "Or would it be better if you told her we were here and asked if she'd see us?"

Livingston shook his head. "She's refused to see anyone except my wife and me and the boy."

"Boy?"

"My grandson. He's five, only child she and my son could have. I think if it hadn't been for him, she'd have given up before this. But she's so tired from refusing to eat, even for Danny's sake, she can't go on much longer. Perhaps the surprise of seeing you will bring her around." He turned to Eb and held out his hands imploringly. "Forgive me for asking, but did you care for her?"

64

"From the first time I saw her." It came from the heart.

"Thank God." Livingston wrung Sears's hand. "Come with me."

Eb looked down at his riding garb. "Shouldn't I get some better clothes? I aimed to buy a suit."

"No, no." Livingston impatiently shook his head. He led his visitors out a private entrance, down a flight of stairs to the street, and across it. "Be what she remembers."

Joel and Eb silently followed the almost-running store owner a few blocks over to a residential area. A large, white frame house sat back in a cluster of trees. Livingston threw open the door and ushered them inside. A sweet-faced older woman rose from a low chair, her hands dripping yarn and bright knitting needles. A dark-haired, dark-eyed child solemnly looked up from his place on the floor at his grandmother's feet. Joel heard Eb's quick intake of breath and knew Danny must be the childish reflection of Lily.

"Mama, this is Eb Sears, an old friend of Lily's," Livingston explained. "The young man is Joel Scott, nephew of the kind young stranger who gave her money and sent her to Colorado Springs."

65

Emotion crumpled the woman's face, and she hastily said, "Danny, go to the kitchen, and ask Hannah to give you a cookie."

"All right, Grandma." The child trotted away.

For a moment, Joel became that child, being sent away while grown-ups talked. He remembered the brown faces of the Mexican servants at the Circle S and how Rosa and Carmelita welcomed a tired, uncertain little boy.

Then, Livingston said, "I'll just take Mr. Sears up first, if it's all right." He looked anxiously from Eb to Joel. "Lily won't know you, Mr. Scott."

"That's fine," Joel said, but he leaned close to Sears and whispered in his ear, "I'll be praying."

Eb gripped his hand. "Come as far as the door in case I need ya." Joel quietly followed the other two men up a flight of stairs, down a comfortable hall to an open door, then stopped. Livingston stepped through with Sears right behind.

"Lily, here's an old friend, come all the way from Tomkinsville to see you."

Joel could see every detail of the airy, wallpapered room and the slender, girlish woman who slowly rose from a rocking chair. Her dark eyes all but filled her thin face. Seldom had he encountered such gulfs of despair and sadness. *God, give Eb the right words.*

"Howdy, Lily." In the strain of the moment, all Sears's insouciance rose to sustain him. "You've been under the weather, huh?" He crossed the room with his hand held out.

She stumbled toward him. "Eb? Eb Sears?" A flicker of life stole into her eyes. "Why, after all these years! You look just the same."

"You don't," he told her frankly. "You're better lookin' now than ya were in Tomkinsville." A blush stained her pearly face, but Eb took her little white hands in his for a moment, then released them. "Sorry about your husband, Lily, but ya sure have a great little buckaroo downstairs. He's a mite puny, though. Now that spring's here, you'll need to be gettin' him out in the fresh air so he can get some color."

Joel had caught the flash of pain when Eb mentioned Lily's husband, but it disappeared into a little frown at the word *puny*. How wise of Eb to get her attention on her son and off her own problems. Concern for Danny could be the first step to her own healing.

"I brought someone you'll wanta see," Eb continued. "Joel Scott, nephew to the Scott

67

who rode in, staked Tomkins, and sent ya out of Tomkinsville." He stepped aside, and Joel came into the pretty room.

"Lily, my uncle Gideon — who called himself Cyrus when he knew you — never forgot you or Eb." Joel quietly explained how Gideon could no longer travel long distances without pain and that he had come in Gideon's place. The growing interest in her face rewarded him. "Most of all, he wanted to tell you how much he regretted failing you."

"Failing me!" Lily backed away and sat back down in her rocker. "Cy— Gideon Scott *saved* me. If it hadn't been for him, I'd never have come here or met Dan or had little Danny or . . ." Her hands tightened on the arms of her chair.

Joel nodded, pleased with her response but noting how tired she looked. "Gideon sent you a special message, but it can wait. You need to rest. We'll come back later if you like." He held his breath.

"For supper, perhaps?" Lily looked at her father-in-law, who eagerly agreed. The three men walked out and back downstairs. Mrs. Livingston stood waiting.

"Mama, she's coming down for supper, and these men will be our guests." Happy tears filled the woman's eyes and overflowed when Livingston brokenly explained, "It will be the first time in more than a month that Lily has left her room." In a wave of thanks and more tears, Eb and Joel finally got away, promising to be back no later than five o'clock.

With one accord, they walked to the livery stable, saddled and mounted Querida and Ranger, and rode for miles, viewing Colorado Springs and the surrounding area.

When they headed back to town, Sears quietly said, "I'm still goin' to get new clothes, but no dud's trappin's. Lily ain't used to me in city clothes." He paused and waited until they reached the stable again before adding, "Joel, ya may have to go lookin' for your daddy without me." His rock-stern expression softened, and he glanced in the direction of the Livingston home. "Somehow, this feels like the end of the trail for this cowpoke. I ain't askin' anythin' of Lily 'cept to be a friend. I just feel I can help her and the buckaroo by stickin' around."

"I understand," Joel assured his friend. "The Double J will always be there no matter what happens."

"Yeah." Eb cleared his throat. "Uh, when ya said that God of yours would help us, I was leery. But we found her, didn't we?" He took a deep breath, held it, then expelled it. "If He makes her well, I'll start ridin' His trail."

"No, *no,* Eb!"

Joel's outcry froze Sears. His face hardened. "Ain't I good enough, after all ya said about Him followin' lost critters?" He laughed bitterly. "Mighta known I was playin' against a stacked deck."

"It's not that." Joel felt compelled as he had never been before. His heart burned. "Everything I said is true, but you can't bargain with God the way you'd horse trade, promising Him this if He'll do that. You know I'd give anything for you to follow the Master, but it has to be everything or nothing. Either you choose to do what you know is right and stick with it *even if Lily dies,* or it's no good, Eb."

The anger faded from Sears's face. A muscle in his left cheek twitched. "That's a mighty powerful prop'sition," he said slowly.

"It can't be any other way. Otherwise, the only reason we'd accept Christ would be for what we could get out of it."

"Isn't that what a feller does anyway?" Sears demanded. "He says yes to God so he can skitter out of gettin' punished for all the mean things he's done."

Joel never wavered. "Some folks do just

70

that, but people who are smart give themselves because they love and appreciate what God did for them, not just to keep from getting what they deserve."

Eb grunted and changed the subject. Joel, however, noticed how thoughtful and withdrawn Eb acted while selecting his new shirt, vest, boots, hat, and pants at the emporium and while shaving, more carefully than usual. At five minutes to five, they knocked on the Livingstons' door, shiny-clean and expectant. A new dignity surrounded Sears, and Joel realized that the selflessness evident in his friend's life had changed a tough rider into a man who would put aside his own desires for the sake of another.

By early summer, Lily had lost much of the shadow in her eyes. Eb simply would not allow her to remain in her room and brood. Time after time, he coaxed her into walking, then riding, "Because Danny needs his mama, not just a roughneck like me," as he said.

Sometimes Joel joined them. He had faithfully delivered Gideon's message, the gospel of salvation, to Lily. In her, he found depths of bitterness that God would allow the husband she had loved to die in a senseless

71

accident. Yet, Lily found gradual healing in the fact that God had lost His only Son — not in an accident, but in the deliberate plan to save His creation. She began to open like a tightly closed rosebud, and by the time Joel rode away in late summer, Lily and Eb both hovered on the edge of committing their lives to their Master.

Joel had intended to follow the trail to Wyoming and Montana that Gideon had taken, but the inner urgency that had prodded him, then subsided, rose sharply. On a clear summer morning, he shook hands with Sears, vaulted onto Querida's back, and turned his face toward Texas.

Well past nineteen, he no longer looked all boy. New maturity firmed his lips except when he smiled. The experiences of the past months showed in his compassionate gaze, a gaze that held more tolerance for those who slipped and fell than when he first left Arizona. Where once he would have condemned, now he stooped to lift. Yet, always in the depths of his heart, fire and ice lived side by side: the fire of his passion to find Cyrus Scott, the icy realization it might never come to pass. The thought made him tremble, and the long miles Querida carried him became hours for introspection. He had never been alone for such an extended time.

First Tomkins, then Sears had provided an older and more experienced influence. Now he rode alone except for the uncanny feeling of companionship he knew must be God.

At times, Joel and Querida were tiny black dots, the only moving creatures in a vast expanse of sky and land. Then it was that Joel missed the mountains, the wilderness. How could anyone live forever in a rolling country that stretched from horizon to horizon in every direction with never having the friendly peak of a jutting mountain to offer encouragement? In sheer desperation, he sought out those riding his way, often veering from his course for the sake of hearing another human voice. After a few times, he gave this up; the naked greed in the eyes of many who he met betrayed their lust for Querida, and he slipped away.

Tired and drooping, Joel trailed into San Scipio country. He was amazed at how much he recognized and was thrilled when landmarks brought the familiar feeling he had been there before.

Almost a year after he left the Double J, the young minister and his faithful Querida, more beloved than ever after their arduous journey, *clip-clopped* into the dusty town that had changed so little that Joel blinked

73

in astonishment. Had San Scipio been asleep these long years? No, for on closer examination, he saw signs of weathering, a few new houses. Yet, the illusion of time standing still persisted, so much so that he gasped in astonishment when he saw the church his grandfather had built now had a small, cozy cabin next to it with smoke curling from the chimney.

Tempted to stop and see who lived there, Joel shook his head. "Not yet," he told Querida. "Just a little longer, and we'll be at the Circle S." Strange that he had not said home, or was it? Most of his life had been on the Double J. "Trot along, Querida. Maybe there will be letters from home."

In response to his voice, the black mare raised her drooping head, pricked her ears, and speeded up while Joel's keen gaze shifted from side to side in his unwillingness to miss any cherished childhood sites. Then they topped the promontory rise that overlooked the Circle S; below lay the ranch, warmed by the late afternoon sun. With a cry, Joel slid from the saddle. He raised his glance to the hills and felt a surge of strength go through him. Surely God would somehow, in some way, lead him to his father. Why else would he feel closer to that unknown man than at any other time in his life?

Stiff from long hours riding, Joel swung back into his saddle and started down to the valley. With every step Querida took, Joel relived childhood days on the Circle S. The cottonwoods he had climbed now rose tall with many years' growth. But the house looked the same — foot-thick cream walls that held heat in or cold out, depending on the season. A red-tiled roof that glistened in the sun. Joel's heart pumped. He had not sent word of his arrival, and mischief tilted his mouth skyward. He would just bet that Grandpa and Grandma would be surprised at how much he had changed from the almost seven-year-old who rode away atop a covered wagon. Yet, when he reached the hacienda-style house and called, "Anyone home?" Joel knew the seven-year-old boy still lived inside him.

The massive front door opened, and a man stepped out. Life's tragedies had silvered his hair, thinned him to gauntness, and carved permanent furrows in his face. But they had not been able to bow the large head or bend the shoulders that were held as erect as Joel remembered. Intent on the similarities and changes in Lige, Joel stayed in the saddle until the booming voice he would have recognized anywhere asked,

"Well, are you going to sit there all day? Light down, Boy." In three giant strides, Lige reached Querida and held out his hand. His ox eyes rolled, still blue as Texas bluebonnets.

Joel dismounted, grabbed the large hand, and felt his eyes sting. He opened his mouth to speak, but a rush of flying feet halted him. A whirlwind with wiry arms and a tear-stained face caught him. "My baby!"

"Don't carry on, Naomi," Lige told his laughing, crying wife. "Let him loose long enough to look at him. He's no baby."

Joel's grandmother pulled back. Although her hair had also whitened, she looked less changed than Lige. Her eyes still snapped in the way he remembered. "Elijah Scott, it doesn't matter if he is half as tall as a mountain, this is my little boy come home." She hugged him again, announced, "Your room is ready," and fled toward the front door. "By the time you're washed up, Rosa and Carmelita will have a meal ready. You look like you could use one! There'll be hot water in your room. See that you use it. I never saw such a dusty rider." She vanished inside after her pronouncements from the porch.

"I guess Grandma will never believe I'm grown up." Joel laughed. The peppery nature that hid beneath her usual calm made him a child again. Strangely, it felt good.

"Mighty fine piece of horseflesh." Lige turned from Joel to the tired mare. "This the one you wrote about when you were a lad?"

"Yes." Joel caught the reins in one hand and headed for the corral. "I need to clean her up. She's carried me a long way."

"Better not risk Naomi's wrath," Lige suggested with the hint of a twinkle in his eyes. "I'll care for — what's her name?"

"Querida — Spanish for *beloved.*"

Lige looked amused but did not say anything, just took the reins and admonished, "I'd step lively, if I were you."

Joel did. He barely wasted a glance on the large hall except to see it had not changed. The polished dark floor and furniture attested to loving care. Bright serapes on the cream plaster walls and matching, woven Mexican rugs welcomed him. So did the courtyard just outside, abloom with late summer flowers. The fountain splashed just the same as the fateful day he and Judith came to the Circle S. He started toward the large room and alcove they had used while there.

"Not there." Naomi appeared at his elbow.

"You'll have Gideon's rooms." Her voice sounded choked. "You are so like him — and your father." The hand she laid on his arm trembled, but the next moment she dashed it across her eyes and crisply reminded him to hurry.

After his long journey from Colorado, Joel found himself content to mosey around the ranch, let Querida rest, and simply soak up the outward peace of the Circle S. Still, after a few days, his youthful resilience overcame his fatigue, and he spent hours riding with Lige. He received a visit from the San Scipio minister, a frank-faced, likable fellow who lived in the little cabin next to the church with his wife and baby.

"I'd be proud to have you preach come Sunday," the minister invited.

Joel hesitated, then caught the perceptible nod from his grandmother and Lige's quickly smothered grin. "I'd be happy to accept," he agreed.

After the visitor drove away, Joel asked, "Do they — the church — know it wasn't Gideon —" He could not go on in the face of the pain that replaced Lige's half smile and his gruff, "They know," before the big man stood and walked out.

"I had to ask." Joel stared at his hands.

"I know, Dear." His grandmother twisted her apron, then smoothed out the folds with painstaking care; Joel's heart twisted at the action. "I don't know how much you remember of that time or what Judith told you, but the Sunday after the message came from Cyrus asking forgiveness, Lige went to church alone. He wouldn't even let me accompany him. Later I learned that he courteously waited until after the sermon had ended, then told the church how unjust he had been to his younger son because of his blind love of the older. He has never mentioned his confession, but I know it must have cruelly knifed his pride." Her hands stilled, and a poignant blue light shone in her eyes. "Joel, there is no man bigger than one who will publicly admit he's wrong, even when the cost is high."

A wave of love and admiration for his grandfather tightened Joel's throat and made his heart pound. He blurted out sympathy and went to find Lige. Before the matter could be closed forever, he must again rush in where wise men would not.

He found Lige standing with one arm resting on the corral fence while he gazed toward the distant mountains. Without turning, he said, "She told you."

"Yes." Joel inhaled a blend of stable and

hay odors. He wanted to cry out his feelings, but Lige had moved to some remote, unapproachable place. Joel's stubbornness rose. "Not many men would do what you did." If he lived as many years as some Old Testament patriarchs, he would never forget Lige Scott's reply.

His grandfather whipped toward him, eyes blazing with sapphire fire. "Boy, any *man* would." Lige strode away, looking even taller to Joel than ever before.

Saturday night at supper, Joel fired the first gun in a private campaign. "Why don't you sell the Circle S and move to Arizona? Gideon can't do all the riding and overseeing of the ranch he'd like to. He sure could use another good hand." He shot a covert glance at Lige and blandly continued, "Grandma, Aunt Judy really needs help with the twins." He chuckled. "Matt and Millie were eight when I left and perfect rascals. I don't know what they're like now, but they're bound to need a firm hand."

"Leave Texas?" Lige's heavy eyebrows met in a forbidding line. "Never!"

"Now, Lige," Naomi began, wistfulness at the mention of the twins softening her face. "My heart's plain hungry to see Gideon and the rest."

Lige shook his massive head as if she had

hit him with a log. "You want to sell this place we've worked to build and go kiting off to Arizona? Woman, are you out of your mind?"

"No." She helped herself to more chili and passed the enormous bowl to Joel. "I just want to see my son." A spasm of pain contorted her smooth face. "We've waited here all these years hoping Cyrus would come back. He hasn't. Must I die without seeing either boy again?"

All the fight went out of Lige. He paled and, for the first time, looked old to Joel, shrunken.

"I don't mean you should sell immediately," he quickly put in. "Why don't you go to Flagstaff for a visit? See how you like the country? Your foreman's run the Circle S for years and can handle things while you're gone."

Lige straightened, and interest crept into his face. "Would you stay here while we're gone — if we go?"

A sickening flood of anguish filled Joel. How could he tell — but he had to say it. "Grandpa, I can't. Ever since I left the Double J, I've felt God had a special mission for me. That's why I'm here, as well as to see you."

Recognition, shock, hope flared in Lige's

81

eyes. "And this mission is —"

Joel licked dry lips. His hands felt cold, his face hot. "To find my . . . my father."

Lige sucked in his breath. Naomi gave a little cry.

Joel leaned forward and planted his hands on the tablecloth before him. "I hope you'll go. There's been too many years between you and my Arizona family." His hands clenched. "Even if you stay, I'll be riding out right after I preach on Sunday."

CHAPTER 5

"Who am I?"

Rebecca Fairfax despairingly stretched her arms out toward the panorama before her, searching for secrets the distant wilderness might hold. How many times had she ridden to this eastern New Mexico vista in hopes it would trigger memories that tumbled in her mind, too ephemeral to hold? Some, Kit Carson and Lucien Maxwell among them, said the scene that lay before her was the grandest in New Mexico. The fan-shaped holdings of the Lazy F ranch lay between forested slopes and rolling plains where the Old Santa Fe Trail and Cimarron River wound into the blue distance. Thousands of acres, broken by a few cattle ranches, spread west past slopes that jutted sharply to glistening, white-peaked mountains. How she loved them! If only —

"Thought I'd find you here."

Vermilion, the mustang that Smokey Travis had broken and given to the girl on her eighteenth birthday just a few months before in December, shied and danced away from the man on foot who had sneaked up on them. Rebecca expertly quieted him, then turned. "What are you doing, creeping up on me, Hayes?" Her usually merry brown eyes flashed fire. Rebellious tendrils of her nut-brown hair had escaped her sombrero and curled moistly around her flushed, angry face. "I told you before to leave me alone!"

Admiration for her charm lightened Clyde Hayes's heavy, sullen face. Bold gray eyes surveyed her from dusty boot tops up her lithe, five-foot, six-inch frame. Hayes doffed his worn Stetson, exposing mousy brown hair. "It's time we had a talk," he announced.

Ugh, how I hate him, she thought. In the last year, he had turned the ranch from a place of freedom to a nightmare. Well, she would not stand for it. "I have nothing to say to you," she retorted.

"Fine way for a woman to talk about the man she's goin' to marry." Triumph leered in his eyes. "Your daddy promised you to me five years ago when I took over as foreman."

Sheer rage threatened to topple Rebecca

from the saddle where she could stick like a cactus on the wildest horse. "Marry you?" She laughed scornfully and rejoiced when an ugly red crept into Hayes's face. "You're thirty-five years old, almost old enough to be my father. Even if you weren't, do you think I'd marry a man I hate with all my heart, especially since you tried to maul me coming home from the rodeo in Raton last fall?"

The red deepened. "Aw, Becky, you know I'd been drinkin' and —"

"And didn't have the decency of a rabid skunk." She dug her spurless boot heels into Vermilion's sides. He snorted, leaped, and Hayes jumped aside, but not before the stallion's shoulder caught him with a glancing blow and sent the would-be suitor flying.

Rebecca laughed again and called back over her shoulder, "Next time I'll run you down. Stay out of our way, Hayes." As soon as they reached level land, she goaded Vermilion into a dead run. Even if Hayes were mounted, he could not catch her. Not a horse for a hundred miles around equaled Vermilion.

Wind whistled past her, and if the girl's sombrero had not been firmly mashed down on her head, the hat would have gone sailing. Her laughter changed to joy, and her spirits rose, but by the time she reached the Lazy F, they drooped again. *Has Father really promised me to Hayes? If so, why?* As clearly as if it had been this morning, she remembered the day the two-hundred-pound man came. Even at thirteen, she had instinctively distrusted him, and she avoided him all she could. Perhaps the change in her father troubled her most. From the moment Hayes took over, Samuel Fairfax lost even the small amount of patience with her that he had shown before.

Now Rebecca wondered, *Does Hayes know something that would discredit Father? If not, why did he lord it over the hands until, one by one, he drove them away?*

Smokey Travis was the exception. Twenty-one, only a few inches taller than Rebecca, he had stuck. Without being vain, she knew the reason — herself. A little smile added sweetness to her lips. She did not mind having Smokey in love with her. It had changed the harum-scarum cowboy from a gambling, drinking man who kept up with the best — no, the worst — of the riders to a considerate, thoughtful protector.

Dark-haired, dark-eyed, and droll, Smokey refused to let Hayes drive him away, and when he could do so without raising Hayes's ire and ending up fired after three years of top service, Smokey unobtrusively saved the girl from encounters with the persistent foreman.

Sometimes Rebecca considered eloping with Smokey. He had never suggested it, but the way his midnight gaze followed her spoke eloquently. If she married him, she would have love and respect, not what she sensed in Hayes — his desire to possess and tame her the way she had seen him tame a wild horse.

"I'm glad he didn't get you," she whispered to Vermilion. The red stallion whinnied. "Smokey used kindness, not mastery. I wonder if real mastery actually is kindness?" She stroked Vermilion's glistening shoulder, uncoiled the lariat she always carried on her saddlehorn, and swung it in a wide loop. It dropped over the gatepost to the corral. Still in the saddle, Rebecca gave an expert tug, and the gate swung open.

"Good girl." The sound of applause from the rider perched on the fence changed her mood again. Smokey Travis's teeth gleamed white against his deeply tanned skin. His dark eyes sparkled. "Where'd you ride? I finished my chores an' looked for you." He shook his head ponderously and put on a long face. "Like looking for a white rabbit in a snowstorm." He doffed his Stetson.

Rebecca rode into the corral, slid from the saddle, and tossed Vermilion's reins to Smokey, the only cowboy the stallion would let groom him. "Will you rub him down, please, Smokey? Father will be a bear if I don't change and get to supper on time."

"How come you're so late?" Smokey cocked a laconic dark eyebrow at her.

All the girl's earlier fury returned. "Skunk Hayes followed me to the promontory."

Smokey jerked straight; his teasing fled. "What'd he want?"

A mischievous devil prompted Rebecca to say, "Me." She regretted it instantly.

Smokey's lips thinned to a slit. His eyelids half closed, and he drawled, "One of these days, me an' Hayes are going to have to have a little talk." His face turned to steel. "Even if he is the boss around here."

A little bell rang deep in Rebecca's mind but not loudly enough for her to figure out why. She grabbed Smokey's checkered sleeve and tugged. "Don't start anything. Please. He'll send you away and —"

"Would you care?" The cowboy stood bareheaded before her, face curiously still.

"You know I would." Her lips trembled. "Sometimes I feel like you're the only friend I have on the Lazy F."

"Good enough for me." Smokey relaxed

and smiled at her.

She pretended not to hear his almost indiscernible "for now" when he led her horse toward the gigantic barn. Rebecca seldom allowed Vermilion the privilege of open grazing. She had seen too many avaricious riders examine her mount's every point and would take no chances on risking Vermilion's loss.

A few paces away, Smokey stopped and glanced back at her. "You know the reason you don't have all the friends you'd like, don't you?" He did not wait for her response. "Your daddy's never cottoned to us cowpokes hanging around."

Red flags waved in her face. "I don't see that it's stopped you," she shot back.

Smokey immediately reverted to his laconic self. "That's 'cause I'm the best shot, the best rider, and the best roper in northern New Mexico."

"Talk about stuck on yourself!" Rebecca made a gamine face at him. "Besides, I can outride you any day."

"Only on Vermilion," he reminded. He scratched his head. "I'll be hanged why I gave away the best horse I'll ever straddle to a braggy girl who thinks she's a real cowpoke."

Rebecca's merry trill brought a sympathetic grin to his rueful face. "Thanks for rubbing Vermilion down," she told him, then ran toward the sprawling log house a hundred yards away.

Formed in the shape of a crude "H," the weathered logs, chinked with thick adobe, had silvered with summer sun until their pale, rounded sides gleamed. Years before, when he took possession, Samuel Fairfax had wisely kept the original house and added to it. Wide porches across the front and west offered a view second only to the one Rebecca saw from the promontory. As usual, she paused and looked back, awed by the magnitude of this part of New Mexico. Could she ever live anywhere else?

Impatiently, she opened the huge front door and stepped inside. No plastered or wallpapered walls greeted her. Just white-washed logs hung with hunting trophies and a smooth floor covered with bearskin rugs both brightened by fantastically designed Indian blankets on couches and chairs.

"Daughter?" Heavy steps from the left arm of the "H" where Samuel had his room preceded her father's entrance into the living area that took up the full front half of the crossbar. Behind it lay an enormous kitchen and Mrs. Cook's quarters.

"Cook by name, cook by trade," the

round-faced woman said when she hired on at the Lazy F shortly after Samuel advertised. "Not for a bunch of roughnecks, though. It's understood that I cook for the family only, plus keep the house clean." She fondly repeated the story during Rebecca's growing-up years. Each time Mrs. Cook grew bolder, though, her boss grew more timid.

The girl loved her too much to admit she had trouble believing her father "just up and lay down and rolled over like a pup," so she merely chuckled and told Mrs. Cook how lucky they were to have her.

"There's plenty of others who'd be glad for my services," Mrs. Cook always said darkly. "Folks who won't be prying into what doesn't concern them."

Rebecca knew it would take an avalanche to uproot their cook/housekeeper, but the threat of her leaving served as an excuse not to ask about a possible Mr. Cook.

"Rebecca?" Samuel stepped into the living room and frowned with displeasure. "Why aren't you ready for supper? I won't have you at the table wearing riding clothes."

With the new awareness that had been growing since she turned eighteen, Rebecca surveyed him through the eyes of a stranger.

Not quite six feet tall, he could be anywhere between forty and fifty; she had learned early not to ask questions. About 180 pounds, with not an ounce of fat, blue eyes, and graying brown hair, he wore the face of an old man on a remarkably strong and healthy body.

"I asked you a question." Not a flicker of love showed, although Rebecca knew she represented the only object in his life that could soften him.

Resentment crisped her reply. "I'd be ready if Clyde Hayes hadn't waylaid me." She ignored the storm signals that sprang to his face. "Why don't you tell him to lay off? I'm not going to marry him, ever, even if you did tell him I would." Color burned in Samuel's face at her well-placed shot, and she incredulously added, "So he wasn't lying." A pulse beat in her throat. "Father, how dared you do such a thing? He's a . . . a snake." She shuddered, as much at the look in her father's eyes as at the grim prospect of ever belonging to a man like Hayes.

"It's not for you to question your father." He retreated into the coldness that normally brought her to heel. "Hayes can run the Lazy F when I'm gone. You can't. You may as well get used to the idea."

Did she dare tell him Hayes had tried to manhandle her on the way home from Raton? She opened her mouth . . . closed it again. If he believed her, he would kill Hayes. No matter how much she hated him, she would not have blood spilled on her account. "I'll go change."

"See that you do," he told her dictatorially.

She turned toward the right arm of the "H" where the western sun sent slanting rays into her room and the storerooms. His voice stopped her in the doorway.

"I don't want you riding out with Travis again. He's in love with you, and I won't have it. Do you hear?"

Rebecca whirled. Her hands clenched into fists, and she planted her feet apart in a fighting posture. "He's the only friend I have on this ranch except Mrs. Cook. Hayes has driven away every cowboy who tried to be nice and friendly. The men barely speak to me. Do you know how it feels to be imprisoned?"

"Has Travis ever laid a hand on you?"

She hated the suspicion in his eyes. "No," she cried. *That's more than I can say for your precious Hayes.* She bit back the inflammatory words. "He respects me too much."

Her father grunted. "Go change your

clothes."

Dismissed, Rebecca felt like a small child being sent to her room. She ran away from her father's presence into the haven of her bedroom and flung herself on the bed. Tears she would not shed before him came in a hot flood. How much longer could she bear his tyranny? Yet — *"Honour thy father and thy mother"* (Exodus 20:12). Where had the words come from? Rebecca believed in God. *Who could live in such a wonderful world and not believe?* But her knowledge of the Bible was vague, although she dimly remembered a woman's voice reading to her. *Had it been my mother? Do the phrases that sometimes spring into my mind have their source in the mists of my past?*

"Rebecca." The muted roar from the living room brought her to her feet. She made a hasty toilet with water, soap, and soft towels that Mrs. Cook must have fetched while Rebecca and her father argued. Then she slipped into a simple white gown, with a modest round neck, that left her arms bare below the elbows. She threw a gaily colored Mexican shawl over her shoulders, opened her door, and started toward the living room. The sound of voices halted her, but she disdainfully went on, dreading but knowing what she would find. Yes, a white-shirted Hayes, with slicked-down mousy hair and reeking to high heaven with pomade, smirked at her from the round table at one end of the living room where meals were served.

She almost fled to her room. Instead, she lifted her chin, gave the unwelcome guest who more and more frequently joined them for the evening meal a cold nod, and slipped into her chair. At least he had not held the chair for her, the lout.

All through the meal she answered in monosyllables, only when spoken to directly. Not by the flicker of an eyelash did she betray that Mrs. Cook's finest roast beef, mouthwatering rolls, and accompanying vegetables tasted like moldy sawdust to her. The moment she choked down the ambrosia pudding, she pushed back her chair.

"May I be excused, please, Father?" She rose, slim and remote in her white gown and gorgeous shawl. "Mrs. Cook promised to show me a new knitting stitch."

"Not very friendly of you to run off when I'm here," Hayes drawled.

His effrontery stung her to quick but guarded speech. She forced a brilliant smile. "But I've already seen you today, Mr. Hayes." She did not dare put him in his place by calling him Hayes as she usually did except when in the presence of her father. "Or have you forgotten so soon?" She laughed maliciously. "Father, would you believe your conscientious foreman took time to ride all the way to the promontory to talk with me instead of making sure the boys got those draws combed?" Before either man could answer the taunt, she vanished into the kitchen, eyes blazing, and carefully closed the door behind her without slamming it. "I just can't bear it," she burst out.

Mrs. Cook looked up from a pan of soapy water. Suds sparkled on her plump hands and glinted from the worn gold band on the third finger of her left hand. Her shrewd, blue eyes held welcome and sympathy. "You always have me, Child."

"I know." Rebecca crossed the kitchen and hugged the housekeeper, heedless of the flying soap bubbles that rose. "If I didn't, I . . . I . . . I'd run away with Smokey Travis!"

"Now why would you want to go and do that?" the buxom woman asked, eyebrows arching almost to her brown hair, dusted with silver that shone in the lamplight. "You're not in love with him, at least not the way you need to be when you marry." She dried her hands on a towel, hugged Rebecca, then held the girl away from her.

"Child, marriage can be wonderful with the right man or miserable with —"

"Hayes." Rebecca's shoulders shook; her face whitened. "Wouldn't it be better to marry Smokey, even if I don't love him the way you say I should, than to be with Hayes? I'd rather be dead."

Mrs. Cook led her to a small table with two chairs. She gently pushed the weeping girl into one of the chairs, then billowed into the other. "And I'd rather see you dead than married to a varmint like him." Her hand, still warm from the dishwater, stroked the girl's hair. "On the other hand, it wouldn't be right or fair to Smokey for you to up and run off with him just to get away from Hayes."

Rebecca looked up and through her tears saw the puzzled expression in Mrs. Cook's face before the good woman slowly said, "I can't understand why your father's so intent about you marrying Clyde Hayes. It's almost as if our foreman knows some secret Samuel Fairfax doesn't want let out."

"Why, that's what I was thinking earlier today." Rebecca straightened and mopped her face with a handkerchief that Mrs. Cook offered her. "Smokey said something funny, too." She wrinkled her forehead, trying to remember exactly what it was. "No use. It's lost. Mrs. Cook, what would you do if you were me?"

For a long time, the housekeeper did not answer. A shadow crept into her blue eyes, darkening them. Finally she said, "First I'd ask God to help me get things straightened out; then I'd keep my eyes peeled every minute and my ears wide open. There's a lot going on around the Lazy F that I can't figure out, but I have my suspicions."

"What are they?" Rebecca leaned forward and whispered.

"It's not for me to say, at least not just yet."

Disappointed, the girl pounced on the first suggestion. "Does God help or even care about me?"

A look of reproach left her feeling scorched with shame when Mrs. Cook quietly told her, "You know better than that. If there's one thing I've taught you in all the years on the Lazy F, it's that God loves everyone and it's up to us to believe it." Her voice changed to a deceptively bland tone. "Of course, it's a lot easier to talk to Him when we know we're His children, and that only comes after we invite His Son to live in our hearts."

Longing rose in Rebecca. "I'm so tired of fighting. I wish I could, but —" A vision of

98

the smirking Hayes danced in the warm kitchen. "He wouldn't want to live in my heart. It's too filled with hate for Hayes," she bitterly said.

"I don't like Hayes, either," Mrs. Cook admitted. "Just remember, we can despise what folks do, but God says we can't hate the miserable sinners who are trying our patience." She stood, looked at a watch she drew from beneath her apron. "Too late for the knitting lesson. Off to bed with you, Child, and don't forget to talk to God."

Rebecca did not answer. It would only hurt Mrs. Cook to know how many times her darling had talked to God and found that He did not answer. She sighed. Perhaps it would not hurt to try again. Things could not get much worse, or she would do something awful.

"God, I'm in the middle of a mess," she stated frankly when she had climbed into a nightgown and knelt by her bed. "I don't even know how to pray." Dissatisfied but void of words, she quickly said, "Amen," and got into bed.

Her outdoor life provided exercise enough to put her to sleep immediately, but first she remembered Smokey's words. *Even if he is the boss around here.* She sat bolt upright. *Why did Smokey think Hayes was boss, not Father?*

CHAPTER 6

Among the hundreds of beautiful places to ride on the Lazy F, one lured Rebecca again and again. The day after her encounter with Hayes, she expertly saddled and mounted Vermilion. Warm spring sun had blossomed the range into meadows of flowers. Cottonwood and willows along the stream born in the mountains that ran through Fairfax's land and never went dry whispered secrets. In the east, the Old Trail continued its never-ending way with its sister, the Cimarron, and the sloping range smoothed into an endless prairie gray. Melting snow patches on the mountains above smiled down on the girl and her horse as they weaved their way up steep sides until they rode through groves of aspens that quivered with every breeze.

Rebecca and Vermilion emerged from the grove onto a promontory. "Whoa." She pulled lightly on the reins and wheeled the red stallion. Never did she take this particular ride without turning to look over the valley floor. The ranch in the distance looked small by comparison with the vast world spread below her.

A Mexican village she seldom was allowed to visit huddled its adobe houses together as if for protection against danger. She remembered a fiesta day, the colorful clothing, strum of guitars, and happy dancing from a year before and laughed at the way she had deliberately slipped away from home in defiance of Samuel Fairfax's orders.

"It was worth being shut up in my room for three days," she confessed to Vermilion, with a toss of her head that dislodged her sombrero and tumbled her nut-brown hair around her laughing face. The merry sparkle left her eyes. "Why doesn't Father want me to visit the village? Or ride to the neighbors?"

Vermilion shook his head, and his reddish mane brushed the girl's gloved hand.

She patted him. "I know you want to go. You're thinking about the lush green grass at Lone Man Cabin." In spite of the warm day, a shiver went through her, but she nudged Vermilion into a trot and climbed the slope to a small pass that lay above her destination. Lone Man Cabin stood in a grove of white-trunked aspens in the heart of a canyon. It had been built years before by a settler who had been killed by hostile Indians before peace came to New Mexico. A shining stream intersected the aspen grove and ran beside the dilapidated shack that, nevertheless, held a morbid fascination for Rebecca. The gobble of a wild turkey, from a thicket to her left, brought a thrill to her nature-loving heart, and she called, "Run, you white-tailed beauty!" to a graceful antelope that sprang from its grazing and bounded away at the crack of Vermilion's hooves on rock.

Minutes later, they paused by Lone Man Creek. Rebecca slid from the saddle, threw herself flat, and drank her fill of the icy water while Vermilion splashed into the stream below her, then lowered his head to drink. Satisfied, he sent up sprays of water, lunged out of the creek, and grazed, no stranger to this haunted, lovely spot.

Something about the place felt strange, not like its usual air of solitude that both fascinated and repelled the girl. She rose to investigate, walked past the cabin, and stopped short.

A fence of peeled poles, still oozing, stretched from slope to slope. A wide, closed gate kept horses and cattle from straying.

"Why, there's never been a fence here before!" Rebecca took an involuntary step toward the gate.

"Stop right there, little missy." Words harsh as the black-browed man who glided out of a clump of aspens froze her to the ground.

"Who are you, and what are you doing on the Lazy F?" she demanded, more angry than frightened. "What's this fence doing here, and why are those horses and cattle penned?"

"Beggin' your pardon, Missy, but that's my business, not yours."

"It *is* my business." Using the quick draw Smokey Travis had taught her, Rebecca pulled the small but deadly weapon she always carried and pointed it rock-steady at the intruder. "I'm Rebecca Fairfax, and this is my father's land."

A curious whistling sound alerted her, but too late. A noose sang and dropped over her head and shoulders, pinning her arms to her side with a tightening jerk that loosened her fingers until the pistol dropped. The next instant, she lay on the ground, securely bound.

The black-browed man leered down at her. "So, Missy, thought you'd hold me up, did you?" He bent, and she flinched from the smell of sweat and his whiskey breath. "Now, there ain't no use of you bellerin', so I won't gag you. Just keep your mouth shut, and you won't get hurt." He blindfolded her and laughed crudely. "My pard's pertic'ler about folks seein' his face."

Deprived of sight, Rebecca's other senses intensified. She strained her ears, trying to hear above the hard pound of her heart. *Who is the second man, the one who roped me and doesn't want to be seen?*

Hayes! The word shot into her brain like sunlight into a dark well. It drove out the fear that had paralyzed her when the evil-looking man stood over her. Bad as she suspected Hayes to be, he would not stand for any man except himself to maul her. So she lay still, motionless except for her cautious exploring fingers behind her back that tried to pick at the knots and loosen the lariat.

If I can get even one hand free, I'll snatch the blindfold off and get a good look at Hayes, she promised herself. Her plan did not work. Hayes, or whoever had tied those knots, obviously did not take chances. She could not budge them. Her mind steadied, considered, and rejected a half-dozen plans. Suddenly, hot blood pumped from her heart in a spurt of determination. She had it! Turning her head to one side, Rebecca slowly rubbed her face against the ground, flinching when dirt imbedded in her cheek but gradually working the blindfold up far enough for her to see.

She had been right. Hayes and the man who had accosted her by the fence stood several yards away in low conversation. Once, Hayes glanced at her, and she stilled and closed her eyes, praying he would not notice the position of the blindfold. He looked angry, yet something in his manner told Rebecca he was pleading with the other man. Again, she listened intensely and managed to catch a few words. ". . . didn't see me . . . you lay low . . . we'll meet. . . ."

Hayes turned abruptly and walked out of her line of vision. Rebecca did not dare move her head, but her keen ears picked up the creak of saddle leather, then guarded hoofbeats that increased into a diminishing drum. She thought of the look the black-browed man had given her and almost called out. Better to take her chances with Hayes than be left here with his partner.

"Sorry, Missy." Cold steel slipped between her wrists and cut the lariat; a rude hand snatched the blindfold from her eyes. "I didn't reckon you were really Sam Fairfax's girl." He laughed uneasily, and something flickered in his eyes. Rebecca knew he had lied. "A feller can't be too careful," he went on.

She stood and brushed debris from her riding habit. "My father will hear of this outrage," she furiously told him. She bit her tongue to keep from flinging out that she knew Clyde Hayes was involved in whatever nefarious scheme this turned out to be.

"I wouldn't say anythin' if I was you." The black-browed man opened his sheep-lined coat and showed a badge of some kind. "I've been appointed to look into the rustlin' that's goin' on, and a purty little thing like you wouldn't want to throw a hitch into my 'nvestigations, now would you?"

Not for a minute did she believe him. Yet, when Rebecca thought of the isolation, she wisely did not argue. Mrs. Cook always said there were more ways than one to skin a cat. Rebecca did an about-face and became the helpless female who is impressed with the law. "Oh, my, I can see why you couldn't have me interfering!" She gave him a dazzling smile that successfully masked her fear and disgust. "Deputy — it is *deputy,* isn't it?"

"Dep'ty Crowley." He half closed his eyes,

and she saw suspicion in their murky depths.

"It's just that I got such a shock, seeing the fence and all." She nodded toward the newly erected barrier. Her frankness lightened the deputy's face, and she went on, "If I'd known you were an honest-to-goodness law officer, I wouldn't have pulled my gun." She almost choked, wondering if he would swallow that, even though what she said was true. "Is the other man a deputy, too?"

"Naw." Crowley spat a stream of tobacco juice dangerously close to his boot. "He's what you might call an intr'sted party." He pulled a plug of tobacco from his shirt pocket, cut off a quid, and stored it in his cheek.

Rebecca wanted to laugh. It made him look like a lopsided chipmunk. Instead, she delicately shuddered. "This has all been most upsetting." She managed a feeble smile that should convince the bogus deputy of her helplessness. "I suppose the corral and the horses and cattle are all part of your plan to catch rustlers?" She hoped her naïve question would disarm him.

"Uh, yeah. That's why it's 'mportant for you to keep mum." His gaze bored into her, and she suddenly felt more afraid than ever.

"I won't tell Father right away," she promised. "You'll probably get your job done soon, and then it won't matter who knows."

A hasty hand to Crowley's mouth half concealed his grin. "You're right, Missy. My job'll be done soon, and it won't matter."

Her cheek smarted from ground-in dirt, and her fingers itched to slap his leering face, but Rebecca chose the better part. "Good-bye, Mr., uh, Deputy Crowley." She turned and walked to Vermilion, who had finished grazing and now stood waiting for her. She put her left foot in the stirrup and swung her right leg across the saddle.

Crowley's voice stopped her. "Say, how about tradin' horses?" His eyes gleamed with the lust for good horseflesh that she had seen dozens of times before when rough men saw Vermilion. "This stallion's too big for such a little girl as you. Now, my mare there —" He nodded at a piebald horse Rebecca would not have ridden to an outhouse. "She's just your size."

What a credulous fool he considered her. Well, that image might just be her best protection. When he stepped in front of Vermilion, Rebecca overcame her desire to ride the man down and cried out, "Oh, be careful! Vermilion only allows me and the cowboy who broke him to handle him." The horse raised both feet in the air to prove her point, and Crowley leaped aside.

"I'd take that out of him," he muttered.

Rebecca brought her horse down and started back through the aspens. "I couldn't sell Vermilion, even to you, Deputy Crowley, but I see you know a good horse when you see one." She wanted to pointedly gaze at the corralled animals but restrained herself. Right now, getting away meant continuing the role she had chosen.

"If you ever change your mind, I'll be waitin'," he called after her.

Thoroughly disgusted, Rebecca did not answer. She used the long miles back to the ranch house to mull over everything that had happened. A half mile from home, the clatter of hooves warned that someone desperately planned to overtake her. A quick glance behind showed Hayes riding bent over the muscular neck of the racing bay he unimaginatively had christened Bay. She fought the impulse to outrun him and composed herself. A little voice inside whispered the significance of this meeting. Under no circumstances must Hayes discover that she had recognized him back at Lone Man Cabin.

"Ho, Becky." He swung up beside her and

110

tipped his Stetson. "Have a nice ride?"

"Splendid. I went clear to Lone Man Cabin. Too bad someone doesn't build a house there. It's the prettiest place around."

"I'll start layin' the foundation tomorrow if you say the word." He pulled Bay closer and laid one hand over hers on the saddle horn where her hand rested. "Say, what happened to your face?"

Rebecca unobtrusively nudged Vermilion with her boot heel, and he danced away, leaving Hayes trying to control Bay, who feared the big red stallion along with most of the other Lazy F horses. "I hit the ground. And I told you I won't marry you."

"Girls change," he doggedly said. "How about forgiv'n' me for last fall?"

Could he really be so thick-headed he thought the only reason she hated him was because of his actions on the way home from Raton when he had been drinking? "Hayes, why don't you find a woman close to your age instead of hanging after me?" she blurted out.

His face darkened, and she knew her taunt had been a mistake. Before he could reply, she innocently asked, "Why, where's your lariat?" She pointed to Bay's saddle horn.

It distracted him, as she had known it would do. Hayes stammered and finally said, "Left it in the bunkhouse, I guess. Yeah, that's right. One of the hands sneaked it out and brought it back soaked. When I find out who, there'll be one less hand on the Lazy F."

She could not resist saying, "I thought we needed every hand we could get. I heard Father telling you to hire all the vaqueros from the Mexican village for spring roundup."

"Maybe I'll wait until after roundup." He lapsed into sullen silence, then asked, "How was everythin' at Lone Man Cabin?"

Rebecca feigned surprise. "Why? Should there be anything wrong?" She saw the quickly hidden but satisfied look in Hayes's eyes and knew it had been his idea for "Deputy Crowley" to swear her to silence about the peeled pole fence, raw in its newness.

"I just haven't ridden out there lately. Guess I should one of these days. Sometimes cattle and horses drift down the canyon by Lone Man Creek." His false laugh could not have fooled Vermilion. "Strange how dumb the critters are. They drift in but not out!"

Not so strange when they are corralled, Rebecca wanted to shout. Instead, she said, "Maybe you and some of the boys should check the canyon. I did see horses and cattle."

They reached the ranch house in time for her to escape more conversation with Hayes. As usual, Smokey Travis waited on the top rail of the corral.

"Travis, why are you sittin' there like a prairie hen on a nest?" Hayes blared, while his nondescript eyes flashed.

Dull red suffused the cowboy's brown face, and he started to speak. Behind Hayes's back, Rebecca shook her head slightly in warning. Smokey's face broke into a smile. "I'm waitin' for you, Boss, an' am glad to tell you we found most a hundred head of cattle up a draw. They must have wandered in there last fall. Anyway, we put the Lazy F brand on at least a dozen new calves and herded the whole kit and caboodle back down with the main herd." His gaze turned to Rebecca's face, and his eyes flashed.

The tension drained from Hayes's shoulders. Overbearing, even crooked he might be, but he loved the range and cattle. "That's good news." He slid off Bay, yanked off the saddle, and gave the horse a slap that sent him whinnying into the pasture nearby. "Fairfax aims to make a killin' on the roundup this spring. The more we sell, the fewer that'll fall to rustlin'."

Smokey had a coughing spell that left him red-faced and teary-eyed. "Sorry, Boss, Miss Rebecca. Must have picked up some dust in my throat." He leaped down from the fence. "I'll take care of Vermilion, if you like," he told the girl.

She started to protest and thought better of it. While she could and did perfectly groom her own horse, she knew Smokey loved Vermilion as much as she did. "Thanks, Sm— Travis," she quickly corrected. She had learned long ago that calling the cowboys by their first names made her father and Hayes furious. No use rousing their ire, especially when she had a secret. The less attention they paid her, the freer she would be to solve the mystery of Lone Man Cabin and the newly constructed fence. She burned to tell Smokey what had happened. She had promised not to report to her father about being waylaid and the developments in Lone Man Canyon but had carefully omitted any promise about not telling Smokey.

How could she get a message to him? When Father was not watching her, Hayes replaced the vigilance. Even when she did not see them, she felt their spying. Well, she could be clever, too.

After supper and dishes, while the two voices rumbled in the big living room, Rebecca covered her white gown with a long, dark cloak that hid every trace of it and allowed her to become just another dark shadow in the night. Praying for luck to find Smokey alone, she groped her way to the bunkhouse and peered in a window. She counted off the hands, from Curly the cook, to Jim, who had been with the Lazy F just a few weeks but long enough to learn that friendliness beyond a nod and "howdy" with the daughter of the house was not permitted. All accounted for — except Smokey.

An iron hand covered her lips. Another jerked her away from the window and into a clump of cottonwoods. "Who're you, an' why're you spying?" someone hissed. Rebecca found herself spun around. *God, help me,* she silently prayed. *If Father or Hayes is holding me, what will happen?*

Strong hands pulled her closer. Miserly light from the edge of the moon that rose over the mountain spilled onto the dark-clad figure, the man who held her. "Rebecca, what are you *doing* out here?"

She sagged in relief and would have fallen if not for his support. "Smokey, thank God!"

"Shh." He picked her up bodily and

stepped deep into the dark shelter of the cottonwood grove. Again, he placed his hand over her lips, but gently this time. Screened by leaves filtering pale moonlight that brightened as Hayes and Fairfax stood smoking on the ranch house porch, she scarcely breathed. She could feel Smokey's deadly calm body coiled ready to spring in her defense. A lifetime later, Fairfax went inside and slammed the door; Hayes marched very close past them. Not until a light came on in the bunkhouse room, which was set apart from the long, tiered-bunk sleeping quarters of the rest of the men, did Smokey remove his hand.

"Sorry. But how'd I know you'd do such a fool thing?"

"I was looking for you," she whispered. In quick sentences, Rebecca told him what had happened from the moment she saw the fence in Lone Man Canyon until she and Hayes reached the corral.

"Why, that skunk!" Smokey shook with rage. "He roped you? I'm gonna call him out right now, and —" He tore free from her involuntary grasp and took a quick step out of their hiding place.

"Smokey, no!" Quicker than a mountain lion, she slid in front of him. "I won't have you kill because of me." She grabbed his arms with hands made strong by fear. "There's a better way to get Hayes. Don't you see? We'll watch and spy and expose his rustling, for I'm sure that's what he's doing."

"Your daddy will never believe it." He stood stock-still in her grip. Enough light sneaked past the trees to show his whitened face and inscrutable dark eyes that could dance with mischief but now looked hard and cold, relentless.

Rebecca shivered. "He will have to. I don't believe Crowley's a deputy any more than you are."

She felt Smokey give a convulsive start before he said in an odd voice, "That's — you'd better go in, Rebecca." His voice changed. "I . . . I'm glad you told me."

"So am I, Smokey. Sometimes I feel the only one who really knows or understands me is God."

He parted branches, checked both ways, then ran with her across the lighted yard to a side door in the right arm of the house where she could slip into a storeroom, then get to her bedroom, unobserved. At the doorway, he leaned down, awkwardly planted a kiss on her forehead, and said, "That's just to let you know God an' me are both on your side." Then he swung away with a remarkably light tread for a man who spent most of his waking hours in the saddle, leaving Rebecca staring after him and feeling less alone now that she had shared her heavy secret.

CHAPTER 7

Sometimes, Joel felt he had been riding forever. Querida scrambled up a game trail and came out on a mesa. Her owner gasped. What a view! Grand country, this New Mexican land. He had been told in Santa Fe what to expect, yet from the backbone of the tableland, between the mountains and foothills, the range curved in a half moon, walled by the Rockies. Dark, timber-sloped gullies joined cedar ridges; a bleached moon cast its pale light. No sign of human habitation for as far as Joel could see; just empty miles unrolling around him.

"We camp out again tonight, Querida." His old habit of talking to his horse and a cheerful whistle brought an answering nicker from Querida, who, freed from saddle and blanket, rolled in spring grass and then contentedly settled to graze.

A crackling fire, a meager meal of toasted biscuits and the last of his dried beef topped off by a treasured tin of peaches, brought a sigh of satisfaction. "Nothing like a meal to lift spirits. Right, old girl?"

Querida raised her head, then went back to munching.

Joel laughed, yet a certain wistfulness shone in his eyes. He washed his few eating utensils, spread blankets on the ground near his fire, and stared into the dying blaze. Now that night surrounded him, even the food could not fend off discouragement. Six months earlier, he had preached in San Scipio with startling results. Now, he rested his head on his saddle and stared at the starry sky, remembering that fateful Sabbath.

For some reason, Joel had struggled with finding a text more than at any other time he prepared a sermon. He considered and discarded a full dozen, settling on one, then another. Yet, all through his study, the words of Jesus in Matthew 5:23–24 remained present. How could he step into a strange pulpit and preach on that text? Yet, how could he deny what he felt led to say?

Refusing breakfast on the gorgeous West Texas autumn morning, he rode to town on Querida, still struggling. Early as he was, a crowd had preceded him. He remembered many of the faces and recognized others' names. One tall, thin, tired-looking woman with straw-colored hair and washed-out gray eyes approached him. She wore clothing more suitable to a young girl than to a woman nearing forty.

"You look just like your dear uncle," she gushed. "Gideon and I were sweethearts years ago." She giggled girlishly.

The grotesque sound, coming from this faded blossom trying to cling to the past, brought a startled, "Really!" from Joel.

"Oh, yes," she chortled, making no effort to lower her voice.

"I'm Lucinda — used to be Curtis. I'm sure dear Gideon has spoken of me."

Joel thanked heaven for the control he had learned over the years that now kept him from laughing at the pathetic woman. Gideon had indeed spoken of Lucinda, sharing how even though he felt sorry for her, she had made his stay in San Scipio as a preacher unbearable with her chasing.

"It's nice you could come, Miss . . . Mrs. . . . ," he managed to say while she pumped his hand up and down.

"Mrs. Baker." She looked skyward and dragged a meek little man forward. "My husband, these past ten years." She gave the man no chance to speak. "Do remember me to your uncle when you see him again."

With an arch smile, she took her husband by the arm. "Come along, or we won't get the front pew." He trotted obediently after her, the way a fawn followed a doe.

"Sweethearts, my eye," someone whispered behind Joel. "Leave it to Lucinda Curtis Baker to kick up a cyclone when there's no more wind than from slamming a door!"

Joel repressed a smile and greeted the next person. After folks stopped coming and every seat was filled and men were standing at the back, the San Scipio minister introduced Joel. "You all remember Gideon Scott, Elijah and Naomi's son. This is his nephew, the Scotts' grandson. I've asked him to bring the Word of the Lord to us today. Brother Joel, you have our careful and prayerful attention."

Joel found it hard to begin. His heart went out to Lige, who sat rigid at the introduction that made no mention of the long-missing real father. Yet Joel had a feeling the text that had been impressed on him was not for Lige's benefit. He opened the worn Bible that traveled on Querida wherever Joel rode. " 'Therefore if thou bring thy gift to the altar, and there rememberest that thy brother hath ought against thee; leave there thy gift before the altar, and go thy way;

first be reconciled to thy brother, and then come and offer thy gift.' " He closed the Bible and leaned forward against the sturdy, handmade pulpit. "I don't know why Matthew 5:23 and 24 has driven all other Scripture passages from my mind and heart ever since I knew I would preach to you." He saw looks of surprise and exchanged glances.

"Perhaps it is because every one of us at times realizes someone, somewhere, has something against us. We may have offended our brothers and sisters years ago and not even recognized it. Or, we may secretly know of times when we spoke unkind words that cut a tender heart." Joel continued preaching in a clear, simple manner, using the thoughts he felt coming. He referred to the healing that comes to both when a child of God seeks out one wronged.

He concluded, "If anything in your life is keeping your gift at the altar from being acceptable to God, make it right." He paused to be sure nothing more needed saying, then sat down.

"Let us pray," the San Scipio minister said. He offered one of the humblest, most beautiful prayers Joel had ever heard and followed it by leading the young guest minister to the back of the church to greet the congregation as they left.

A good half hour later, everyone except Lucinda had gone after having shaken Joel's hand and wishing him Godspeed. Even the meek Mr. Baker silently shook hands, then slipped out.

"Why, Lucinda, you're still here?" The minister turned.

Red-eyed and swollen-faced, the woman said, "I must talk with the Reverend Scott."

Joel cringed. He hated being called Reverend and set apart as some holier-than-others being. He also did not care for a private interview with the woman. Yet, none of her former kittenish attitude remained. His heart went out to her, as it did to anyone in trouble. "Tell my grandparents I'll be home soon," he said to the minister. The other man nodded and left, closing the door behind him.

"What is it, Mrs. Baker?"

Fresh tears poured. "I . . . I've done something terrible." She pressed her hands to her twisting face. "All these years, I should have spoken." The hands fell and revealed a tragic face filled with regret. "I knew, but I didn't want to . . . and then he was gone, and I hated Judith for marrying Gideon. . . ."

He could not make sense of her broken

confession. "What is it you know?" he gently asked.

"Cyrus Scott. He . . . he . . ." The cloud-burst came again.

Joel had always thought novels that said someone's heart stood still were the height of stupidity. Now, he experienced that very thing. He could not speak. He could not breathe. Not until hope for a long-hidden clue to his father's disappearance loosed him to action could he do more than stare at the repentant woman. "What do you know of him?" he inquired hoarsely.

She blew her nose and raised her head. Remorse lent depth to the gray eyes. "The night before he . . . he left, I saw him." Dying sobs still racked her thin frame. "I . . . I thought he was Gideon, and I called out. He was riding toward the ranch. He wheeled his horse, and when I saw who it was, I asked him to tell Gideon how thrilled the town was with his preaching." She sniffed.

"What did he say?" Joel's head spun. Had this vindictive woman held the key to Cyrus's whereabouts all these long years?

"He . . . he laughed in that hateful way he had and said he wasn't a messenger boy for his brother. When he turned back toward the ranch, he laughed again, mocking me, and said, 'Besides, I'm off to Albuquerque.

125

Too bad I can't take Gideon with me and get him away from simpering females like you.' " Anguish filled her voice. "I made up my mind I'd die before helping him or ever telling anyone what he said." She crossed her arms over her thin chest and threw back her head. "I kept that promise until today. But when you read those verses, I knew God meant them for me." Her voice trailed to a whisper.

Hot anger over her silence melted into pity. Her eyes showed long-held pain and what it had cost her to speak. Joel put a warm, strong hand on one of her cold ones. "Mrs. Baker — Lucinda — all we can do to atone of the things we do or leave undone is to repent. That's the wonder of God's grace, that He forgives. Now, you must forgive yourself."

"Should I stand up in meeting next week and confess?"

He knew she would do it but shook his head. "No. I will tell my grandparents, but it would only cause more pain to have San Scipio hashing it over again. Tell your husband, and then accept God's forgiveness."

Something akin to glory gradually crept into her face, and when Lucinda Curtis Baker walked out of the church to her patient, waiting husband, Joel swallowed hard. Thank God for His power that had changed the foolish woman who entered church that day into the new creature who went out.

He shook his head at his musing and, with a glad heart, raced Querida back to the Circle S. His shocking announcement precipitated a crisis. Life flowed back into Lige Scott's face, and he nearly reneged on his promise to take Naomi west.

"Don't you see," he protested, "now we have something to go on, a starting place. Naomi, how can I go to Arizona when Cyrus may be alive and needing me?"

"Your younger son needs you, too, Lige," she quietly reminded. "Will you again choose Cyrus over Gideon?"

He flinched as if she had struck him, and Joel stepped in.

"Grandpa." His face shone with boyish eagerness. He gripped Lige's brawny arm. "If Cyrus is alive, I mean to find him; I vowed that when I left Flagstaff. Gideon needs you. All these years he's longed to see you and blot out the anger between you when he left. We don't know that my . . . my father is in New Mexico. He may have changed his mind or drifted there and gone elsewhere. Can't you trust me to seek him

127

out?" He licked dry lips. "I believe God will help me."

The moment stretched into infinity before Lige bowed his head to a force greater than his own. "Son, I trust you. Naomi and I will catch the train from El Paso as soon as we can get there."

"Do you want me to take you?" Joel offered.

Lige shook his massive head. "No. The sooner you go, the better." He lifted both arms and let his huge hands drop on Joel's shoulders. "Go with God, Joel."

The howl of a distant coyote calling for its mate roused Joel from his reverie. He threw more wood on the fire and pulled his blankets closer against the cold spring night. The long day of riding should have left him weary. Instead, he remained sleepless, even when he closed his eyes against the display of stars hanging low in the sky. How high his hopes had been when he departed from the Circle S a few hours after Lige and Naomi boarded the stage for El Paso!

With youthful exuberance, he ignored the interminable years that stretched between Cyrus's flight from the discovery of his cruel deception and Joel's return to the ranch. He debated leaving Querida on the Circle S and going by train to New Mexico but discarded the idea immediately. He had no guarantee his father had ever reached Albuquerque or that it had not been merely a picturesque stopping place.

While Joel disconsolately reviewed the history of New Mexico, frost gathered and sparkled the range with diamond dust. Cyrus had ridden away in 1874, the same year that opened the bloodiest years of western history in eastern and central New Mexico. Between then and 1879, more desperate and vicious men than could be counted terrorized the land. Three hundred men died in the Lincoln County War that pitted rustlers, desperadoes, and cattlemen, honest and crooked, against each other. Billy the Kid boasted twenty-one killings. Sentenced to be hanged in April 1881, he killed two deputies, escaped, then was killed by Pat Garrett in July — at the age of twenty.

Geronimo, one of the last of the hostile Apache chiefs, added to the terror until his surrender in 1886. During the late 1870s, the territorial governor, General Lew Wallace, called on martial law and used troops to end the bloodbath.

Gloom dropped like a tarpaulin over Joel. Could Cyrus, with his wild love of adventure, have escaped the violence and death of those turbulent New Mexico territorial days? Or did his bones lie in some unmarked grave on the "lone prairie" along with countless others who lived and died by the sword?

In the dark hour between the waning moon and the gray dusk that heralds the dawn, when bodies and minds are at their lowest ebb, Joel Scott faced the truth. He might not be able to keep his vow. He had planned every bright bit of color concerning his father, only to have it turn to fool's gold, dross, in his hands. Most of the old-timers he talked with had never heard the name Cyrus Scott. One or two had scratched grizzled heads and admitted seeing young fellers now and then with "goldy hair and blue eyes like you'n," but they couldn't recollect any such name as Cyrus.

Joel ranged far and wide, stopping over at ranches and leaving word that if anyone knew of the man he sought, to contact Gideon Scott in Flagstaff; a reward would be forthcoming. Periodically, Joel lighted long enough to send and receive letters. So far, there had been no takers on the reward offer — just two or three false leads that roused great hope and petered out like all the others.

Joel wintered on a ranch not far from

Santa Fe. He won the admiration of the hands with his range skills, the gratitude of plain folk and Mexican families with his preaching on Sundays. When spring came, they reluctantly bid him farewell.

Joel had left the Double J in Arizona in late summer of 1888. In some ways, spring 1890 found him no closer to a solution of the mystery.

Still wide awake, Joel's lips twisted in a wry grin. A few weeks from now, on April 30, he would be twenty years old. He felt at least thirty and far removed from the excited boy who set off to reclaim his father and win him for the Lord. A fierce attack of homesickness assailed him. What he would give to see the Double J, spar with Lonesome and the boys, marvel over how much Matt and Millie, the twins, had grown. When dawn broke, why should he not just saddle Querida and head west? He had acted on the advice of a cowboy from the ranch where he wintered to "ride east into as purty a country as you'll ever see" and ended up agreeing. The hand had added, "I useter work on a swell spread called the Lazy F. Wish I'd never left." Longing softened the planes of his face.

"Why did you?" Joel's keen gaze bored into the other's open, honest countenance.

"Huh, got driv' off by the owner." Amber fire flashed in the cowboy's eyes. "All I did was try an' spark the daughter." His face reddened, but he continued to look directly at Joel. "I only smiled an' talked with her a coupla times. Never even touched her. But Fairfax's foreman, Hayes, told the boss I was sweet on Rebecca. I was," he admitted. Hardness thinned his lips. "At least I didn't mean bad by her."

"Who did?"

The cowboy buttoned his lip, shook his head, then unslitted his mouth just wide enough to say, "I ain't sayin', but I sure feel sorry for any girl Hayes gets his hands on." His oblique, meaningful glance finished the story.

Joel felt pity for the unknown Rebecca and something else. "What's this Hayes like?" he demanded sharply.

"Mean. Mid-thirties. Loco over the girl. Mousy brown hair, gray eyes that make you feel like he's hidin' somethin' all the time. Big jasper, tall as you." He measured Joel with a glance. "You weigh in about 160?"

Joel nodded.

"Hayes has a good forty pounds on you." He cocked his head to one side. "If you ever just happen to mosey up that way, tell Smokey Travis howdy from Jeff."

"I will." Joel's hand shot out. But when he finished packing his saddlebags and mounted Querida, Jeff stepped closer.

"In case you should end up at the Lazy F, keep your eye peeled an' don't never let your horse run loose."

Joel's spine snapped to attention. "Hayes?"

"I never said nothin' a-tall." Jeff half closed his eyes and grinned.

"Thanks for nothin' a-tall," Joel mimicked and turned Querida in the direction the inscrutable cowboy pointed.

Mile by mile, he headed through incredible and varied country until he knew he must be near the Lazy F. The sun yawned, opened its eye a crack, and peered over a mountain. Joel still had not slept. He had to make a decision . . . go or stay. Head home in defeat and take up his lifework of preaching or aimlessly search when every clue had died. Lige and Naomi had fallen in love with the Double J, and the last thing Joel had heard was that they had ordered their foreman to sell the Circle S. Why not join them and forget the father who had never known he had a son?

Still undecided, Joel broke camp. Before he did much more riding anywhere, he needed supplies. He remembered Jeff saying a Mexican village lay on the Lazy F. He could replenish his food, get oats for Querida for a change, and look over the ranch. Time enough then to head out.

Late afternoon found him riding through range inhabited by cattle as far as he could see. Hundreds, no thousands, must be on this rolling, endless, grazing land. He finally reached the line of cottonwoods he knew bordered the stream that ran through the ranch and lay below the ranch house.

Coarse jeers and curses rent the still air, and Joel circled to avoid meeting a group of riders face to face. Something in their hard faces warned him they would not welcome a stranger. Yet, his overdeveloped sense of curiosity forced him to investigate. Admonishing Querida to silence, he slipped from the saddle and led his horse around a willow thicket.

Dear God, no! Thirty feet away, a cowboy who could not be more than a year or so older than Joel straddled a buckskin horse that nervously shifted. The man's hands were tied behind his back. With a thrill of terror, Joel saw the noose around the white-faced cowboy's neck, the big man with a taunting smile who stood with hand upraised to hit the buckskin's flank. *Hayes!* He fit Jeff's description to the last detail.

"Got anythin' to say?" a mounted rider called.

"A lot!" the doomed cowboy yelled. "Hayes knows I'm no rustler. Ask him the real reason he framed me."

"Shut up!" Hayes snatched a Colt from his holster and pointed it.

"Let him talk, Hayes." A murmur of assent ran through the assembled men, and Joel took heart. Evidently, they were not as eager for a hanging as the Lazy F foreman was.

The courageous cowboy whose life hung by a thread shouted, "Ask him about Lone Man Canyon an' a bogus deputy that calls himself Crowley an' how they roped and tied Miss Rebecca —"

In the heartbeat before Hayes moved, guilt blackened his face. The riders froze. "You lyin', thievin' —" Hayes swung his arm high, opened his palm. It exploded with a horrid crack on the buckskin's flank.

The buckskin leaped. A shot rang out and severed the tightened rope. The cowboy, still bound, fell to the ground and lay stunned.

Joel, a gun in each hand, one still smoking, stepped from the thicket and confronted the paralyzed men.

CHAPTER 8

"Howdy, boys." Joel kept his revolvers trained square on the slack-jawed Hayes, whose face had gone a dirty yellow. "Drop the gun, Mister."

Hayes slowly let his unfired Colt drop from his fingers.

Joel shot a lightning glance toward the huddled group of staring riders, stopped at the one who had demanded that the condemned man be allowed to talk, and ordered, "You, there. Untie the boy."

"What is this, a holdup?" Hayes recovered his voice and some of his shaken arrogance. He took one step toward the newcomer.

"Don't you move." Joel's eyes flashed blue fire. He waited until the man on the ground dazedly sat up and rubbed circulation back into his wrists where the rope had cut into them. "What's your name, and what's this all about? Where I come from, we don't hang folks without a mighty good reason."

The contempt in his voice sent angry red into Hayes's face and shame to the still-mounted riders' countenances.

The reprieved cowboy sprang to his feet. Tossed dark hair and scornful dark eyes highlighted his deeply tanned face. "Thanks, Stranger. I'm Smokey Travis. Clyde Hayes is foreman of the Lazy F — you musta seen the brand on a lot of cattle no matter which way you came. He's hated me an' tried to drive me away like he did every hand who's protected Miss Rebecca from him —"

"Jeff, for instance? I rode with him down Santa Fe way, and he said to tell you howdy." Joel's revolvers never wavered, but he caught the pop-eyed look on a half-dozen faces. "Now, you boys lay down your guns real nice and easylike."

A slight movement from Hayes sent steel into Joel's eyes. "I wouldn't try anything if I were you."

"Do as he says," Hayes's hoarse voice bellowed.

Joel waited until the men disarmed, then said over the pounding of his heart, "All right, let's have it." He sheathed his guns.

Smokey stepped up beside him and glared at Hayes. "He's crookeder than a mountain goat trail. Rebecca Fairfax found it out weeks ago an' told me. He's running some

137

kind of double cross on the boss, who thinks so all-fired much of him he won't believe anything but good."

Joel's lips curled. "And the rest of these men?"

"Aw, we sure didn't know anything about a crooked deal — until just now," the cowhand who untied Smokey protested. His clear eyes attested to his honesty, but the dark faces of some of the others indicated that they had known and were neck-deep in the plot against Samuel Fairfax.

"What do you have to say?" Joel wheeled back toward Hayes.

"Lies. Travis has been a burr under the saddle ever since he rode in. I'm goin' to marry Becky, and he's jealous." Hayes spat on the ground.

"That's not what she says," said Smokey.

Joel's lips involuntarily curved upward in sympathy with Travis's mocking smile.

"It's what her daddy says that counts. Now get off the ranch. You're fired. If I ever catch you sneakin' around again, I'll run you in." Hayes stooped to pick up his Colt.

"Hold it." Like magic, Joel's revolvers sprang from his holsters in a draw so fast the crowd of men gasped. "Smokey, pitch those guns into the willow thicket. The men can get them back after we're gone."

"Just who are you, anyway, to come ridin' in where it's none of your business?" Hayes frothed at the mouth.

A slow smile of pure enjoyment crept across Joel's face. He could feel it stretch the skin across his cheekbones. "Why, saving folks is my business. I'm a preacher."

"Huh?" Hayes's exclamation mingled with Smokey's loud, "Whoopee!"

"You mean a preacher got the drop on us?" the clear-eyed cowboy demanded. "Haw, haw!" He rolled on the ground in a paroxysm of mirth.

Hayes screamed, "You're fired, too, Perkins! I knew you wouldn't last when I hired you." His colorless eyes flamed.

Perkins leaped to his feet. "Too late, Boss. I quit when Smokey said you lassoed Miss Rebecca." He looked each of the other riders in the eye. "If any of ya are men, you'll come with me." He waited a moment, but no one moved. "I'd rather ride with a herd of polecats than you. C'mon, Smokey, let's hit the trail. Half-a-dozen ranches around here'll be glad to get us. Preacher, how about comin' with us?"

Joel hesitated. Should he take the safer trail and leave with Smokey and Perkins? Or — he shook his head. "Jeff told me a lot about the Lazy F. I'm hankering to meet this Samuel Fairfax. Once I do . . ." He shrugged.

"Whaat?" For the third time, Joel's coolness shocked Hayes. "You think bein' a preacher's goin' to save your skin? Better get out while you can."

"You just gave me the best protection of all," Joel defied him. "Now, if anything such as an unexpected accident happens to me, Perkins, Travis, and the rest of the men will have to swear they heard you threaten my life." He strode back to Querida, calmly mounted her, and rode back to the others.

Hayes changed his tune instantly. Greed etched itself on his face and in his eyes at the sight of the black mare. "Maybe I was hasty," he half apologized. "I didn't mean anythin'." He cleared his throat with an obvious effort. "Where'd a preacher get a horse like that?" His quivering forefinger pointed straight at Querida.

"I sure didn't steal her," Joel sarcastically told him.

Smokey and Perkins went off into convulsions of laughter. Hayes glared at them but pressed his lips tight before saying, "Looks like you came a long way."

Something in his inscrutable eyes blocked Joel from frankly admitting his journey and the reason for it as he had done at other ranches. His years among rough men had not been in vain; they had given him insight into human nature. Now, he weighed Hayes and found him wanting: mean enough to be dangerous but a coward at heart. The kind of bad man without the nerve to be thoroughly bad. Followed by rustlers but never respected. Ruthless but more likely to shoot a man from ambush than meet him in a fair fight, evidenced by the way he had framed Smokey Travis on some flimsy charge, then rushed through a hanging to rid himself of a trouble spot.

"Hayes, I'm riding up to the ranch house with Travis and Perkins so they can get their gear from the bunkhouse without any interference." He lowered his voice. "I wouldn't be too anxious about following close behind if I were you." His gaze included the rest of the riders. His sunny smile flashed. "On the other hand, I guess we don't have to worry about it, do we? Smokey's horse took off for parts unknown, so he'll have to borrow yours." He thought Hayes would explode before Smokey vaulted to the saddle of Hayes's horse and rode out of sight, closely followed by Perkins and Joel.

Hidden by the willow thicket and a stand of close-growing cottonwoods, Smokey reined in Hayes's horse and motioned for his comrades to stop. His dark eyes danced, and he said in a low voice, "I'm a mighty curious galoot, an' I bet if a feller or fellers were to creep back up on them rustlers, why, it just could be interesting."

Joel slid to the ground and tossed Querida's reins to Perkins. Smokey followed suit. "Keep the horses quiet," Joel ordered.

Disappointment filled Perkins's face. "Aw, why can't I go, too?"

"We may need those horses in a hurry," Joel replied. "If you hear us yell, come running." He ignored Perkins's grunt and followed Smokey's stocky frame back to the willow thicket. A few rods away, they took cover, close enough to hear but far enough away to avoid being seen. Smokey pressed Joel's hand for silence when the crashing of brush and curses nearby told them the men were retrieving their guns.

"I'll get Travis and Perkins and that goldy-haired rider who says he's a preacher." Hayes's furious voice came clearly. Joel felt a thrill go up his spine. Without hesitation or thought of the consequences, he had rushed in to save Smokey. Now, he would have to face the consequences.

"While you're at it, I bet you'll get your hands on that black mare, too, huh, Hayes? I seen how ya looked at her."

A start went through Joel's tall frame, and only Smokey's powerful hand dragging him back down kept the sometimes reckless young minister from betraying their hiding place.

Hayes's unpleasant laugh sawed its way into Joel's brain, and his words beat red-hot and searing. "The way I see it, a dead man don't need a horse."

A burst of raucous, threatening laughter followed, then the scrambling in the brush ceased. After an altercation on who would ride double, a lot of grumbling, and Hayes's loud remarks on the subject, the steady cadence of hoofbeats faded and died in the distance.

"Thought we were goners there for a minute." Smokey sat up. "Preacher, you've gotta learn to lie still when there's danger around, no matter what." He stood, offered a hand to Joel, and sternly added, "What's your handle, anyway? Jim — that's Perkins — an' me can't keep calling you Preacher."

"I wouldn't want you to." Joel brushed leaves from his clothes, and they retraced their steps to Jim and the horses. "My name's Joel. Uh, what will Hayes do now?"

"Make up some story on why he fired the Lazy F's two best hands," Jim put in sourly. He clamped a worn Stetson down on straggling brown locks.

"Let's beat him to it." Joel bit his tongue to keep from laughing at the amazement in the cowboys' faces.

"What'd ya say?" Perkins demanded, face reddening.

"Here's what we'll do," Joel said. "The way I figure it, after what happened, Hayes won't head straight for the ranch. Instead, he and his men will circle and come in later from another direction. He'll count on us being gone by the time he gets there. According to what you and Jeff said, whatever reason Hayes gives for firing you two will be swallowed whole by Fairfax." He drew his brows together. "Wonder why a man smart enough to own a spread like this doesn't have enough savvy to see through Hayes?"

"He plumb don't want to," the loquacious Jim put in. "I ain't talked much with Smokey about it, but even in the short time I've been here, it 'pears Hayes has some hold on the boss."

"Any idea what it is?" Joel mounted Querida, waited until Smokey clambered aboard Hayes's horse, and started up the trail.

"Not eggzackly, but I'm workin' on it." Jim suddenly clammed up, as if realizing how freely he'd talked to a stranger.

"What . . . uh . . . what's a preacher doing riding around in eastern New Mexico?" Smokey asked with a keen sidelong glance.

Joel deliberated for a full minute, then laid his cards on the table. "I'm looking for a man. I heard that Samuel Fairfax had been in these parts for a lot of years. Thought maybe he would have known of or have heard of my man."

"He might at that," Smokey said ponderously. "Did this feller do you wrong?"

"He doesn't even know I exist." A feeling stronger than himself prompted Joel to tell his story in a few brief sentences.

Jim, the more talkative of the two, spoke first. "That's the most peculiar tale I ever heard." He shook his head. "I never knew any Cyrus Scott." He scratched his cheek. "Never heard the name Cyrus, even."

"Smokey?"

"Naw. Beats me why you want to find your daddy, seeing he never knew you were born an' all that." He sounded doubtful.

"If he's still alive, I can't let him die without knowing about the Lord and that he's forgiven," Joel murmured.

A new constraint fell between them, broken only when Smokey pointed to the ground at a fork in the trail. "You predicted right. Hayes and the men are heading away from the ranch house." A grin split his likable face. "Whoopee! This is gonna be fun." He goaded his horse into a gallop. "Race you to the corral."

Jim followed with a yell. Querida, trained to be in front in any race, leaped forward and stretched out full length until she became a flowing machine that ate up the trail in enormous gulps. She flashed past Jim, overtook Smokey in spite of his lead, and pounded ahead of the others until Joel took pity on them and slowed her so they could catch up. Then, he leaned forward, called into her ear, "Go, Querida!" and she put on a burst of speed that brought her to the Lazy F ranch house and corral in time for Joel to slide off her back and perch on the top rail of the fence until Smokey and Jim arrived.

"Snappin' crocodiles, if Hayes ever sees that mare run, your life won't be worth a dead cactus," Jim panted, admiration written all over him.

"She doesn't even look winded," Smokey complained after keenly observing Querida contentedly munching grass, reins over her head.

A trill of laughter, sweeter than the song of a meadowlark, broke into their conversation. Joel glanced toward the ranch house about a hundred yards from the corral where he sat. A slender, running figure had covered about half the distance. Joel had seen Indian girls run with the same fleet grace. He jumped down from the fence, bared his head, and waited for the girl, who could only be Rebecca Fairfax.

Clad in boys' jeans, a blue blouse, and red kerchief, her riding boots barely touched the ground. What little hair he could see from under her sombrero curled nut brown, almost the same shade as her merry eyes. Red lips parted over even, white teeth. "Smokey Travis, whose horse — why, it's Hayes's!" Blank astonishment obliterated her smile. She raced straight to the three men, then on to Querida. "Oh, you beauty!" She whirled. Fear replaced her natural joyousness. "Jim, Smokey, what — ?" A slim, tanned hand went to her throat, and her cheeks paled until the wild roses faded.

"Aw, it's nothing," Smokey mumbled.

"Don't lie to me." The brown eyes sparkled dangerously.

"Miss Fairfax?" Joel courteously began. "Is your father home?"

"Why, yes," she faltered. The fear in her eyes intensified.

"May we see him?"

"Of course, but —" She trotted alongside the men toward the ranch house.

"We'll explain everything," Joel reassured her. Some of the girl's trouble melted, and he heard her sigh of relief.

The quartet finished the walk to the large, porched, log home in silence. Joel noted the "H" shape, different from most ranch houses. They reached the bottom step, with Rebecca in the lead. The massive front door burst open. A tall man with graying brown hair and cold blue eyes stepped onto the porch. He fastened his gaze on Rebecca. "Didn't I tell you to keep away from the hands?"

"Father, something's wrong. Smokey came home riding Hayes's horse, chasing this stranger."

Joel could have sworn a look of actual relief brightened the intense blue eyes. Samuel Fairfax ignored his daughter's stumbling explanation and turned toward Joel. His mouth dropped open. He took a backward step as if hit by a battering ram.

Joel's heart leaped. This man must have somewhere encountered Cyrus! From babyhood, Judith and Gideon told him he was a replica of his father. Consternation brought Joel's spirits to earth with a resounding thud. Some tragedy lay between Samuel and

148

the long-missing Cyrus. Could they have met, quarreled, and settled their differences in the time-honored western tradition that added bodies to Boot Hills throughout the land? It could account for Hayes's stranglehold on Fairfax. If he knew . . .

Joel's imagination ran riot.

"Who are you, and what do you want?" Fairfax demanded.

Face-to-face with a possible end to his long search, Joel could not speak. Jim Perkins mercifully introduced him.

"Boss, this here's Joel Scott, and if he hadn't come ridin' in at just the right minute, well, ol' Smokey here'd be pushin' up the daisies."

"What's that?" Fairfax roared and turned his full attention to Perkins. Yet, the pallor of his first sight of Joel remained.

"Hayes rigged up some phony evidence to show Smokey was rustlin'," Jim explained. "Even fooled me. Wasn't even goin' to let Smokey speak up in his own defense, just roped him and got ready to hang him." Memory of the tense moments brought his story alive. "Hayes slapped Smokey's horse and left Smokey danglin', but quicker than a roadrunner, Scott steps out from a willow thicket, hauls out his guns, and cuts the rope with the best shootin' I ever saw. Then he up and covers us, makes Hayes crawl, finished the party by tellin' us he's a preacher, and beats Smokey and me in a race home ridin' that black mare over there."

Fairfax ignored Jim's pointing finger, his daughter's quick gasp of horror. "Travis, if Hayes says you were rustling, you were. Now get out of here. You're fired. You, too, Perkins."

"Too late, Boss," Jim said cheerfully. "Hayes done did that. We just rode in to get our gear and 'cause Scott here said you had the right to hear what really happened 'fore Hayes comes in with his lies."

Joel grinned at his audacity but not for long. Fairfax turned back to him, accusingly. "If you're some kind of preacher, why aren't you doing your job instead of sticking your nose in where it ain't wanted?"

"I'm looking for a man," Joel said for the second time that day. "Have you ever heard the name Cyrus Scott?"

"Kin of yours?"

"My father." Joel had difficulty forming the words.

Samuel Fairfax crossed his strong arms and stared. The logs of the ranch house behind him looked no stronger than their owner. "Why come sniveling to me? What did he do . . . this . . . what's his name? Oh yes, Cyrus Scott." His face turned even stonier.

"He married my mother using his brother's name, ran out on her before she found out she would bear his child, then fled from Texas when he learned of her death." Joel did not budge an inch.

"All that?" A sardonic smile accompanied his question. "Doesn't seem to me that you or anyone would chase around trying to find a man who'd do those things."

Joel took in a deep breath, held it, then let it go before he said, "If he's dead, I want to know it. If he isn't, he needs to know he's forgiven by God and his family." Truth rang in his voice. He saw something flicker in the cold eyes and added, "So is the man who killed him, if Father died by violence. God's love covers even that."

For a moment, Samuel Fairfax stood rigid. For an eternity, he stared into Joel's eyes. Smokey coughed, and the spell broke. Fairfax unfolded his arms and said, "If this Cyrus Scott is as foolhardy as his son, he probably died years ago." His boot heel ground into the porch when he turned and went back into the house. But before he closed the door, he called, "The best thing you can do is ride out with Travis and

151

Perkins. There's nothing on the Lazy F for you."

Was his glance at Rebecca, followed by a meaningful look back at Joel, meant as a deliberate warning? His mouth tasting like ashes, the young minister watched the door close. Its slamming sounded a death knell to his search — and his hopes.

CHAPTER 9

"Mr. Scott, I apologize for Father." A strong but shapely hand lightly touched Joel's arm and released him from his stupor.

He looked into Rebecca Fairfax's upturned face, dusky red from her efforts not to cry. Something in her troubled brown eyes reached out to him. Joel inhaled sharply; his humiliation at the hands of her father vanished. For some insane reason, he wanted to shout, to listen to his pumping heart instead of the common sense that told him to leave. He glanced at the hand still resting on his sleeve. *What would it be like to take that hand . . . and its owner . . . and ride away?*

Joel felt the blood rush to his head at the preposterous idea. He had known Rebecca Fairfax less than an hour. He ignored the little voice inside that demanded, *So what?* "It's all right, Miss Fairfax." He looked deep into her lovely eyes. "We'll meet again."

The assurance in his words set new red flags waving in Rebecca's face. "I . . . I don't see how," she faltered.

Smokey Travis and Jim Perkins had been standing silent during Joel's altercation with the owner of the Lazy F. Now, they stepped forward, Stetsons in hand. Smokey half closed his keen dark eyes and drawled, "A preacher preaches, doesn't he? If I know Samuel Fairfax, an' I do, even he won't kick up a dust storm 'cause his daughter wants to go to a meeting."

"That's how I see it, too," Jim eagerly assented, his boyish face opening into a wide grin. "Pards, we'd better get out of here." He pointed to a distant band of dark riders heading toward the ranch house. Pure devilment shone in his eyes. "But we could pervide a welcomin' committee."

"You'd better go," Rebecca told them. A shadow swept over her sweet face. "Smokey, thanks for being my friend. Good luck, Jim." But her gaze fastened on Joel. "Goodbye, Mr. Scott. God help you in your search for your father." She stepped back.

"Will you be all right?" Joel hurriedly added, "Hayes is going to be in a nasty mood."

"God and Mrs. Cook, our cook, will look after me!" Her red lips twitched. "The worst

Father can do is send me to my room."

"An' your window's big enough for ya to climb out if ya had to," Perkins observed.

Rebecca looked startled at the thought, then nodded.

Five minutes later, Joel on Querida, Smokey on the buckskin that had come straight back to the ranch, and Jim on a trim pinto that he said was his rode away. Rebecca waved good-bye to them from the ranch house porch.

"Kinda hate leavin' her here to face Hayes," Jim growled.

"She'll be all right. I used to think someday I'd up an' marry her," Smokey said somberly. "Get her away from Hayes."

"Why didn't you?" Joel could not keep the words back, but when Smokey's face darkened, he wished he had kept still.

"Rebecca thinks a whole lot of me, but it's like the brother she never had but should have." Smokey stared ahead at the path wide enough for them to ride three abreast. "At least I was her friend, as much as Hayes and Fairfax allowed." He turned toward Joel. "I never was good enough for her. Perkins here or the other hands aren't, either. Now, a strapping young feller like you might just —" He never finished what he started to say. His buckskin chose that moment to shy away from some real or imagined danger and execute a dance that kept Smokey busy and Joel and Jim laughing at the horse's antics.

But the young minister did not forget the gleam in Smokey's eyes. If he could win the cowboy's confidence, he would have a loyal friend for life. The same held true with Perkins, witnessed to by the way he stood up to Hayes back by the willow thicket.

"I need supplies." Joel shoved aside meditations and spoke. "I suppose I can get what I need at the Mexican village?" He intercepted the quick glance Jim sent Smokey, the lifting of eyebrows before Jim drawled, "We've seen ya ride and shoot. Can you rope?"

"A little." Joel stifled a grin, glanced around, and selected a cottonwood stump off to their left. He uncoiled his lariat from the saddle horn, swung it in a wide loop, and dropped it over the stump with an expert twist of his wrist.

"Yup, ya can rope . . . a little." Perkins waited until Joel twitched the lasso, recoiled it, and put it back in place. "Why don't you 'n' me 'n' Smokey get jobs t'gether? Like the fellers in that book."

"The Three Musketeers?" Joel's heart lifted at the thought, and a pang of lonesomeness for his comrades back on the Double J went through him. "Think anyone will hire a preacher?"

"Sure, if you're with us. Right, Smokey?"

"Haw, haw!" Smokey grabbed his hat and slapped it against his leg. His horse went into another spin.

"What's so funny, ya bowlegged galoot?" Perkins demanded as soon as Smokey got the buckskin quieted.

Tears of laughter streaming down his dark face, Smokey choked, "I reckon any rancher who sees what our new pard can do won't worry about him preaching on his own time." He wiped his eyes with a bright neckerchief. "Say, Joel, how about playing a joke on the Bar Triangle? That's the next biggest spread to the Lazy F an' always wanting good riders."

"What kind of joke?" Joel looked at Smokey suspiciously.

"We'll ride in, ask for jobs, an' not let on you're a preacher."

"Naw," Jim chimed in. "That ain't no good. When they find out, they'll think Joel's ashamed of it."

Smokey's jaw dropped. "I never thought about that." He ruefully shook his head. A moment later, his dark eyes twinkled again. "Well, how about just not telling how fast his mare is?"

Jim sat up straighter; mischief filled his lean face. "Then, when the Mexican village holds their fiesta day, Joel c'n enter his horse — what's her handle, anyhow?"

"Querida. Spanish for *beloved*."

"Kayreeda'll purely outrun ev'ry horse in New Mexico," Jim predicted.

"Not Vermilion." Smokey glared at Perkins.

Jim snorted. "Think old man Fairfax'll let Rebecca ride in any race? Not 'til all the dogies come home wearin' ribbons in their ears." He rolled his eyes.

Joel, the peacemaker, asked, "What kind of horse is Vermilion? I've yet to see an animal beat Querida, given an equal start."

"He's the purtiest, best-tamed, brightest-red mustang you ever saw," Jim admitted. "Smokey caught him an' babied him an' gave him to Rebecca on her eighteenth birthday last December." He pushed his Stetson farther back on his head. "Smokey, I'd lay even odds on Vermilion an' the black."

Smokey jealously eyed the beautiful mare. "She might win a short race, but Vermilion can't be beat in a long one."

Joel smothered a grin. The longer the race, the better Querida performed. "No sense arguing about it. When does this fiesta day come off, anyway?"

"After roundup. The whole country comes."

"Who won the horse race last year?" Joel inquired.

"Hayes." The corners of Smokey's mouth turned down. "His big bay's a grand horse." He laughed gleefully. "I did enjoy riding him today. He ain't no match for your horse or Vermilion, though. Is it a deal? We keep mum an' surprise folks at the race?"

"Why not? We won't be lying or anything."

"I wouldn't ask a preacher to lie." Smokey sent his buckskin into a run and left Joel staring after him.

"Did I say something wrong?" asked Joel.

"Don't pay no 'tention to Smokey," Jim advised. "He's taken a shine to ya, but sometimes he's plum' peecooliar about things. Love does that to some fellers." Jim shook his head and looked wise.

"Do you have a girl?" Joel asked curiously.

Perkins's blinding smile burst forth again. "Sure. Conchita's the most beautiful gal in the Mexican village. Soon's I save a little money, I'm gonna hawg-tie her an' marry her before some long-legged jasper beats me to it." A thundercloud drove away his sunny look. "An' if Hayes don't quit hangin' around her all the while he's playin' up to Fairfax, intendin' to marry Rebecca, there's gonna be trouble like you never saw."

A cold breeze of foreboding blew across Joel's heart. "You mean that rustler's actually —"

Jim nodded and looked far older than his young years. They had nearly caught up with Smokey and the buckskin, who waited for them where the road forked. "Don't say nothin' in front of Smokey," Jim cautioned in a whisper. "He hates Hayes the polecat enough already."

If ever a range were white and needing harvest for God, this wild New Mexico land fit the description! Joel silently followed his new friends. Miles later, the Bar Triangle cattle with their distinctive brand replaced the herds of Lazy F stock.

With his first view of the Bar Triangle house and outbuildings, Joel's heart beat faster. Unlike the Lazy F, the original Bar Triangle owners had built of adobe. In many ways, the main house reminded Joel of his grandparents' hacienda. Low, long, and cool, the splashing fountain in the courtyard merrily welcomed the dusty, tired riders. The owner, Ben Lundeen, practically greeted them with open arms.

"Travis, Perkins, I figured someday you'd

come riding in looking for work. It's a wonder you lasted so long as you did on the Lazy F, 'specially you, Smokey. Everyone knows Fairfax don't cotton to younger riders." His firm grip and keen look measured Joel. "Who's your pard?"

"Joel Scott, an all-round ridin', ropin', shootin' hand, plus he's a preacher," the irrepressible Jim bragged.

"Whaat?" Lundeen's eyes bulged in his strong face. Doubt crept into his voice. "I don't know about hiring a preacher. What'll the men say?"

Quick-witted as a ground squirrel in danger, Joel replied, "Why not let them decide? Put me on for a week, then ask your outfit if they want me to stay." He glanced away from Lundeen long enough to catch Smokey's delighted grin and the way Perkins put one hand over his mouth.

"Fair enough." Lundeen nodded. "You boys know where the bunkhouse is. Go stow your gear." His eyes gleamed, and he casually added, "You can do as you like about telling the men about your interrupted necktie party."

"How'd you know?" Jim belligerently placed both hands on his hips in a fighting stance.

Again, that curious gleam filled Lundeen's

161

eyes. "You'll find an old friend in the cook-house. He rode in earlier today with an interesting tale for my ears only. Said he couldn't stand living with the kind of men Hayes has been hiring and that he reckoned the only two worth much wouldn't be staying."

"So, you knew all the time we were coming!" Chagrin fell on Smokey's expressive face.

"I didn't know young Scott was a preacher," Lundeen admitted. "I guess that little fact got by Curly. He spilled the other to me, and I told him to keep quiet." Trouble brooded on the lined face. "The men will hear of it soon enough. You know range talk." His gaze bored into his new riders. "It's up to Scott to prove himself."

"He will," Smokey predicted.

"Yeah, but if anythin' happens an' Joel don't stay, we go, too," Jim loyally added.

"Fair enough." Lundeen's rare smile lightened his countenance, and he looked years younger. "Go get settled." He wandered down toward the corral with them to where they had tied their horses. His steps quickened, and he headed straight for Querida. "Whose mare is this?" He stroked her soft nose.

"Mine." Pride of ownership and the long,

faithful trail they had ridden together underlined the word.

"She's a beauty. You wouldn't want to sell her."

"No."

"I wouldn't, either, if I owned her." He patted Querida again, and his eyes flashed. "Good thing you're here instead of on some of the ranches. Your horse is safe on the Bar Triangle." His unspoken words, *but not on the Lazy F,* hung in the quiet air until Lundeen said, "Tomorrow we'll see what you can do, Scott," and trailed back up to his house.

It took less than a week for the Bar Triangle crew to accept Joel Scott. His range skills showed up with the best and won the respect of both men his age and much older. Lundeen just grunted at Joel's display of hard work and expertise.

True to their pact, Jim, Smokey, and Joel did not breathe a word about Querida's fleetness, even when some of the hands said a trifle too nonchalantly, "Bet she can run. Are you going to ride her in the fiesta race?"

"I might." Joel lounged on his bunk, as he had done dozens of times on the Double J. In spite of being the adopted son-of-the-house, once he had learned to ride with the outfit, he spent a lot of time in the bunkhouse and kept a bedroll there.

"Sure will be some race," some of the boys sighed enviously. "Sure hope Hayes don't win again. He wouldn't, if Fairfax'd let that girl of his ride her red horse," seemed to be the general agreed-on opinion.

"Once, when I was separatin' our cattle from the Lazy F's, I saw her racin' across the range," one cowboy said. "Never will forget it. She rode just like an Indian, bent forward in the saddle 'til her and that Vermilion looked like one critter."

"Hey, Travis, how come Fairfax's so all-fired anxious to get her hitched up with Hayes?" someone called out.

Smokey's pupils dwindled to pinpoints of blackness. "Crazy, I reckon." He breathed hard. "Beats me."

A frank-faced, young rider confessed, "I'da got me a job there in hopes of sometimes seein' the girl, but, even for that, I couldn't stomach Hayes. One of these times, he's gonna get his." Cold steel rang beneath the idle words.

Joel spent Sunday afternoon propped against an ancient oak, considering his future. He knew he had passed his trial at the Bar Triangle; he also felt at home. Yet, how could range work be related to his two missions: finding his father and preaching? A burst of song from the bunkhouse brought a sympathetic smile to his carved lips. Jim must be getting duded up to go call on Conchita. On impulse, Joel left his tree friend and ambled back to the bunkhouse. "Perkins, mind if I ride to the Mexican village with you?"

"Not atall." Jim's face was flushed with the efforts of pulling on boots shined almost as brightly as his eyes. His Sunday-white shirt and colorful scarf pleasantly added to his excited, handsome face. "Just don't ya get no ideas about her."

"I won't," Joel promised and turned to Smokey. "Are you coming?"

His friend looked up from a magazine he was reading, disgust etched into his face. "Might as well." He threw the magazine aside, stood, and stretched. "The feller who wrote the story I was reading has never been west of Boston! According to him, all us cowboys sleep in our chaps an' don't eat nothing but beef an' beans. Too bad he doesn't come out here for a spell an' see the meals Curly turns out for us poor, miserable punchers."

"Better of him if he don't come," Jim said sagely. "It'd be too bad if a feller like that got the outfit turned loose on him."

165

Joel laughed, but on the way to the village, he asked, "Do you think some of the men would come if I found a place to preach some Sunday?"

"They might," Smokey said after a sidelong look at Jim that Joel duly noted. "There's a padre in the Mexican village an' a little church, but not many of the ranchers go to Mass an' none of the hands." He pondered for a minute. "Now that we're on permanent-like at the Bar Triangle, ask Lundeen if it would be all right to hold a meeting there. He's honest all the way through; so's his wife. Kids are all grown and gone."

"Good idea," Jim seconded. "Maybe Rebecca Fairfax would ride over an' you could see her . . . horse Vermilion."

Joel knew exactly what Jim hinted and could not keep color from rising until he sarcastically thought, *I must be the same shade as the wonder horse they keep praising.* It made him feel hotter than ever.

"You better forget her an' keep your mind on Conchita," Smokey told him. "If you don't marry her pretty soon, I'll up an' beat you."

"She wouldn't look at the likes of ya," Jim loftily told his partner.

"Why not? I'm better looking than some

166

people around here," Smokey retorted. "Even if I don't have a brand-new shirt an' a kerchief I could use to scare off a wild bull."

They good-naturedly wrangled all the way to the Mexican village, heaping mock insults on each other and appealing to Joel for support, and looking disgusted when he would not take sides.

The Mexican village resembled similar ones he had seen in his travels. Adobe buildings, strings of red and green peppers, the tang of dust and horseflesh, guitar music from a cantina, laughter, and the after-siesta relaxation of a Sunday.

"Conchita lives with her married sister," Jim explained when they stopped before a cream building with the inevitable red-tiled roof. Green vines grew up and over, giving an illusion of coolness Joel knew would be present even on the hottest day.

The door stood open. They dismounted and hitched their horses to a crude rail fence. Perkins's spurs jingled musically when he led the way up a path made of flat stones.

"Pard, ain't that Hayes's bay?" Smokey crouched and pointed toward a tethered horse grazing nearby, barely visible through a clump of cottonwoods.

Jim stopped in midstride. His face whitened, then a look that sent fear crawling through Joel spread across Jim's face. In the frozen second before Perkins leaped for the open doorway, a low cry came from inside the house.

Like a speeding bullet, Jim bounded inside. Smokey and Joel raced after him. The trio burst through an empty room toward the sound of a voice that pleaded, "No, no, Señor!"

"That dirty scoundrel!" Smokey choked. He and Joel crowded through the door to the small courtyard until they stood side by side with Perkins. A man with mousy brown hair stood with his back to them. An ashen-faced Mexican girl, whose disheveled dark hair and terrified eyes told the whole story, struggled in the man's arms. A ruffled white blouse sagged over one brown shoulder, and the red rose in her hair drooped in bizarre contrast to her distorted face. Hayes's fingers dug into her soft arms, and he jerked her closer. She screamed.

"Hayes!" Perkins's low, deadly voice loosened the man's hold. Hayes reached for his gun and whirled. Revolver half out of his holster, the livid-faced man faced the three men. He stared straight into Perkins's face — and saw death from the steady Colt

168

covering him, the trigger being slowly squeezed.

CHAPTER 10

Horror so deep he could neither pray nor move engulfed Joel. Then, Smokey struck up Perkins's gun with one hand, while keeping Hayes covered with the Colt in his other. Perkins's shot fired harmlessly into the ceiling.

"Drop it, Hayes!" Smokey ordered.

Hayes's revolver clattered to the floor. His mouth worked helplessly; rage and wonder mingled. Long scratches on his cheeks oozed blood. He finally burst out, "You!"

"Why'd ya do it?" Jim Perkins cried. Anger still mottled his face. "The dirty skunk don't deserve to live an' ya know it! Why didn't ya let me kill him?"

Joel shrank from Smokey's bitter laugh. "Think I did it for him? Naw. He ain't worth spilling blood for." He laughed again, a wild sound that turned Hayes's face even grayer. "Besides, someday he's going to hang." He waved toward the door with his gun. "Get out, Hayes, an' don't come back here — ever. I reckon I saved your life; now I'm telling you, the next time . . ." He choked, and his dark eyes glittered.

Hayes did not say a word. He stumbled past Joel, who stepped aside from the doorway and let him go through.

Joel was sickened by the violent scene he had just witnessed, a scene that nearly led to death. His ears rang, and a few moments later, he heard hoof-beats, and he knew Hayes had fled.

"Conchita, are you all right?" The Jim who knelt by the girl bore little resemblance to the cowboy who, but for Smokey's interference, would have killed Conchita's attacker.

"Yes." She pulled her blouse back onto her shoulder. Great drops made her black eyes look like twin lakes at midnight under New Mexican stars. "He come, grab me. I fight." She extended broken-nailed hands that still trembled. "Hayes is bad." Conchita leaned against Jim.

Smokey jerked his head toward the doorway and walked out. Joel followed, conscious of shame. Not only for men like Hayes, who sank so low they made girls' and women's lives on the frontier a nightmare but for his own inadequacies. He, a minister of God, had stood speechless and powerless in the face of peril. Thank God Smokey had not.

Humbled by his lack of ability to act when necessary, a shortcoming Joel had not known he possessed, he hoarsely told his new friend, "It's a good thing you were here." He shuddered; drops of sweat sprang to his forehead. "Hayes can't help being grateful that you . . . after what he tried to do . . ."

Smokey's look of contempt stopped his stuttering. "Like I said, it wasn't for Hayes. I just couldn't stand for Jim to have a killing on his head. It would always be between him an' Conchita, for one thing. For another, Hayes's time is getting short on this range. That Lone Man Canyon business shows that." An unpleasant smile twisted his lips. He glanced back at the house, then at all sides of the wide porch where they had stopped to wait for Jim. "You look like a feller who could keep things under his hat."

"I am." Joel braced himself for the startling revelation he felt coming.

Smokey again checked to make sure they were not observed before he pulled back his vest just far enough for Joel to catch a flash of silver.

"Smokey Travis, you're a —"

"Shh. Don't tell Jim," the shorter man warned in a whisper when heavy footfalls and lighter steps announced Perkins and Conchita's arrival.

Perkins's arm lay protectively around her waist. Tearstains could not disguise the Mexican girl's beauty. Her eyes glowed with happiness that reflected in her sweetheart's face. "Joel, you're a preacher. Will ya marry us?"

Jim's question drove the thought of the deputy marshal's badge that Smokey wore clean out of Joel's head. "Why, yes," he stammered. "But —"

"Pard, how can you get married?" Smokey demanded. "Where are you going to take Conchita if you do?"

A look of doubt did not change Jim's dogged determination. "We'll ride out an' find a job somewhere. Connie's willin' to work at cleanin' or cookin'." His mouth tightened. "Snappin' crocodiles, Smokey, ya don't expect me to leave her here, do ya?"

Smokey pondered. "It ain't none of my business, but if it were me, why, I'd just pack up Conchita an' her duds an' take her back to the Bar Triangle with us." A smile, singular in its sweetness, crept to his face. "Mrs. Lundeen'll take care of her 'til you get a place, especially when she hears what

Hayes tried to do."

"Connie, will ya trust me an' my pards an' go?" Jim's poignant question set Joel's heart to pounding. So did the love in Conchita's liquid eyes when she said, "Yes," and pressed her face against Perkins's still-fresh white shirt. She raised her head, smiled mistily at Joel and Smokey, and ran lightly back inside.

Smokey, the coolest of the three, snickered and asked, "Do you have any money?"

"Money?" Jim stared at him.

"Yeah. Pesos, cartwheels, simoleons, good old American dollars."

"Not much." Jim spread out a pitiful array and turned deep red. "Uh, what do I need money for?"

Smokey threw his hands up in exasperation. "How're you going to get Conchita to the ranch? Does she have a horse?"

Joel laughed out loud at the comical look on Jim's bewildered face. "Don't worry. I've got plenty." He laughed again when his comrades gasped at the bills he pulled from his shirt. "Buy her a horse, Jim. Get a pack mule if you need it."

"I can't take your money," he protested.

"Call it a wedding present."

"Whoopee!" Smokey yelled. Jim rushed back inside. He returned wearing the grin

Joel had come to associate with his light-hearted companion. "Connie says she doesn't need a pack mule. All she has is her clothes an' we can stow them in our saddlebags." His eyes glinted when he awkwardly added, "Thanks . . . both of ya." His face reddened. "I'm just glad we got here when we did."

"Thank God for that," Joel soberly agreed. "Wonder how Hayes is going to explain to Fairfax what happened? The Lazy F's bound to hear range gossip."

Smokey fixed a warning gaze on Joel. "You can bet your life that snake'll come up with lies enough to make himself out an angel an' the rest of us devils," he darkly prophesied. Conchita peeked out the door, and by unspoken consent, they dropped the subject. Just before dusk, the three men and a tired Conchita, unused to hours in the saddle, dismounted at the Bar Triangle.

"Pards, come with us," Jim begged. They nodded and trailed Jim and his drooping bride-to-be inside the adobe ranch house.

If Joel had ever entertained qualms about Perkins's sincerity, they vanished when Jim manfully told the surprised Lundeens, "Conchita and me aim to get married soon as I can fix a place for her. My pards and me got to her place today just in time to save her from Hayes." His eyes flashed. "Smokey said he thought you could look after her. She's willin' to work hard."

Not by a flicker of an eyelash did either Ben Lundeen or his kindly wife betray shock. Mrs. Lundeen stood, took both of Conchita's hands in her own, and said in a genteel voice, "How nice to have a girl with us again! Now that our daughter's gone, I just get hungry for another woman's company." She smiled and added, "Come, Conchita. You'll want to freshen up from your long ride."

Joel's eyes stung. The woman's acceptance and unfailing hospitality reminded him of Judith; so would she have taken in a stray.

Lundeen waited until the ladies disappeared, then inquired, "How's Hayes?"

Joel shuddered at the implication. Womenfolk in the West were to be protected and those who transgressed, punished. *God, will the day ever come when law and order other than the law of retribution rule this land?*

"Hayes'll think twice before he gets in our way again," Smokey slowly told Lundeen. His eyes shone like molten metal. "That's the second time our paths have crossed."

Joel silently added, *I pray to God there won't be another.*

■ ■ ■ ■

During the days that Joel proved himself at the Bar Triangle and settled into the outfit, Rebecca Fairfax had troubles of her own. A strange restlessness filled her, stemming from the two different versions of the attempted hanging of Smokey Travis.

Samuel made sure his daughter was present when Hayes rode in with his story of catching Smokey in the act of rustling. She noticed how he downplayed the young minister's part in it. All he said was, "Fool stranger interfered, and the men and I let Travis go after firing him and that mouthy Perkins." Yet, the girl hugged to her heart the clean blue fire of Joel Scott's eyes, his waving corn silk hair, tanned skin, and, most of all, the look in his face when he quietly said they would meet again.

How? She considered the question from her favorite range viewpoints, in her bed at night. Other comments haunted her, including Jim Perkins's laconic observation about her window being large enough to climb through if she had to.

One tense day followed another. Her father grew more taciturn and unapproachable than ever. If it had not been for the faithful Mrs. Cook, Rebecca could not have stood it. More and more, she spent free time in the kitchen, one of her few refuges away from the ever-present Clyde Hayes, who had renewed his pursuit of her, no, intensified it. Sometimes, she felt she would eventually be forced to marry Hayes simply because her father commanded it.

Yet, every time she thought of it, she cried out, "Never!" She also began to heed Mrs. Cook's lessons about trusting in the Lord and asking for His protection and help. Verses in the Bible that Rebecca had not known existed now offered comfort.

Late one Sunday night, she and her father sat reading in the big living room, a rare occurrence. Usually, if he came in before dark, Samuel buried himself in papers concerning the ranch. Tonight, she stole glances at him from behind a well-worn copy of *The Pilgrim's Progress,* a book Mrs. Cook said would help Rebecca forget her own troubles. How old and worn he looked, as if life had effectively stamped out any happiness he had ever known.

Rebecca impulsively left her chair and went to stand before him. "Father, what is it? You seem so sad." He didn't speak for such a long time that she wondered if he had heard her. When he did speak, his words left her stunned.

"Rebecca, if you don't marry Clyde Hayes, I am ruined." He spread his hands wide, expressing defeat as she had never seen him do before. His eyes pleaded. "Daughter, will you save me?"

She almost fell to her knees and promised. Then the memory of Hayes laying hands on her stilled her voice. Marriage with him would be torment until death mercifully freed her. "Father, I —"

The door flew open and slammed back against the wall with a mighty bang. Clyde Hayes strode in, glowering. Red welts stood out on his pale face, and his colorless eyes flamed with triumph. Rebecca shrank away from him.

"Hayes? What happened to you? Looks like you tangled with a wildcat."

"Might as well have." He dropped heavily into a chair without being invited. "That's what a man gets for tryin' to help a woman he don't care about."

"What are you talking about?" Fairfax dropped the book he still held.

"I rode into the Mexican village. Found Travis and Perkins attackin' the girl called Conchita. I challenged them, and they vamoosed with their tails between their legs. They sneaked back up on me, and I pulled

179

my gun. Next thing I knew, the girl was all over me, scratchin' and spittin'. Last time I'll mix in."

Rebecca stared in disbelief. The part about Conchita scratching was obviously true. The rest she did not believe.

Neither did she believe it when Hayes contemptuously added, "That kid who calls himself a preacher was there, too. Didn't do any showin' off this time, though. Too scared, probably."

"It's an outrage when things like this go on right here on our range," Fairfax shouted. "I've a mind to get the outfit and ride down there myself." Rebecca noticed the fear in Hayes's face before he quickly said, "It ain't worth it. Besides, the girl's gone. I hid in a clump of cottonwood and watched them ride out. The men had scared up a horse for the girl, and the four of them rode off. I followed a spell, and they were headed for the Bar Triangle."

"Mighty strange they'd go that way." Samuel's eyebrows met in a frown. "The Lundeens and their ranch that's getting bigger all the time are a cactus spine in the leg, but they're decent folk. They won't put up with them."

Hayes glanced at Rebecca, whose heart nearly burst with indignation. "Oh, those men'll have some story," he carelessly said. "I just wanted you to hear what really happened."

She almost retorted, "If we want the truth, we won't get it from you," but bit her tongue and edged toward the door.

"Where are you goin'?" Hayes arrogantly demanded.

It took all Rebecca's control to say, "I rode a long way today, and I'm tired. Good night, Father, Mr. Hayes." She whipped out of the room and ran to her own.

Later, after she heard the front door close and knew Hayes had gone, she crept noiselessly down the hall and peered into the living room. Her father sat before the dying fire, graying brown head bowed as if in despair. Pity stirred her. A burning stick snapped; Samuel Fairfax groaned. Rebecca leaned forward and strained her ears to catch his low words. "God — is there no end to it?"

She wanted to go to him, but fear held her prisoner. If she did, he might ask her again to become the purchase price for his — what? Freedom? Life? Peace of mind? On hesitant feet, Rebecca stole back to her room, only to lie sleepless for hours and watch the mysterious night, shadowy and filled with uncertainty, just like her life.

Morning brought relief. No matter what, she could never marry Hayes. She avoided being alone with her father, unwilling to start another bitter argument. With Smokey no longer on the ranch to protect her, Rebecca sometimes felt herself to be a prisoner. She dared not ride far from home for fear of encountering Hayes. Not that she stood in awe of him. Vermilion could outrun Hayes's bay, and Rebecca could defend herself ably with her marksmanship. Yet, if she were forced to do so, would Father believe what she said or listen to Hayes? She could not risk finding out.

The morning after he rode in, Rebecca had privately told Hayes's story to Mrs. Cook. Her shrewd blue eyes and round face showed how little stock she put in anything Hayes said. "Looks to me like what probably happened was the other way around," she said and punched down the bread dough as if she had Hayes on the well-floured board. "If I know folks — and I do — neither Smokey nor young Perkins would have dishonorable intentions toward any girl. As for that young preacher, I only got a glimpse of him, but what I saw is in his favor."

A few days later, Mrs. Cook said, "Mrs.

Lundeen sent word over there'd be a meeting on Sunday at the Bar Triangle. She invited us to come Saturday and stay over. Want to go?" Her eyes sparkled. "It's been a long time since we had a visiting preacher come through."

"I don't suppose Father will consent," Rebecca said despondently, while her heart beat fast at the idea of an outing and the chance to see Joel Scott again.

"Let me ask him," Mrs. Cook suggested.

"All right, but it won't do any good."

Rebecca's pessimism held all that day but miraculously left at supper when Mrs. Cook said, "Mr. Fairfax, the Lundeens are holding a meeting on Sunday and asked us to come over Saturday and stay. I think we should go, all of us. Rebecca needs to be with folks other than us."

Samuel laid his fork down. "You do, do you?" He frowned.

"Yes, I do. It pays a body to let the neighbors know he's friendly."

Fairfax jerked at the word "he," took a mouthful of beefsteak, chewed it thoughtfully, and swallowed. "Might not be a bad idea. I've been meaning to talk to Lundeen about roundup. This is probably as good a time as any."

Mrs. Cook reverted to her humble servant

role. "Thank you, Sir." But, when she went to bring in the dessert, she lifted her eyebrows in a victory signal behind the master-of-the-house's back.

Rebecca could scarcely believe it. She wanted to mention the jaunt to her father but held her tongue. To do so might cause him to change his mind, and she simply had to go.

On Friday before the meeting, a second messenger arrived from the Bar Triangle. "There's gonna be a weddin' tomorrow night," he told Mrs. Cook and Rebecca. "Bring your fanciest clothes." He looked at the girl admiringly. "Uh, Smokey Travis sends greetin's."

"Is Smokey getting married?" Mrs. Cook gasped.

The rider shook his head. "Nope. It's that pard of his." He glanced at Rebecca again. "All the boys at the Bar Triangle are jealous. Lundeen's done fixed up a little cabin for the newlyweds." He grinned. "This is sure a big weekend for the preacher."

Before Rebecca could ask why, the rider shifted in the saddle. The girl followed his glance toward her father riding in.

"Gotta go. See y'all tomorrow." He spurred his horse and rode off with a cheerful wave and a tip of his hat to Fairfax.

184

"Who was that, and what did he want?" Samuel demanded sharply when he reached the house and slid from the saddle.

Mrs. Cook placidly said, "Mrs. Lundeen sent word we'd get in on a wedding as well as preaching and to bring our good clothes."

"Wedding? Whose?" The words shot like bullets out of Samuel's pinched mouth.

"Why, I don't rightly know, except it isn't Smokey Travis. Kind of sounded like it might be the young preacher himself."

Fairfax stared at her, dumbfounded. An odd look covered his face, one Rebecca had never before seen. "Scott? Who's the bride?"

"I don't know that, either," Mrs. Cook admitted. "Maybe one of the girls from the Mexican village."

Anger contorted Samuel's features. He brushed past the two women, slammed into the house, and let the door crash behind him.

"My stars," Mrs. Cook gasped. "What did I say to set him off? He sounded like he actually cared who the preacher married!"

He isn't the only one who cares, a wicked little voice inside Rebecca taunted. She raised her chin defiantly and said, "What does it matter? Come help me decide what to wear, will you, please?" Yet, all during the choosing of just the right gown and press-

185

ing and carefully packing it before the wedding, Rebecca's heart lay cold and heavy in
her chest, making it hard for her to breathe
and talk normally.

CHAPTER 11

One look into Conchita's innocent, dark eyes put to rest forever any suspicion Rebecca carried concerning the Mexican girl's reputation. An hour after the Lazy F contingent reached the Bar Triangle, the two maidens giggled and chattered as if they were long-separated sisters — especially when Conchita blushingly confessed she had been in love with "Señor Jeem" ever since young Perkins first visited the village.

Why should a great burden roll off Rebecca's shoulders? Her face rivaled the pink rose tucked in her nut-brown hair.

Later, Smokey managed to whisk Rebecca out of her father's vigilant scrutiny and whisper, "How come Hayes showed up? Did he trail you?"

Rebecca made a sound of disgust; a frown marred her pretty face. "I couldn't believe it when he said he reckoned he'd mosey along." Her eyes flashed. "I overheard

Father tell Hayes privately there had better not be any trouble."

"An' what did Hayes say to that?" Smokey's intense, dark gaze never left her face.

"He told Father he wouldn't start anything but if —" She hastily swallowed Hayes's derogatory "those three snakes" and substituted, "If anyone started trouble, he'd see that he finished it." She caught Smokey's rigid arm with one hand. "For Conchita's sake and mine, keep away from him."

"I can't back away if he comes looking for me," Smokey protested. Storm signals waved in his face. Rebecca could see he was torn between wanting to please her and following the range law that demanded a man answer an insult.

She lowered her voice. "It's just that every time Hayes gets mixed up in something, Father pushes me more to marry him. I can't, Smokey, I just can't. If only we could prove how rotten Hayes is and get him sent away!"

A curious expression rested on the cowboy's lean face. "Keep holding out. Maybe one of these days, we'll nail Hayes." He grinned, and mischief lurked in his eyes. "My new pard's been looking forward to seeing you again."

Rebecca could not stop the rich blush that mantled her face. "Oh? How strange, since Jim's marrying Conchita tonight."

"My other pard. The long-legged galoot duded up ready to perform the ceremony who's leaning against the door frame an' watching us." He raised one hand, motioned Joel to join them, and whispered in a woebegone voice, "Since you only care for me like a brother, you couldn't do better than Scott. He may be a preacher, but he's a real man, too. I sneaked around an' listened while he practiced preaching. He talks 'most as well as he rides an' ropes an' shoots."

"We meet again, Miss Fairfax. I'm glad." Joel's eyes glowed like blue jewels. In spite of obvious attempts to make his blond hair lie down, it lay in waves and looked even more golden in contrast with his suntanned skin. His blinding smile set Rebecca's heart to beating.

"It's nice to be here," she said noncommittally and held out her hand. It lost itself in Joel's strong one, but she noticed he made no effort to hold it longer than courtesy allowed, unlike some riders who used introductions as an excuse for extra friendliness.

"Excuse me, but I'd better hunt up Perkins an' make sure he hasn't got cold feet."

Smokey abruptly abandoned them. Rebecca found herself at a loss for words and felt horrified when she heard her own voice asking, "Mr. Scott, why did you and Smokey and Jim bring Conchita here?"

The blue gaze turned to steel. "No gentleman speaks to a lady of what would have happened to her if we hadn't arrived just when we did. Thank God we came."

His heartfelt prayer filled in all the blanks left by his refusal to discuss what she had suspected all along — that Hayes had been the villain.

A little later, Conchita confirmed it. While dressing in the beautiful white gown and Spanish lace mantilla Mrs. Lundeen had kindly lent her for her wedding, she told Rebecca in a few broken whispers how Hayes came, took her by surprise, and attacked her. "He is bad," she finished. "Señorita, never let him find you alone." It took all Rebecca could do to change the fear in the bride-to-be's eyes to the joy that rightfully belonged to her on her wedding day.

Conchita had shyly asked Rebecca to stand up with her, along with Smokey, who flanked the eager groom. Glad that she had heeded Mrs. Cook's advice not to wear white and rival the bride, Rebecca's rose pink gown swished around her ankles and made a perfect background for the dark-haired girl who turned toward Perkins in perfect trust. Quite a crowd of neighbors had ridden to the Bar Triangle for the event. Admiration of the young women's beauty rippled through the small crowd.

Rebecca could openly observe Joel throughout the simple but touching ceremony. His face shone with goodness. He spoke of the responsibility Jim and Conchita faced and the happiness they could find in one another by becoming part of God's plan for husbands and wives since time began. When he came to the question, "Do you, Conchita, take Jim . . . ," Rebecca thought, *What would it be like, promising to take a man for better and worse, in sickness and health; mutually agreeing to be his companion; promising to keep yourself for him and from all others until death?* How much love she would have to feel before consenting to such solemn, irrevocable vows!

She glanced to the side and caught Hayes's stare. How terrible to be linked with him. Not even to save her father could she face life as Hayes's wife. The curl of his lip showed his contempt for the sacredness of the vows that Conchita and Jim made before God and these people. Rebecca forced herself to look steadily at Hayes for a moment, refusing to show the fear that crawled in her veins, then she deliberately turned back to watch Jim place a simple gold band on his bride's finger and salute her with a quick, boyish kiss.

You couldn't do better than Scott. Smokey's satisfied announcement rang in her ears. Her heart fluttered, but a wave of people, determined to greet the bride, washed between them. Not until the new Mr. and Mrs. Jim Perkins fled to the privacy of the cabin that the Lundeens provided did Rebecca get to speak to Joel again. She found herself tongue-tied once more.

"They'll be happy," Joel said. He looked both ways and lowered his voice. "This is my first wedding."

"It was beautiful," Rebecca murmured, wondering how a man like this had escaped feminine wiles. Smokey had mentioned that Joel had passed his twentieth birthday a few months before this early summer wedding. "I look forward to hearing you preach tomorrow."

Humility replaced Joel's smile. "It's been some time since I gave a sermon, not since I left Santa Fe." He expertly guided her to a small bench partially secluded from the party that had spilled out of the adobe ranch house into the yard. "I know the Lord will help me give the right message, though. He always does." Moonlight silvered his fair hair.

"Mr. Scott — or do I call you Reverend?" She laughed and nervously pleated her soft pink gown.

"Just Joel, please."

Encouraged, she asked, "Would you tell me more about your search to find your father?"

One of Joel's best skills lay in his ability to paint vivid word pictures. He told the pathetic story of his mother in a way that brought a mist to Rebecca's eyes. He mentioned his long trail to find those his uncle Gideon longed to reach with the gospel for Jesus Christ. A happy laugh crinkled his face when he said, "Just today I got word from Colorado Springs that Eb Sears and Lily are going to marry. Little Danny will have a father again, but the best thing is that Eb and Lily have decided to follow the Master. Eb is going into the store with Livingston, Lily's father-in-law, who loves her and Danny and can't bear to lose them."

"A sad tale with a happy ending. Mr., uh, Joel, do you think God has a happy ending for everyone?"

He remained quiet for several moments,

then slowly replied, "I believe everyone who accepts Christ and walks in His path will have the happiest ending of all — eternal life. I also feel God gives His children what He knows is best for them, although it may not be what we think will make us happy."

"Then, even if you don't find your father, you won't feel cheated?" It suddenly seemed vitally important to know. Rebecca clasped her hands, looked up at him in the moonlight, and added, "You won't feel that God let you down?"

"I'll be disappointed," the young minister admitted. "I still believe someday I will find Father. If I don't, God must have a reason."

Rebecca felt bitterly disappointed. "Mrs. Cook always says the same thing, that God must have a reason. If this is true, why can't He let us know?" Her fingers clenched. "I've tried to trust Him, but when I see Father growing old and going somewhere inside himself away from me, it's hard. I don't know how long it's been since he's laughed."

"Is Hayes responsible?"

The sympathetic question opened the floodgates. "He has to be. Father never was boisterous, but before Hayes came, he smiled and rode with me. Now, most of the time he just broods and lets Hayes run things. Run them down," she added. Her lips twisted. "Smokey said cattle are disappearing from the Lazy F. Then, that episode at Lone Man Cabin —" She put her hand over her mouth.

"It's all right. Smokey told me what happened."

Relief at having someone else know left her weak. "I promised not to tell Father, but I had to tell Smokey." A puzzled feeling went through her. "He said something funny tonight about maybe nailing Hayes."

Joel took her hand and pressed it. "Miss Rebecca, will you trust Smokey and me and most of all God? I have a feeling things will work out."

"Sometimes I don't think there is a way out," she said.

His fingers tightened. "There is always a way up." He freed her hand and smiled at her. "Now I'm getting into my sermon for tomorrow."

She felt her lips quiver into an answering smile but sobered when a heavy voice demanded, "What are you doin' out here?" Hayes stood at her elbow with a scowling Samuel Fairfax just behind him.

How much have they heard? Rebecca frantically wondered before she sprang to her feet. "I can't see that is any of your concern."

195

"It's mine." Fairfax pushed past Hayes and confronted her. "Get in the house." He turned a scorching gaze on Joel. "If I catch you around her again, I'll horsewhip you. Like father, like son."

Rebecca gasped at the sneer in his voice, the satisfaction on Hayes's face made grotesque by waving shadows that crossed and recrossed it with every movement of the rising breeze.

"I wouldn't try that if I were you." Joel leisurely got up, planted his feet apart, and did not give an inch.

"Who do you think you are!" Hayes fairly frothed at the mouth.

"Shut up, Hayes." Smokey Travis stepped from behind a cottonwood. His wedding clothes had been replaced by work shirt, pants, and vest. His Stetson rode on the back of his head, and moonlight glittered in his eyes.

Had he been playing watchdog? Rebecca felt herself go cold. "Father, Smokey, please. Don't spoil Conchita's wedding."

"That woman? I'm surprised even Perkins'd marry her," Hayes jeered. "But, he's no better than she is."

"Liar!" Smokey bellowed and dove head-first into Hayes's stomach like a barreling cannonball. The unexpected attack knocked

196

the taller, heavier man to the ground and winded him enough so that Smokey could get in a half-dozen pounding blows on Hayes's face before Fairfax could pull him off.

"Look out!" Rebecca screamed.

Hayes had recovered enough to reach for his gun, black death in his face.

Rebecca screamed again and flung herself in front of Smokey. In the same instant, Joel, unarmed, drew back one foot and sent the gun spinning. "You rotten coward!" he said.

Smokey tore free from Fairfax and towered over Hayes on the ground, nursing a bruised hand from the powerful kick. "Next time I see you, you'd better see me first, Hayes." He whipped around toward Fairfax. "If you aren't as crooked an' yellow as this coyote, you'll kick him off the Lazy F before there ain't no Lazy F left." Rage overcame caution. "While you're at it, ask him about hawg-tying your daughter at Lone Man Cabin an' having a phony deputy who calls himself Crowley make her swear she wouldn't tell you what happened."

Father, be a man, Rebecca silently prayed — in vain. Samuel licked dry lips, sent a furious glance at the huddled figure of Hayes, cursed him, and ordered, "Get back to the ranch." His daughter saw hatred beyond belief in his face, but not a word came concerning Smokey's charge.

"I told you to get in the house." Fairfax glared at Rebecca. With a little cry, she gathered her skirts around her and ran, but not before hearing Joel Scott's accusation, "Samuel Fairfax, the meanest animal alive protects its young. God forgive you for standing by and letting this vile man near the sweetest, purest girl God could create!"

His praise warmed the fleeing figure's cold heart. She slowed down before she reached the main body of merrymakers. Incredible as it seemed, they laughed, talked, and evidently had not been aware of the fight. Rebecca paused and smoothed down her hair, hoping she did not look as distraught as she felt.

"It's about time to start the shivaree," someone called. Rebecca had never been allowed to participate in the mock serenade with which cowhands often celebrated weddings. They would keep the young couple awake with their hollering, beating on pans, and demands for food.

But Rebecca could not face it now. Mrs. Cook stood a little apart, and she went straight to her. "I'm really tired. Do we have to go?"

"My stars, no, Child. Let the cowboys do

the noisemaking. We'll go on to bed. You sure looked lovely tonight. That new preacher could barely stop looking at you long enough to get Jim and Conchita hitched." A wistful look that reminded Rebecca of long-forgotten feelings crept into her face. "Joel Scott would be a solid foundation a woman could build love and a home on and know they would stand."

First Smokey, now Mrs. Cook. Rebecca wondered if she had fallen into a conspiracy to throw her into Joel's arms. The idea sent a glow through her, and long after Mrs. Cook slept, Rebecca lay awake reliving those moments on the little bench until Hayes and his evil crept into her patch of Eden.

Before daybreak, shouts and hoofbeats awakened Rebecca.

"What is it?" Mrs. Cook sleepily rose on one elbow.

Rebecca ran to the window and threw it wide open. Smokey's voice cut through the murky dawn. "Roll out, men! One of the night guard just rode in, shot to pieces. The red-and-white herd in the south pasture's gone."

"Gone?" Was that Jim Perkins's voice?

"Yeah. Gone. Vamoosed. Disappeared. Every hide an' horn of them. We're riding."

"What's going on out there?" Rebecca

recognized her father's bellow.

"Rustlers." Smokey's succinct reply brought action.

Ten minutes later, Rebecca had dressed, told Mrs. Cook she was going to Conchita, and joined the pale, deserted bride on the tiny porch of the cabin. Together, they watched the group of riders vanish into the predawn mists, Conchita openly crying. Rebecca's heart muscles contracted. Even the mists had not hidden a certain sunny head, bare of covering for a moment when Joel doffed his sombrero and rode away. Would there be a preaching after all? Or would some of those grim-faced riders not return? Rebecca strained her eyes until the moving black dots disappeared from sight.

"Why do men rob and kill?" Rebecca burst out. "Sometimes I hate this country."

"They have not the love of God in their hearts," Conchita sadly replied and wiped her eyes.

God. A vision of the world as it could be rose with the New Mexican sun. The day came alive in a burst of glory that failed to lift the spirits of those who watched. By mutual consent, Mrs. Cook, Rebecca, Mrs. Lundeen, and Conchita spent the waiting hours cheering one another.

"It's a shame your wedding had to be followed by something like this." Mrs. Lundeen stabbed a bright knitting needle into the ball of yarn in her lap and sighed. "Men ride off, women wait."

Conchita pressed her lips tightly together and did not answer; neither did Rebecca. Yet, time after time, one of them went for a drink of water or outside for a breath of air, but always in the direction that faced the trail that had swallowed the pursuing party.

Curly, the former Lazy F cook who now reigned in the Bar Triangle cookhouse, added fresh horror when he reluctantly crossed to the ranch house and told them that the night herder had died. "Not any older than Smokey," he said. His face contorted, and his lips thinned. He barely resembled the jolly man Rebecca remembered. "I hope they get the skunks who did this and hang them on the nearest cottonwood." His eyes slitted. "I'da gone, too, but the boy needed me worse." His shoulders sagged, and he looked straight into Rebecca's face. "Be careful, Miss," he whispered when the others considerately turned away. "Hayes didn't go with the others."

A thrill of fear shot through her. "Why not?"

"He says . . ." Curly paused. "He says Fairfax told him to keep his eyes peeled and

201

stay here." The cook made a rude noise with his mouth.

"Do you believe him?" Rebecca demanded, hands icy with foreboding.

"Sure, just like I b'lieve the sun comes up in the west." Curly gave her another warning look and waddled back toward the bunkhouse where Hayes stood on the porch watching.

"What're you tellin' her?" Hayes held his hands menacingly close to his holsters.

"Whadda y'think I'm tellin' her?" Curly retorted. "The kid died, didn't he?"

Even with the distance between them, Rebecca could see Hayes relax. He put his hands on his wide hips and stared at her. She gave him a look of unutterable scorn and went back inside.

Yet when the men had not come back by dusk, she could no longer stand being cooped up. "I think I'll go into the courtyard," she told the others. She glanced both ways, and relieved that Hayes had ridden off earlier on some pursuit of his own, she idly walked around the flower-bright area. The perfume of roses heavily scented the evening air; the dimness before moonrise, broken only by light streaming from a few windows into the otherwise dark garden, offered respite to her aching heart. Somewhere in the vast range or forest her father, Mr. Lundeen, Smokey, and the others tracked a band of murderous rustlers who had killed once and would not hesitate to kill again. Joel rode with them, with his angelic face that could change to righteous anger, the way it had done when he defended her against her father.

Perhaps Samuel Fairfax really was not her father. If he were, how could he sacrifice her to Hayes? Or, after today, would he no longer insist she must marry against her will to save him? Surely, even though he failed to rebuke his foreman, his blind eyes must have been opened to Hayes's wickedness. Rebecca, while gazing at the splashing water in the fountain, tried to piece together the scraps of her past and Hayes's hints, the way Mrs. Cook pieced patchwork scraps until she had a complete quilt.

Lost in concentration, she forgot Conchita and Curly's warning that Hayes presented unseen danger. Suddenly, a stealthy step behind her triggered an alarm in her brain — but too late. She opened her mouth to cry out, but a rag, stuffed in her mouth, stopped her. Strong arms lifted her, too tightly for her to struggle. *God, are You there?* She clung to Joel's faith; her own was too weak to help.

CHAPTER 12

Fury flowed through Rebecca like flood-waters in autumn. How could Hayes dare to manhandle her like this? Now, she must put her anger to work and get out of this predicament. She had been warned against him but never dreamed he would be bold enough to snatch her out of the courtyard. She tried to think with his brain. Next would come a wild ride to some deserted cabin. She refused to consider anything further.

To her amazement, Hayes made no attempts to ride off with his captive. He merely carried her to an unlighted room at the far end of the sprawling ranch house and whispered in her ear, "Promise not to yell, and I'll take the gag off."

She nodded, eager to get rid of the rag or scarf or whatever it was that nearly choked her. Hayes set her down and yanked the gag. In a twinkling, Rebecca darted toward the door through which they had come. She had not promised not to escape.

"Here, none of that!" Her enemy caught her with strong hands that dug into her shoulders. She silently fought, but her 120 pounds, although range-trained to strength, could not overpower Hayes's 200 pounds. He forced her into a chair and tied her down, hands behind her back, feet crossed.

Rebecca's eyes had adjusted to the faint light that crept in through the window even before Hayes had carefully closed the shutters, struck a match, and lit a lantern. She saw he had brought her to a storeroom. Her lip curled. "I see you prepared for this outrage." She nodded at the lantern, strangely out of place among the neatly stacked boxes of supplies.

"It's time we had us a little talk," he announced. In the lantern light, he loomed taller and meaner than ever, and she hated the triumph flaming in his eyes. Had he looked like that the day he caught Conchita alone? Rebecca forced herself not to shudder. Once she showed fear, he became the master.

"There's nothing for us to discuss. Ever," she defied him, even while her bonds cut into her delicate wrists as she surreptitiously moved them to try to free herself.

Hayes lost any semblance of courtesy. "When you know everythin', you'll come crawlin' to me, beggin' me to marry you." She just stared at him, and he added, "Now you and me are goin' to settle things right now. When I rode into the Lazy F and saw you, I arranged with your daddy that we'd be married. I've kept my mouth shut waitin' to let you get used to the idea. No more. Samuel's actin' like he's about to go back on our deal and take what comes." Hayes fixed his gaze on Rebecca and laughed harshly. "It's been worth waitin'. You were a purty kid, but you're a better-lookin' woman. Too good for Travis or that young preacher."

She started, and he laughed again. "I saw him lookin' at you."

"Why don't you just say what you have to say and let me go?" Rebecca's brown eyes flashed fire, but she deliberately yawned. "I find this whole conversation tiresome."

Had she gone too far? In spite of her determination not to cringe, she could not help shrinking back when Hayes's long arms reached out as if he would shake the living daylights out of her.

"You and your haughty ways," he cried, keeping his voice low, which made it even more frightening. "Why, you ain't even

Fairfax's kid! He picked you out of some hole-in-the-wall run by outlaws, made a deal to meet your own daddy here, then murdered him, brought you to the ranch, and claimed it with some kind of paper."

Rebecca felt the blood drain from her face. Her mind churned. "It isn't true."

"You callin' me a liar? Then listen to this. If Samuel Fairfax is so pure and lily-white, how come when I rode in and accused him to his face, he turned the color of ashes and begged me to forget it?" Passion contorted Hayes's features into those of a monster bent on devouring its prey. "He offered me the foreman's job and said someday when I married you, the Lazy F would be all mine. There, that takes some of the pride outa you, doesn't it?"

It could not be true. Yet, if Hayes was lying, why had Father given him full rein over the ranch? Why did he not question the firings and unexplained cattle losses? Fairfax was not the kind of man to take such things without protest unless, as Hayes said, he had a terrible secret he feared would be discovered. Yet, something in the whole situation smelled rottener than a dead skunk. Rebecca slowly raised her chin a notch and quietly demanded, "If you're supposed to get me and the ranch anyway, just why have you been running off cattle and horses and hiding them in Lone Man Canyon?"

Hayes's face turned dirty white in the lantern light. "Who says I did that?" he blustered. "Why would I, when it's all gonna be mine real soon?"

She went cold at his confidence, but her intense gaze never wavered from his guilty face. "I worked the blindfold free, Hayes." Her voice cracked like a teamster's bullwhip. "I saw you and confirmed what I suspected when you roped and tied me. There's not an outlaw in New Mexico who'd dare touch Samuel Fairfax's daughter." Her voice broke. Perhaps she was not his daughter at all. Much as she feared to admit it, the ring of at least some truth underscored Hayes's story.

The man's gall held. "Wives can't testify against their husbands," he gloated. "Now, when that preacher comes ridin' back in . . . if he does . . . we'll have us another weddin'." He smiled.

Rebecca wondered how a smile could look so evil. Yet, with keen insight born of desperation, she saw something else. Clyde Hayes, wicked to the core, loved her. Not in the tender, gentle way she dreamed of when she thought of love, but with a love that caused him to take risks beyond belief to possess her. A flicker of an idea tickled her mind and grew. Could she play on that feeling, change it to the kind of love that would put her happiness above his own?

She stared into his face, searching for a clue, a hint of relenting or pity. She found none.

"I won't have to make you promise not to talk about this with anyone." Hayes laughed suggestively. "Men who kill in cold blood end up danglin' from a tree limb."

"The way Smokey Travis almost did — and for nothing," Rebecca bitterly accused. "Thank God Jo— Mr. Scott came when he did."

"I'll get that preacher one of these days," Hayes threatened as he untied her. "You've got 'til noon tomorrow to make up your mind whether I spill the beans and your daddy hangs." He bowed low and mockingly, swung open the door, stepped outside, and checked the courtyard. "Sleep well, Becky." His menacing laughter followed her as she ran.

Somehow, she managed to get back into the courtyard and remain long enough to gather her wits before Conchita came looking for her. The new bride's despair drove some of Rebecca's problems away when Conchita confessed, "I fear for — the men."

"Nothing too bad could have happened," Rebecca automatically consoled, noticing how large her friend's eyes looked in her pinched face. When Conchita showed no signs of being cheered, Rebecca took a deep breath and added, "We must trust in God. He is everywhere, and He can take care of Jim and Father and the others." Joel's image sprang to mind.

At last Conchita responded. Her brown fingers pressed Rebecca's tanned hand. "Gracias." But as more endless hours limped by, the strain continued. Husbands, father, friends — somewhere in the night chasing desperadoes. How could one bear it? Yet, what could not be changed must be endured. Rebecca felt she put away the last of her childhood and became a woman during the waiting time that left her too numb to even face Hayes's revelations.

The clock struck midnight. Rebecca thought she would shriek if something did not happen soon. A faint sound in the night air brought her out of her chair. "Listen!" She threw the front door wide; the steady clatter of hooves increased. Rebecca raced into the yard, closely followed by Conchita, Mrs. Lundeen, and Mrs. Cook, who had absolutely refused to go to bed while the others watched for the men.

Aware of Conchita's hard breathing beside her that echoed her own, Rebecca held her breath when a band of horses and riders swept toward them. She frantically glanced from horse to horse, then caught her throat with one hand. "Oh, God, no!"

Three of the horses wore empty saddles. One was her father's.

Joel Scott had not been asleep when the fatally wounded night herder rode in. For hours he had lain awake wondering, *Can love come this way, in two brief encounters?* Yet, he felt he had known Rebecca Fairfax always, that she had lurked in the dim recesses of his heart until he found her in reality. Everything about her pleased him. Her merry brown eyes, which could fill with horror or pain or comfort. Her tanned skin and nut-brown hair. Her sturdy form, tall enough for the top of her head to reach his lips, as she had reached his heart.

He laughed to himself. Such flights of poetry for a range-riding preacher! Yet, the intensity of her questions, when she asked if God had happy endings for people, had shown real searching for answers about God. Suddenly, his fresh-born love gave way to a higher feeling. Joel bowed his head and prayed for the girl whose rose pink gown had been no fairer than the one who wore it. His fingers strayed to the wilted rose that had dropped from her hair when she fled from her father's wrath and the ugly scene with Hayes. He had absently picked it up when the others left and tucked it in his pocket. Now he held the crumpled flower to his nose; its perfume remained intact, as alluring as Rebecca in all her innocence.

Joel still held the rose petals when the sound of a running horse shattered the predawn. One of a grim-faced group of men, he rode away to — what? Possible death, for sure. Rustlers were not known for their willingness to be captured. Memory of Rebecca's and Conchita's fearful faces when he waved to them rode with him. "God, be with us this night," he prayed, then nudged Querida closer to Samuel Fairfax and his mount. No matter what the man hid, and Joel felt sure he had a dark secret, this was still Rebecca's father. Perhaps in the long hours ahead, a time would come when he needed a friend; Smokey, Perkins, and even Lundeen seemed to have little use for Fairfax.

Smokey spurred his buckskin up alongside Joel and mumbled low enough so Fairfax could not hear, "Do you find anything funny about Hayes staying behind an' not riding with us?"

"I do." Jim Perkins must have ears like an elephant to have heard Smokey, Joel marveled. The just-married cowboy crowded close on the other side of Smokey. "Mighty peecooliar, ain't it?" He pulled his Stetson down over his forehead, and even in the pale dawn, his usually happy-go-lucky face shone sober. "Also strange that rustlers knew just what time to steal the cattle. Word didn't get sent to folks 'round here concernin' the weddin' 'til just a few days ago."

"Then someone who knew tipped the rustlers off, told them there'd just be a few cowpokes night herding," Smokey put in. This time he did not bother to lower his voice.

"What's that you say?" Fairfax spoke for the first time since they had left the Bar Triangle. "Are you accusing someone, Travis?"

"Nope. I know what it's like to be accused an' tried an' convicted when I didn't do anything." Smokey's words dropped like a shroud over the conversation. Fairfax snorted and swung away from the other three, his back stiffer than a ramrod.

Joel saw Smokey cock his head toward Jim, lift his eyebrows, then follow the owner of the Lazy F. He prodded Querida, and

Perkins's sorrel trailed after them.

"Fairfax, hold up."

The tall man reined in and glared. "What do you want?"

Smokey waited until the rest of the riders swept by before opening his coat and showing the silver badge he wore. Rays of the rising sun reflected off it.

"You? A deputy marshal?" Fairfax roared. A gray shadow crept over his face in spite of the sunlight bathing the little group huddled together.

"Shh." Smokey glanced up the trail, then back at Fairfax. "What I said last night is true. Your daughter discovered a passel of Lazy F an' other cattle an' horses all tucked away in Lone Man Canyon behind a new fence."

"Leave my daughter out of this," Fairfax ordered furiously.

"Ump-umm. Not when she ain't safe from being lassoed an' hawg-tied by crooks like Hayes an' that fake deputy Crowley."

Fairfax looked like he might explode. He licked his lips and looked sick. "I can't believe Hayes would do that! Why, when he —"

"When he thinks he's gonna get the whole kit 'n' caboodle by marryin' your daughter," Perkins tossed in.

Obviously shaken, Fairfax resorted to sarcasm. "When did you get on the side of the law, Travis?"

"About a week after Rebecca told me what happened at Lone Man," Smokey said quietly.

"I don't understand," Joel burst out. "All the time, when Hayes tried to hang you, why didn't you show your badge then?"

An unaccustomed red crept into Smokey's face. "Aw, I got so mad at Hayes, I yelled out what he had done to Rebecca instead of telling the boys I'd got myself appointed deputy marshal."

"You no-good dumbhead," Perkins yelled, face redder than Smokey's. "I oughta beat the stuffin' out of you here 'n' now."

Joel stopped impending hostilities by demanding, "Mr. Fairfax, I meant what I said last night. Your daughter needs protection from Hayes. If you won't give it, we will, but it's hard to believe you'll let that snake walk in and take over everything you own."

"I have no choice. If Rebecca ever finds out what Hayes knows, she'll never forgive me. You think I care about the ranch? I'd ride out with my daughter in the middle of the night if I didn't know Hayes would follow and spill everything. How can a man go so far wrong?" He laughed wildly and without mirth. "Every day since Hayes rode in, my life has been miserable!" His granite face worked.

"But you don't have to go on," Joel exclaimed. Pity for the hard man suffering before him reached inside the young minister and demanded his best. "No matter what you've done, God forgives — and I believe your greathearted daughter will, too."

All the fire went out of Fairfax and left him a beaten, old-looking shell of a man. "If I could believe that, I'd . . ." He shook his head. "It's too late."

"It's never too late, Man." Joel could not let this opportunity slip away, perhaps never to come again. Yet, fate thought otherwise; the swift return of one of the posse broke into the trembling moment.

"C'mon. The tracks are leadin' to Lone Man Canyon, an' if they've got provisions, the rustlers can hole up there 'til Judgment Day!"

"Are you with us, Fairfax?" Smokey half closed his eyelids. "I got a feeling we'll find some mighty interesting things in a little while. Maybe enough to put Hayes away or hang him."

Hope flared in Fairfax's eyes, making

them bluer than usual; then it died. "I'm with you, but no matter what Hayes is accused of, it won't keep him from talking before he gets what's coming to him."

"Well, no," Jim Perkins drawled. A cheerful grin tilted his lips. "I don't reckon nobody's gonna believe much of what some rustler sez, right, Smokey? I know I wouldn't."

"Me, either." Smokey's dark eyes flashed. "Hayes can do all the crowing he wants an' just get in deeper. Trying to blackmail a well-known rancher on some trumped-up charge won't hold much water."

"If I thought that, I'd fall on my knees and thank God," Fairfax murmured. Joel saw that the tortured man really meant it. But his blood ran cold when Fairfax added, "He's insanely in love with Rebecca. It's the only thing that's kept him silent this long."

"If ya think you've been in misery, get it into your noggin that marryin' Hayes would put that daughter of yours in a whole lot more," Perkins snapped. "And she ain't done nothin' to deserve it, whether you have or not." He spurred his sorrel. "Now, ride!"

Querida leaped ahead. Joel glanced over his shoulder at Smokey and Fairfax. They followed and soon caught up with the rest of the Bar Triangle men.

"They got a head start," one angry cowboy said. He pointed to the beaten earth that bore mute evidence to the passing of a large herd of cattle. "Our man hadta ride clear back when he wasn't in no condition to do it. This ain't gonna be no Sunday school picnic." His face reddened. "Sorry, Joel. No offense 'ntended."

"None taken. Besides, sometimes even rattlesnakes come to Sunday school picnics." In an attempt to lighten the atmosphere, he added, "That's my sermon for the day, men, since we won't be home in time for the meeting."

"Haw haw." The cowboys and Lundeen roared. A faint smile even crossed Fairfax's set countenance, but the following hours wiped away everything except the knowledge that a hard and dangerous job lay ahead.

Lundeen was aghast when he saw the trail the rustlers had made no attempt to erase; he also advised caution. Once the posse reached the entrance to Lone Man Canyon, the men were to move softly and keep their eyes and ears wide open. "If we can sneak up on them all inside Lone Man Cabin, we'll order them out with their hands up. Wish we had a law officer with us." He sighed.

"We do." Smokey showed his badge. The others gasped, but Lundeen's face broke into a grim smile.

"All right. If they won't come out, we'll burn the shack. It's old and dry as tinder. Not even a rustler's gonna hang out in there once it starts smoking."

"Easy as fallin' off a horse," Perkins muttered. "But it won't be." His prediction came true. A lookout, at the top of a bluff above the canyon, sent a volley of shots down like hail.

"Take cover!" Lundeen bellowed.

Joel dove for shelter, heard heavy, running steps behind him, and twisted around. Fairfax almost made it to the screening underbrush; then he stumbled, fell. More shots rang out. To Joel's horror, Fairfax rose, twitched, and fell back. Heedless of his own safety, Joel leaped from cover and zigzagged the short distance to Samuel. He snatched him up, staggered under the heavier man's weight, and made it back to safety, vaguely conscious that Smokey and Jim had stepped into the open and emptied their rifles toward the unseen shooter.

"Is he all right?" Lundeen slithered across the needle-covered ground.

"I don't know." Joel gently laid down his burden, looked at the bright red stains that covered his hands, and shuddered. Samuel Fairfax lay broken, unconscious, and bleeding at his feet. If he died, anything he might have known about Cyrus Scott would die with him. A thought, so grotesque it made Joel's heart skip a beat, bored into his brain. *What if Rebecca wasn't Samuel Fairfax's daughter after all? What if Cyrus Scott had been that father and Fairfax knew it?*

An even more startling idea insinuated itself into Joel's mind. If such a thing proved to be true, Rebecca could never be his wife — she would be his sister.

CHAPTER 13

Lundeen examined the unconscious Samuel Fairfax with strong, sure hands, then grunted. "Ahuh. Good." He ran one finger along a shallow groove on Fairfax's head. "Creased him just enough to knock him out. Head wounds always bleed bad." He ripped his kerchief off, made a pad of it, and pressed it against the bullet wound. "Give me another scarf, someone."

Joel grabbed his from his neck and handed it over. Lundeen tore it into strips, knotted them, and wound them around Samuel's head to hold the pad in place. When he stood, his face looked stern. "All right, men, let's round up the dirty, thievin' skunks and head home. Haven't heard no more out of that sharpshooting jasper, so he's either dead or out of commission. Joel, you stay with Fairfax. It won't do for him to wake up and not know where he is. Might thrash around and start his head bleeding again.

Smokey, Jim, ride with me. The rest of you scatter and surround Lone Man Cabin. By now, I'd guess that pack of coyotes are holed up in there."

Leaving their horses tied nearby, the posse slipped through the shelter of bushes and behind trees near the cabin. Joel had not realized they were so close. By almost closing his eyes and straining, he could glimpse the dilapidated shack in the distance and hear men yelling in the clear air. He divided the eternity of waiting between checking Fairfax, who had not yet regained consciousness, and the stealthy figures closing in on the cabin.

"Come out of there with your hands up!" Lundeen's stentorian yell could almost have been heard back at the Bar Triangle.

A volley of words from the cabin answered him; a hail of bullets sang past the well-concealed posse. "Let 'em have it, boys," Lundeen roared.

A burst of gunfire and a high-pitched cry from inside the cabin brought Joel to his feet. Why was he here while Smokey and Jim and the others fought the enemy to all decent people? A terrible choice loomed. If he left his post and joined the others, in all probability he would be forced to kill, something he had vowed never to do. Sweat beaded his forehead. "God, those rustlers are vile!" Yet, Jesus had died for such as them. *What had Smokey told him so long ago?* He wrinkled his forehead. Oh, yes. He had been ready to leap up and pummel Hayes, but Smokey dragged him back into hiding and later warned, *You've gotta learn to lie still when there's danger around, no matter what.* Was God admonishing him to lie still now?

A low moan brought Joel to his knees beside Fairfax, whose hand went to his head. Joel caught it before he could disturb Lundeen's bandage. "The lookout creased you. Take it easy."

Samuel's blue eyes glazed with pain and something else. He reached toward Joel with shaking fingers.

The young minister had tended enough pain-racked persons to recognize distress. "You can talk later."

Samuel shook his head vehemently, then winced at the movement.

Sensing the fallen man's need to speak, Joel leaned close and stared straight into Fairfax's eyes. "Remember, whatever you've done, no matter how guilty you are, you can be forgiven."

A curious blend of shame, hope, and poignancy went through the watching eyes before Samuel mumbled, "Guilty . . . as . . . sin," then turned his head and closed his eyes.

Joel's heart felt like a rock. He had hoped beyond hope Fairfax would prove to be Hayes's victim and not criminally guilty. What chance did Rebecca have for the happy ending she had so wistfully confessed she dreamed of?

Lundeen's shout pierced Joel's thoughts. "Come out, or we'll burn you out," he bellowed. A sneering laugh and another round of shots served as an answer.

Joel's gaze fixed on a running figure, who carried a torch made from a dry, pitchy, pine branch. Smokey. "God, no!" Joel froze, unaware of his prayer.

The figure zigzagged toward the cabin, nimbly dodging bullets and using the cover of his comrades' heavy firing to near the cabin and toss his torch in a fiery arc that left it on the bone-dry roof and sent flames licking the tinderlike debris. Smokey veered to one side when the Bar Triangle men cheered. The cheers turned to dismay when a defiant shot from the cabin found its mark, and Smokey fell.

Hatred overrode all of Joel's caution. Heedless of the consequences, he leaped up and ran with all his might toward Smokey.

If those murderers had killed him, Joel would personally see to it they paid — unless the posse beat him to it.

Shots, dense smoke, coughing, then a loud, "We're comin' out, hands up."

"Keep them high," Jim Perkins ordered at the top of his lungs.

By the time Joel reached Smokey, seven dark-faced men, led by the so-called Deputy Crowley, had stumbled into the open, tears streaking through the soot on their faces.

"Tie them, or better yet, hang 'em," a cowboy called.

"Naw." Smokey's voice sounded surprisingly strong for a man who had been shot. He struggled to his feet, right hand pressed over his left shoulder, left hand reaching inside his coat and flashing his badge. "We'll haul them in an' let the law take care of them."

"Smokey, you're all right?" Joel grabbed his friend's arm.

"Easy, Pard. It ain't much more than a scratch, but it's sore." He scowled at the men being bound, and a wicked glint flashed in his eyes, brighter than the sun on his badge. "Play along with me," he whispered into Jim's ear, then loudly announced, "Too bad, Crowley an' the rest of you. We know who's behind our red-an'-white herd disappearing an' ending up here." He nodded past the cabin to steers crowded behind a sturdy, new-looking fence, now roiling and bellowing from the shooting. "Yeah, you notice Clyde Hayes ain't riding with us."

"Last I saw, he was standin' on the bunkhouse porch watchin' us ride off." Perkins tightened his rope around a pasty-faced Crowley.

"It wouldn't s'prise me if he's clean outa the country by the time we come ridin' in with you fellers."

"He's just the kind who'll leave someone else to take the punishment," Joel confirmed.

"That's what he thinks," one of the rustlers snarled. "He planned the raid, told us most everyone'd be up at the marryin'. I ain't takin' the blame so he c'n go free!"

"Me, neither," another put in, and a ripple of assent flowed through the group.

Crowley broke under the pressure and to save his own skin. "Hayes said Fairfax'd started actin' funny. He was afraid the old man'd go back on his word about that daughter of his, so he hired us to steal all the cattle we could before Hayes waylaid the girl and rode off with her."

Flames danced in Smokey's eyes. "You skunk! We oughta hang you right here for being part of such a scheme." He yanked out his revolver with his right hand; blood dripped down his left sleeve. Crowley's eyes looked as if he was staring death in the face.

"Get them outa here," Smokey barked and sheathed his gun. "Somebody bandage me up an' see who's hurt or dead."

Lundeen turned doctor again, while Jim and the others finished tying the outlaws in the saddles. A few minutes later, he returned to report, "One rustler's dead. Our outfit's not even scratched 'cept for Smokey 'n' Fairfax. I sent a rider up the bluff to check on the sharpshooter." That rider returned with the news the lookout man had evidently died in the exchange of shots early in the fray.

Lundeen strode back to Samuel Fairfax, who had again drifted into unconsciousness. "Hmm. It's a long ride back. Joel, you stay with him. The rest of us'll take in our prisoners and get a wagon back here as soon as we can."

"I reckon I'll stay, too," Smokey said.

"What? Let a little scratch keep you waiting for the wagon?" Lundeen joshed in his heavy manner.

"Ump-um." Unperturbed, Smokey shook his head. "Reckon you're forgetting something — Hayes." His succinct reminder snapped the men to attention. "The way I see it, soon as you ride in an' he sees his pards all trussed up like a Thanksgiving turkey, he's going to hop on the best horse he can find an' come a-running."

"He won't come this way," Joel protested. "That would be stupid."

"Naw," Perkins butted in, lean face grim. "Smokey's right. Hayes'll figure we figure that'd be just what ya said — stupid. So he'll do a double double cross and go where he ain't s'posed to be a-tall." He looked longingly at Smokey and Joel. "Lundeen, can't I stay with my pards?"

Lundeen deliberated. "You better come with me, Perkins. Just in case any of these rustlers get some funny ideas about trying to escape. With Fairfax, Joel, and Smokey missing, it leaves us shorthanded, and we've got a herd to drive, too."

"Okay, Boss." Jim heaved a big sigh, bent toward his friends, and warned, "Keep your eyes wide open. It's gonna take time to get a wagon back here. You got plenty of water from the creek. Kinda short on grub, though." He brightened. "Hey, Boss, when we knock down that fence and start the herd toward home, want me to leave a beefsteak on the hoof behind?"

Lundeen nodded. "Hurry it up. The sun

won't stick around all night, and we've got a long way to ride." The big man knelt by Fairfax, lifted an eyelid, and grunted. "He will be okay. Probably sleep and wake up a half-dozen times before we get back."

In a short time, silence replaced the cowboy yells, hoofbeats, and clouds of dust that marked the exodus of the Bar Triangle riders with their prisoners and herd.

Smokey gazed after them. "It coulda been a whole lot worse," he said significantly. He gingerly fingered his left arm. "Good thing I hit the dirt when I got winged. Say, how about some of that beefsteak? Jim hacked off a coupla hunks before he left." Smokey nodded toward the charred shack. "Lots of good embers there."

Reaction set in. Joel gulped. "I don't think I can eat anything . . . at least for awhile." He fought nausea and dropped to a downed tree trunk to hide the way his knees buckled.

"I understand." Smokey's face turned grim, and he looked older than the mountains surrounding them. "You've got to look at it this way. Let rustlers alone, an' they get bolder an' bolder. First thing you know, they start picking off honest ranchers and cowpokes, just like they did with the boy who rode out to take night watch, singing an' never knowing he'd come back all shot up." He planted both hands on his hips. "I hate killing, too. Sometimes I think a man oughta move somewhere away from every critter there is." He slowly shook his head. "Guess it wouldn't do any good. There's decent folks an' skunks no matter where you go." He grinned. "At that, let's wait awhile before we eat." He yawned. "I didn't get much shut-eye last night. Mind if I crawl under a tree an' conk out?"

"Go ahead. I'll stay with Fairfax." Joel knew he had slept even less than Smokey did, but the day's events left him wide-eyed. Besides, Fairfax might awaken and talk.

"If Hayes shows up, I'll come running," Smokey promised. "Never did sleep sound, an' since I got to be a poor, lonesome cowpoke, as Perkins calls us, I wake up real easy." He yawned again, stretched, and headed for a tall cottonwood that provided shade. Five minutes later, Joel heard snoring. He grinned. Smokey might wake easy, but he slept sounder than he admitted.

Joel gradually settled down. He drowsed until Fairfax awakened again. "Have some water." He held a canteen. Samuel drank deeply, and once more, that poignant blue light brightened his life-weary eyes. Encouraged by it, Joel asked in a low voice, "Do you want to tell me the whole story?"

Fairfax recoiled, and Joel quickly added, "About Rebecca."

The other man hesitated, then nodded. The water seemed to have cleared his mind. He brokenly began, "Rebecca's not my daughter."

Joel slowly iced in spite of the warm afternoon. What he had suspected changed to certainty. The girl he had fallen in love with must be his sister . . . and Samuel Fairfax had somehow done away with Cyrus Scott, Rebecca and Joel's father.

"I met her daddy years ago, partnered with him until he got tangled in with a band of crooked men. Hayes was one of them."

Joel's mouth dropped in astonishment, and Fairfax managed a grim laugh. "Oh, he knew me long before he came to the Lazy F. You know how he threatened to expose me. I had done nothing wrong, but I couldn't prove my innocence. Hayes only knew part of the story."

Innocence? Joel remembered the agony in Samuel's face when he had whispered, "Guilty as sin." He opened his mouth, but Samuel had already picked up the threads of his story.

Rebecca's mother had died, and her father had no choice but to keep her with him. He worshipped her, as he had worshipped her mother. "Besides, they had no kinfolk near." Fairfax reached for the canteen and drank deeply again. He glanced at the still-sleeping Smokey and lowered his voice. "When he got in so deep with the outlaw again, my pard came to me in the dead of night. He told me to take Rebecca and ride out, to get away from the breaks and head for northeastern New Mexico. Sometime before, he'd arranged to buy a ranch."

"The Lazy F." Joel could almost see Fairfax and young Rebecca fleeing in the dead of night. What must that wild journey have been like to her? His heart throbbed with sympathy.

"The Lazy F," Fairfax confirmed. He lay quietly for a moment, so still that the quivering cottonwoods' secrets traveled back and forth from leaf to leaf, as portentous as those Samuel had revealed. "The man I'd ridden with loaded me with money and gave me ownership papers to claim the ranch. I reasoned that even though he probably got it from stealing or worse, the girl should have a chance. Besides, he said he'd sneak away when he could and come. He'd be able to travel better alone than if he had Rebecca with him; she'd be the first person the outlaws would look for when they followed — and they would. He never said he helped himself to their cache, but I figured it out." Fairfax laughed grimly. "I'd found my chance to be partners, half owner of a ranch in a grand country I fell in love with years before when I rode through it. We came. Rebecca loved it, the same as me. In time, she quit asking when her daddy would come. Long before that, she'd crawled into my heart the way a son or daughter of my own would have done."

Fairfax's lips twisted. "In time, I think she forgot she wasn't mine, at least most of the time. Then, Hayes came." The man's voice changed. The look of granite returned to his face, and his eyes lost their poignant blueness. "I learned Rebecca's real daddy had been killed the very night I rode out with her! Hayes had spent all the time in between looking for me. He'd quit the gang, suspecting the truth — that I had the loot. He wandered from place to place and finally tracked me down. Said he'd swear I killed my pard to get the ranch.

"I couldn't stand for Rebecca to know her own daddy had turned outlaw or that the home she loved so much had been paid for with tainted money. I bribed Hayes to keep his mouth shut, told him he could marry Rebecca and one day own the Lazy F. He saw to it the cowboys couldn't get near her and drove them away — until Smokey came and stuck." Fairfax groaned and struggled to a sitting position, then dropped his head in his hands. "I knew she hated him, but I didn't see any other way. Then you came."

Joel held his breath and endured the searching gaze.

"You rode right in on that black horse of yours, braced me, called me, and made me look at myself. I didn't like what I saw, but I had no choice. Either I kept my word to Hayes and lost Rebecca or broke my promise that she'd marry him and lost her — forever."

"And now?" Joel leaned forward, tense as a bowstring.

"I'll go to jail, but she won't marry Hayes." Manhood flowed back into the nearly beaten man. His shoulders straightened. Some of the greatness that must once have been his came into his features. His blue eyes shone.

"That isn't necessary, Fairfax," Smokey said softly from behind them. His dark face wore a smile, blinding in its unexpected sweetness.

"What did you say?" Samuel got up from the ground, held his head, and tottered toward the cowboy. Joel's heart contracted at the look of hope that dawned in Fairfax's eyes.

"Hayes is the one going to jail for a long time, maybe forever. I've been snooping around since I got to be a deputy marshal, an' I've discovered some mighty interesting things. Such as a warrant out for the arrest of a man named Hill, who bears a curious resemblance to Hayes."

"Warrant? For what?" Fairfax shook his blood-stained head and looked bewildered.

"For the murder of Seth Foster years ago."

"Seth Foster?" Fairfax blanched and gave an awful cry. "But that's him, the man Hayes claims I killed. My pard, who bought the Lazy F under the name Samuel Fairfax!"

"Correct." Smokey grinned, took the makings from his shirt pocket, and rolled a cigarette. He stuck the brown paper cylinder into his mouth, lit it, and puffed once.

Joel felt he had wandered into a never-ending maze. Seth Foster . . . Samuel Fairfax . . . Hayes who was really Hill. He shook his head. Once, he had been caught in rolling, red floodwaters. Their turgid undercurrents had threatened to suck him under and hold him until life fled. Now he felt caught the same way, tossed by dark currents he could neither understand nor fight. "Then Rebecca Fairfax is really Rebecca Foster?"

"I took his name to claim the ranch, the way he insisted. The transaction had been through another party, one who knew nothing of Seth's real name." Fairfax clutched his head and sat back down on the ground. "Can you see why I didn't want Rebecca to know all this, when I could prove nothing except that I traveled under a dead man's name, had that man's daughter, and lived on a ranch he owned?"

A million questions danced in Joel's beleaguered brain. Yet foremost, relief underlined each. Rebecca was not his sister. Gladness like a prayer winged into Joel's heart.

"Hold the confab," Smokey warned and ran toward a vantage point to return a few minutes later wearing a broad grin. "It's okay. Thought I heard something."

"They won't get a wagon back before tomorrow," Fairfax predicted. "Did I hear something about beefsteak, or was I dreaming?"

"I fry a mean piece of meat," Smokey admitted. "Pard, you feel like eating now?" he asked Joel.

The young minister only nodded. All his questions had come down to one burning thought, something between him and Fairfax, not even to be heard by the faithful

Smokey. With a keen glance, that worthy individual grinned and walked away to fry his steak.

"Mr. Fairfax, no, that isn't your name, is it?" Joel tried to find his way out of the maze. "Oh, hang it all, if you aren't Fairfax, who are you?" His voice sounded loud in his ears, but he knew it would not carry past the first tattletale cottonwood. "And what do you know about Cyrus Scott? *I have to know.*" He braced himself for the truth, prepared for anything — except Fairfax's answer.

Quietly, without fanfare, the older man stared straight at Joel. "I am Cyrus Scott, your father."

CHAPTER 14

"I am your father," the man that Joel had known as Samuel Fairfax repeated.

"God forgive me."

Faced by the shocking end of his long search, the younger man could only stare. All these weeks, the father he had sought for months, right here. "But you said he probably died years ago," Joel stammered.

The poignant light he had come to recognize but never understood crept again into the Lazy F's owner's eyes, turning them so blue, Joel wondered how he could have failed to identify this man as a Scott.

Joel felt his own eyes burn when his father said, "I tried to bury Cyrus Scott years ago after I discovered your mother died. If I'd only known about you!" The anguished cry tore into Joel's heart.

"You couldn't know. Judith was afraid you'd take me."

Cyrus flinched. "Once, I would have." He

raised a shaking hand. "Can God forgive me? Can you?" His eyes looked like those of a dog Joel once rescued from a beating.

Everything the young minister believed about forgiveness battled with his long-standing hurt and anger at what Cyrus had done. He had prattled of the need to forgive without knowing the depths of his own resentment or the difficulty of doing so. Now, his father's question nailed him to the cross of memories. If he could not forgive, Cyrus would never believe God could, either.

Slowly, almost of its own volition, Joel's hand extended, and for the first time, he touched his father . . . tentatively, then with a hard grip of hands that promised much. Joel felt Cyrus's fingers tremble. A look of near-glory cut years off Cyrus's face until he resembled Gideon. Joel took a sharp breath. A flood of pent-up emotions roared through him.

"Hey, steaks are done an' burning," Smokey called.

After another mighty squeeze, the two men's hands parted. Shoulder to shoulder, they headed toward Smokey. When they reached him, Joel threw back his head and announced, "I'd like you to meet my father."

Smokey gave them an inscrutable look. "I know."

"What?" Joel leaped toward him and glared. "You know?"

"Sure. When I got to nosing around, I put a few facts together an' figured it out." His maddening smile drove Joel wild, especially when he added with a grin that stretched clean across his face, "The way I see it, 'til your daddy got ready to talk, it was up to me to button my lip an' keep it that way."

"Thanks, Smokey." Cyrus offered his hand to the cowboy he had driven off his ranch.

In the greatheartedness that set Smokey apart from the common herd, he responded and shook heartily before complaining, "If we don't eat, this beefsteak's gonna be tougher than saddle leather."

The three men fell to and finished every scrap of the enormous steak, then chafed at the bit until the wagon from the Lazy F arrived. Lundeen and his men had taken the two dead rustlers' horses and the one Cyrus had ridden back to the ranch with them. Now, Smokey on his buckskin and Joel on Querida trailed the team and wagon, along with Jim Perkins, who had changed horses and come back.

"I'm glad we ain't hauling Rebecca's

daddy back worse hurt than he is," Smokey muttered. He cocked an eyebrow. "Say, Pard, since she won't ever love me the way a woman should, I hope you get her."

Joel marveled at the unselfish loyalty of the man whose life he had saved. "I do, too."

Smokey yawned. "Me for the bunkhouse soon as we get there." The next moment, he straightened out of his slumped position. "Dust cloud over there."

Jim glanced in the direction Smokey pointed. "So what?"

"That's the direction of the Lazy F, Dumbhead," Smokey retorted.

Perkins pulled his Stetson farther down over his eyes. "He's had just about enough time to get to the Lazy F and back."

"Who?" Joel sensed significance in the exchange. "You mean Hayes?"

Jim snorted disgust. "I ain't the only dumbhead around here even if you are a preacher." He narrowed his eyelids and cried, "Will ya look at what he's ridin'?"

Joel concentrated on the distant moving dot.

"By the powers, if that's not Vermilion!" Smokey snapped his spine straight and raced to the wagon driver. "Hayes is heading back toward Lone Man riding Vermilion. Tell the boss we're following him." He wheeled his buckskin and galloped the way they had come. "Come on, pards. We may be able to head him off. Joel, we've been wanting to see what that Kay-reeda horse of yours can do. Now's the time!"

A thrill of adventure shot through Joel. Querida responded to the change of directions with her usual grace. Jim and Smokey could not have kept up if Joel had not held Querida in. She might need her magnificent reserve of strength later rather than at this moment.

Taking advantage of a line of cottonwoods in between, the three riders managed to stay out of Hayes's sight until just before they reached Lone Man. They flashed into the open, then saw Hayes look their way, check the big red stallion that fought him, and take off toward the north.

"I knew Vermilion'd never stand for that skunk," Smokey yelled. "Rebecca an' me are the only ones he takes to."

"Good." Perkins's mouth opened in a wide grin. "Ride 'em, cowboys!" He bent low over his horse's neck and urged her closer, taking care not to crowd Querida with her flying hooves.

A long, straight path lay before them, with Vermilion racing straight for the mountains. Hayes had evidently mastered the stallion temporarily and put him into a dead run.

Smokey sped up until he could shout to Joel, "We can't catch him. Maybe you can. He ain't taking time to use his rifle. He probably cleaned out all the cash an' jewels he could find at the Lazy F an' figures on hiding out. Querida, show your stuff!" He snatched the sweat-stained Stetson from his head, leaned over, and cuffed Querida's flank.

Unused to being struck, the soot-black horse whinnied in protest, gathered her muscles, and gave a mighty spring. She came down stretched out and already into the gliding run that won admiration from anyone who saw her race.

Joel heard the loud "Whoopees" from Smokey and Jim. He looked over his shoulder at them pelting along behind as fast as their mounts could carry them, then slipped into his forward thrust position and called in Querida's ear, "Go, Beloved!"

A half mile later, Joel knew he had gained on Vermilion and Hayes, but not much. Another half mile and the distance between them shrank, but infinitesimally. At the end of two miles, Querida's flowing stride narrowed the space between them until Hayes rode glancing back over his shoulder every few minutes.

Joel knew Querida and Vermilion were equally matched. Under the same conditions, the outcome of the race would be a toss-up. Today, Querida had the advantage of nearly a day's rest and grazing against the long ride Vermilion had already made from the Lazy F.

Now, Joel came close enough to see Hayes's hate-filled face and the way he rudely raked the red stallion's sides with his spurs. "Don't do it!" he wanted to shout. Obviously, Hayes did not realize what such treatment of a high-spirited mustang would do, a horse that had never known spur or whip and had been tamed with love and kindness.

In desperate straits, with Querida closing in on him and Smokey and Jim galloping nearer all the time, Hayes lost his wits completely. He spurred Vermilion again. At the same time, he transferred the reins to his left hand and reached with his right to his rifle scabbard to jerk out his weapon.

With a horrid scream, Vermilion retaliated. Instead of running faster, he leaped into the air, whirled, and came down on stiff legs. It jolted the rifle from Hayes's hand. He snatched for it, missed, and threw himself off balance.

For the second time, Vermilion bucked,

jerking the reins free of Hayes's restraining grip and getting his head between his knees. Humped like an upside down "U," the red horse came to earth in a series of bone-crunching leaps and dislodged his rider.

To Joel's horrified gaze, Hayes fell heavily — but his left ankle twisted in the stirrup. He kicked frantically, trying to free himself. Joel screamed at Querida to run; Smokey and Jim thundered behind them, too late.

Not until Vermilion worked himself free of the dragging man, did he, at Smokey's urgent whistle, halt and stand trembling while the cowboy he loved calmed him down and tethered him to a nearby cotton-wood.

"Hayes?" Smokey asked, his face gray.

"Dead." Joel turned away from the man who had plotted against others, murdered Rebecca's father, and now lay at their feet, a victim of his own evil. Sick of it all, he buried his face in Querida's sweating side and stayed a long time. When he turned, he saw Jim slip a roll of greenbacks into his saddlebag with the comment, "Reckon Fairfax'll be glad to get this."

Joel shuddered, but Smokey looked first at him, then at Jim, last of all at the red stallion that stood quietly, his nose nudging Smokey's shoulder. "We have to tell folks

Vermilion threw Hayes." The gray shade had not lifted from his face. "He's no killer horse, though. An' if Rebecca knows just how Hayes died, she won't ride or trust Vermilion."

"No reason she should know, is there?" Jim's intent gaze bored into Joel.

Joel shook his head, unable to believe the docile creature that trotted after Smokey like a pet dog could have been transformed into a whirling cyclone from sheer pain and mistreatment.

"Then we don't tell her a-tall." Jim sighed. "You'll have to let Querida race Vermilion sometime, Joel, or folks won't believe she beat him."

"It wasn't a fair race," Joel quietly told them. "Vermilion had been ridden miles and miles before it began." He stared at the long, still figure covered by a tarp from Jim or Smokey's saddle. "How do we get him back? I doubt that Vermilion will stand for carrying him."

"The buckskin will." Smokey and Jim hoisted the tragic burden to the horse's broad back and secured it. "I'll ride Vermilion soon as he gets his wind."

Drained by the revelations and events of the past few days, Joel simply let the reins lie loose and left it to Querida to follow the trail home. Smokey and Jim rode behind him, but the minister who no longer felt young did not look back. Behind him lay the ghastly reminder that the wages of sin is death. Only by looking forward could he rid himself of the bloodshed and violence. No wonder Jesus wept over the world and commanded His followers to tell others of Him and free them from darkness.

Hours earlier, when the clock at the Bar Triangle struck midnight, Rebecca heard hoofbeats, and the waiting women ran into the yard. A gang of horses and riders swept toward them. Three of the horses wore empty saddles; one was Samuel Fairfax's.

"Oh, God, no!" Rebecca caught her throat with one hand. "Father?"

"He's gonna be all right, Miss Rebecca." Jim Perkins leaped from his sorrel, gathered a sobbing Conchita in his arms, and smiled at Rebecca over the bowed, dusky head.

"But where is he?" She frantically checked the group of men surrounding a sullen-faced band of bound men. "And Joel? And Smokey?"

"All right as sunshine in the mornin'." Nothing daunted Perkins for long. "Your daddy got creased, head wound. Made him too dizzy to ride. We're sendin' a wagon for him soon as it gets light. Joel 'n' Smokey stayed with him."

"You're sure Father isn't badly hurt?"

Jim shoved back his Stetson, and the light streaming from the open doors behind them shone on his face. "Lundeen says he's okay, and Lundeen knows about doctorin' — he patched up your daddy's head." The reassurance in his voice gave way to a sudden frost. "Where's Hayes? Turns out he's behind all this mess."

"I heard a horse goin' out as we were comin' in," a cowboy sang out. "Want us to go get him?"

"Naw. He won't know for sure if we're onta him." Perkins gave a mighty yawn. "It ain't long 'til daybreak. Get some shut-eye, and we'll go chasin' Hayes tomorrow." He turned Conchita toward their new home, and they walked away, his arm around her shoulders, hers on his waist.

Rebecca watched them through a mist of envy. If God ever allowed her to walk that way with Joel . . . She shook her head, and when she got back inside, went to her room, unwilling to talk even with Mrs. Cook. The shock of seeing that riderless horse and noticing Joel had not come home had unnerved her.

"God," she prayed. "You win. Even if

Father is hurt worse than Jim said or if Joel never loves me, You can help me. No one else can. No matter what happens, please, accept and be with me." Surprisingly enough, she fell into such a deep sleep that she never heard when the wagon went for her father but awakened to sun streaming into the room and a feeling of hope inside her.

The hope wavered when she saw how worn her father looked, the bloody bandage around his head. Not until he held out a hand and said, "Daughter, as soon as I get cleaned up, I want to talk with you," could she believe he really would get well. Yet, the following talk — in which he freely confessed his wild youth, real identity, and how her own father had died — brought her pain beyond belief for the white-faced man who spoke, for the weak, easily led father, for the mother she could barely remember.

Cyrus finished by telling her, "Joel has forgiven me. I believe God will, too." He turned his face toward the west. "One day, we'll go find Gideon and Judith and my parents." His voice faltered, and he brushed his hand across his eyes. "Joel says they forgave me long ago. Can you? My only excuse is that I loved you as the child I longed for."

Tears gushed. She flung herself into his arms as she had longed to do since childhood. "You're the only father I've ever known. The name doesn't matter."

"Especially when it appears to me a certain young minister and newly discovered son of mine intends to convince my adopted daughter that Rebecca Scott's a much nicer name than Rebecca Foster-Fairfax!" His blue eyes twinkled, and color returned to his gaunt face.

"Rebecca, you run along now and let your daddy rest," Mrs. Cook ordered from the doorway. If she had heard Cyrus's comment, she chose to ignore it as well as the rich blush that crept into the girl's fresh face.

Banned, Rebecca fled to her room, then sallied forth to watch for Joel, Jim, and Smokey. Her heart had flip-flopped when the driver of the wagon carrying Cyrus told her sourly, "Those three took off like skeered jackrabbits after Hayes. They should be 'long most any time."

Any time stretched into hours, but at last Rebecca's peering from the window rewarded her. Three drooping horses with tired-looking riders rode into view. Conchita, who had joined Rebecca's vigil, exclaimed, "There are four horses. What —"

Rebecca did not wait for the rest of her sentence. She bounded outdoors in spite of the dress she wore in place of her usual riding clothes. She had put it on, refusing to admit even to herself how much she longed for Joel to notice and approve. "Vermilion?" She halted just outside the corral. "Smokey — what — who — ?" She mutely pointed toward the tarpaulin-covered figure the men slid to the ground.

Smokey waited until they finished, then doffed his hat. "He took all the cash he could find at the Lazy F. Thought he'd get away, probably leave New Mexico territory."

"What happened to him? You didn't shoot him, did you?" Rebecca clenched her hands and looked pleadingly from Smokey to Jim to Joel. He looked at her with such compassion in his eyes that she suddenly felt afraid. "Smokey, tell me."

"Aw, he couldn't handle Vermilion. Tried to run away from Querida, who was fresh." Smokey awkwardly turned the big hat in his hands. "Vermilion threw him and he landed bad."

Relief flowed through her. "Thank God! I couldn't stand for you to have killed him." She shuddered and involuntarily looked at Joel.

A beautiful light dawned in Smokey's tired

face. "We appreciate that. Now, we're three dirty tramps who need baths. If you'll excuse us, I reckon we'll see you later." He limped off, bearing evidence of long hours in the saddle. Jim followed, but Joel lingered.

"Have you talked with . . . your father?"

She smiled tremulously. "My adopted father has told me everything." She remembered Cyrus's final statement and turned rosy red.

"May I see you later?" he asked in a low tone.

"Why, of course." Her traitorous heart nearly gave her away.

"In the courtyard, perhaps?" His blue eyes so like his father's eloquently presented his unspoken cause.

"Not in the courtyard." She bit her lip. "Last night Hayes caught me there and . . . and threatened me." Later, she could tell him the whole story. Now, she moved in a daze through the hours between his homecoming and the end of the supper hour. Clad in white, a rose tucked in her hair, Rebecca glimpsed herself in a mirror, gasped, and leaned closer. *Had love made her beautiful?* Her usually merry brown eyes had softened; her skin glowed. The curves of her red lips looked fuller. *Or had surrender to her Lord added the finishing touches?*

Joel led her away from the lighted ranch house, down toward the river that rippled in the starlight. Columbine and bluebonnets bent their heads when the couple passed. A knowing moon cocked one eye and turned Joel's blond hair to glistening silver; it reflected in Rebecca's eyes.

Joel found a smooth stump, brushed it clean, and seated her. "Rebecca," he said softly. "I think I've been looking for you all my life. Could you ever care for me?"

A rush of unworthiness filled her. "I . . . I can never be good enough for you, a man of God." Her voice sounded small and forlorn in the big night. "Though now I know you're right . . . no one can live and be happy without Him." She drew in a long breath and released it. "I told Him that today before you came home." She ignored his involuntary start and quickly added, "I didn't bargain. I just . . . accepted."

"I am so glad." Joel hesitated. "Love isn't a matter of being good enough. It's sharing and growing. I love you more than anything on earth. Do you care at all?"

"I care." Her low whisper reached his ears. He caught her close, never to let her go. She nestled in his arms, heard his heart beat, and felt more protected than ever before in her life.

Later would come all the explanations, the long trip back to San Scipio and the Circle S, and a much longer trip to the Double J, their new home in Arizona. For now, green leaves fluttered above them, whispering in the wilderness their secrets of love and joy and the gospel of Jesus Christ that they would carry.

But Perkins, the incorrigible, had the last word. Walking with his new wife in the moonlight, they paused and observed the charming tableaux that Joel and Rebecca made posed under the cottonwoods. Jim tightened his arm on Conchita's shoulders and whispered, "Snappin' crocodiles, looks like we'll be havin' another weddin'. Say, Connie, how'd ya like to see Arizona? It's a shame for pards like me 'n' Joel 'n' Smokey to get broke up." He snickered real low and added, "Besides, I bet some Arizona gal's just waitin' to meet some cowpoke like Smokey. Ain't it our duty to see she ain't disappointed?"

Conchita dragged him away and left the night to Joel, Rebecca, and the still-whispering trees.

Dear Readers,

I hope you enjoy reading *Whispers in the Wilderness,* the second title in the FRONTIER BRIDES series as much as I enjoyed writing it. My parents had a deep love for reading and western history. They passed it on to my brothers and me. One Christmas during hard times Mom splurged and bought Dad twenty Zane Grey books. The $14. gift provided many happy hours reading by kerosene lamp light.

After World War 2 ended and money wasn't so tight, we camped all over the western states and saw places we already knew from Zane Grey's accurate descriptions. Those trips strengthened my desire to write western novels "someday."

"Someday" came years later when in 1977 I felt called to walk off my government job and write full-time. Now, with six million copies of my 140+ "Books You Can Trust" sold, I marvel. God chose an ordinary logger's daughter to help make the world a better place by providing inspirational reading.

May the FRONTIER BRIDES series bring

a smile, a tear, inspiration, and hope to each of you.

In His Service,
Colleen L. Reece